THE DUTY TO PROTECT

THE DUTY TO PROTECT

Ethical, Legal, and Professional Considerations for Mental Health Professionals

EDITED BY

James L. Werth Jr.

Elizabeth Reynolds Welfel

G. Andrew H. Benjamin

American Psychological Association

Washington, DC

Published by
American Psychological Association
750 First Street, NE
Washington, DC 20002
www.apa.org

To order
APA Order Department
P.O. Box 92984
Washington, DC 20090-2984
Tel: (800) 374-2721; Direct: (202) 336-5510
Fax: (202) 336-5502; TDD/TTY: (202) 336-6123
Online: www.apa.org/books/
E-mail: order@apa.org

In the U.K., Europe, Africa, and the Middle East, copies may be ordered from
American Psychological Association
3 Henrietta Street
Covent Garden, London
WC2E 8LU England

Typeset in Goudy by Stephen McDougal, Mechanicsville, MD

Printer: Sheridan Books, Ann Arbor, MI
Cover Designer: Watermark Design Office, Alexandria, VA
Technical/Production Editor: Kathryn Funk

The opinions and statements published are the responsibility of the authors, and such opinions and statements do not necessarily represent the policies of the American Psychological Association.

Library of Congress Cataloging-in-Publication Data

The duty to protect : ethical, legal, and professional considerations for mental health professionals / edited by James L. Werth Jr., Elizabeth Reynolds Welfel, and G. Andrew H. Benjamin. — 1st ed.
   p. ; cm.
Includes bibliographical references and index.
ISBN-13: 978-1-4338-0412-0
ISBN-10: 1-4338-0412-3
   1. Mental health personnel—Professional ethics. 2. Mental health personnel—Legal status, laws, etc. 3. Dangerously mentally ill. I. Werth, James L. II. Welfel, Elizabeth Reynolds, 1949- III. Benjamin, G. Andrew H. IV. American Psychological Association.
   [DNLM: 1. Duty to Warn—ethics. 2. Duty to Warn—legislation & jurisprudence. 3. Dangerous Behavior. 4. Mental Health Services. W 700 D981 2009]
   RC455.2.E8D88 2009
   174.2'9689—dc22   2008026716

British Library Cataloguing-in-Publication Data
A CIP record is available from the British Library.

Printed in the United States of America
First Edition

To my clients who inspired me; my students, who challenged me; and my colleagues, who supported me
—*James L. Werth Jr.*

To Fred and Brandon, who keep me smiling
—*Elizabeth Reynolds Welfel*

To Nan, whose warmth and loving support nurture my days
—*G. Andrew H. Benjamin*

CONTENTS

CONTRIBUTORS

Bob Barret, PhD, University of North Carolina at Charlotte

G. Andrew H. Benjamin, JD, PhD, School of Law, University of Washington, Seattle

Christiane Brems, PhD, ABPP, Behavioral Health Research and Services, University of Alaska Anchorage

Lynn S. Dowd, PsyD, University of Massachusetts Memorial Medical Center, Worcester

Jim Evans, PhD, RPsych (AB), private practice, Edmonton, Alberta, Canada

Joanna Fava, MA, Department of Psychology, Fordham University, Bronx, NY

Michele Galietta, PhD, Department of Psychology, John Jay College of Criminal Justice, New York, NY

David A. Jobes, PhD, ABPP, Department of Psychology, The Catholic University of America, Washington, DC

Mark E. Johnson, PhD, Behavioral Health Research and Services, University of Alaska Anchorage

Michelle Keeney, PhD, Department of Homeland Security, Washington, DC

Le'a Kent, JD, University of Washington, Seattle

Samuel Knapp, EdD, Pennsylvania Psychological Association, Harrisburg

Leslie Kooyman, PhD, Montclair State University, Montclair, NJ

Mark M. Leach, PhD, Department of Psychology, University of Southern Mississippi, Hattiesburg

Stephen S. O'Connor, MA, PhD candidate in clinical psychology, The Catholic University of America, Washington, DC

Marisa R. Randazzo, PhD, Threat Assessment Resources International, LLC, Sparks, NV

Jessica M. Richmond, MA, The University of Akron, Akron, OH

Alan Rosenbaum, PhD, Department of Psychology, Northern Illinois University, DeKalb

Barry Rosenfeld, PhD, ABPP, Department of Psychology, Fordham University, Bronx, NY

Bruce D. Sales, PhD, JD, Department of Psychology, University of Arizona, Tucson

Skultip Sirikantraporn, MA, Antioch University, Seattle, WA

John Sommers-Flanagan, PhD, Department of Counselor Education, University of Montana, Missoula

Rita Sommers-Flanagan, PhD, Department of Counselor Education, University of Montana, Missoula

Derek Truscott, PhD, RPsych (AB), Department of Educational Psychology, University of Alberta, Edmonton, Canada

Leon VandeCreek, PhD, ABPP, School of Professional Psychology, Wright State University, Dayton, OH

Barent Walsh, PhD, The Bridge, Worcester, MA

Elizabeth Reynolds Welfel, PhD, Department of Counseling, Administration, Supervision & Adult Learning, Cleveland State University, Cleveland, OH

James L. Werth Jr., PhD, Department of Psychology, Radford University, Radford, VA

ACKNOWLEDGMENTS

We would like to thank the contributors for their excellent work and for conforming to our guidelines for chapter length and content. We appreciated their timely responses and willingness to engage in useful dialogue in response to our own and the reviewers' comments.

We also appreciate the efforts of the staff of American Psychological Association Books Department as they worked with us to move this book through the publication process. The obvious ethical and legal components required additional review and diligence as well as the resolution of varying issues. We are proud of the final product and thank the staff for working with us, especially Genevieve Gill, who was our intermediary in more than one instance.

Finally, we each want to recognize individuals who were important to us as we worked on this book and the ideas that led to our wanting to collaborate on such a project.

Andy gratefully acknowledges the mentoring of Bruce Sales. Andy's first contribution in this area was encouraged by Bruce when the mental health professionals of the great state of Washington were afflicted by judicial activism that had run amok. Legislation was drafted and run; the new statutes replaced the unrealistic common-law standard. Finally, his wife Nan Herbert has provided 39 years of stalwart support that remains a vibrant constancy. Thank you!

Liz wants to acknowledge the wisdom about the complex ethical issues in mental health care that her students and fellow psychologists have shared with her in classes and workshops and to express her appreciation to her colleagues at Cleveland State, who have encouraged her in this and other research projects even when she ought to have been doing a larger share of administrative work. Most important of all in this list of acknowledgments is her family, her husband and son, who have taught her the most about integrity, commitment, and ethics.

Jim wants to thank his clients for trusting him to raise difficult issues, his students for asking questions and inspiring him to learn more, and his colleagues for their patience as he devoted time to this project and requested consultation on topics. He also wants to especially express his gratitude to Dr. Randolph B. Pipes, who inspired him to begin exploring issues associated with the duty to protect during his first year of graduate school and who supported him even when these explorations led to controversial conclusions.

I

FOUNDATIONAL ISSUES

1

INTRODUCTION TO THE DUTY TO PROTECT

ELIZABETH REYNOLDS WELFEL, JAMES L. WERTH JR.,
AND G. ANDREW H. BENJAMIN

Most psychologists, counselors, social workers, and other clinicians in the United States and Canada have heard of the *Tarasoff* case (*Tarasoff v. Regents of the University of California*, 1976) and the term *duty to warn*. Unfortunately, the depth of their knowledge appears limited. For example, on the basis of our collective experience, a review of relevant research, and case law in the 64 jurisdictions of the United States and Canada, most mental health professionals do not seem to know the following facts (all of which are discussed in detail in the chapters that follow):

- The duty to warn established in the 1974 *Tarasoff* ruling was vacated by the California Supreme Court when they ruled again in 1976. It was replaced by the term *duty to protect*. So by 1976, the original language identifying a duty to warn was no longer applicable even in California as the sole means to protect a third party at risk of violent action from a current psychotherapy client.
- *Tarasoff* applied only in California and only until the California legislature passed legislation that changed the common law created by the state Supreme Court.

- Thirty-two states currently mandate a duty to protect regarding professionals' responsibility with dangerous clients.
- Eighteen states or provinces do not mandate any particular action when clients disclose violent intent to their therapists. They permit a breach of confidentiality but do not require it.
- The law of 14 jurisdictions remains silent as to whether a duty to warn or protect exists. In some jurisdictions, a duty to protect (as opposed to duty to warn) also exists with clients who are dangerous to themselves.
- A few jurisdictions specify different duties depending on the discipline of the professional.
- The codes of ethics of the American Psychological Association (2002), the American Counseling Association (2005), the National Association of Social Workers (1999), and the American Psychiatric Association (2008) do not mandate breach of confidentiality with dangerous clients.
- Some jurisdictions also require action when clients make threats against public officials or are engaged in domestic violence.

In fact, a recent study suggested that as many as 75% of psychologists are misinformed about their legal duties with clients who are dangerous to others (Pabian, Welfel, & Beebe, 2007). What is even more troubling is that they seem unaware of their error—90% of the same sample was confident of the accuracy of their legal knowledge of their responsibilities with dangerous clients. Prior research has shown similar, although slightly less discouraging, results (Givelber, Bowers, & Blitch, 1984; Kramer, 1997; Leedy, 1989; Lingefelter, 1997). By definition, the duty to warn applies to the circumstances in which case law or statute requires the mental health professional to make a good-faith effort to contact the identified victim of a client's serious threats of harm and/or to notify law enforcement of the threat. The duty to protect applies to situations in which the mental health professional has a legal obligation to take action to protect a threatened third party, but the professional usually has other options in addition to warning that person of the risk of harm, frequently including actions such as hospitalizing the client or intensifying outpatient treatment. The duty to protect allows for the possibility of maintaining the client's confidentiality, whereas the duty to warn necessitates a disclosure of confidential information to the alleged victim.

These findings are also consistent with our experience as lecturers and consultants on this topic. Two of us have practiced in Ohio, a state with a duty-to-protect statute that allows intensification of outpatient treatment or voluntary hospitalization as viable options with clients who threaten violence, yet in our continuing education workshops the vast majority of practicing professionals are convinced that they must carry out their duty by warning third parties. Such a misunderstanding might be less significant if clinicians could diagnose dangerousness with very high levels of accuracy, but we know from a substantial body of literature that accurate predictions of dangerousness are difficult to make (Haggard-Grann, 2007; Mossman, 1994; Otto, 1992, 2000; Scott & Resnick, 2006). Moreover, warning third parties of a danger from a client does not guarantee their safety or the client's safety. The person who is warned may disbelieve the information, get so panicked that she or he is immobilized and unable to engage in self-protection, or may take violent action against the client. Consequently, exercising a duty to warn may lead to inappropriate breaches of confidentiality that risk client trust and participation in further treatment and cannot guarantee anyone's safety. In certain circumstances, warning is the most prudent and appropriate course of action, but for most professionals in many situations, it is not the only option.

Professionals' misinterpretation of their legal and ethical duty to protect is problematic in still another way. Case law and state statutes are continuously evolving. Ohio, for example, has revised its duty-to-protect laws twice since 1991. An Ohio clinician who was following the rule in effect before 1999 would be acting inconsistently with the current statute. Other states show similar variability. Recently, a California Appeals Court case resulted in an expansion of a clinician's legal responsibilities with dangerous clients, moved the duty closer to the original *Tarasoff* obligation, and eviscerated legislative efforts at clarifying the duty for mental health professionals (*Ewing v. Goldstein*, 2004). As the chapters to follow clearly illustrate, nearly every jurisdiction has a different interpretation of the duty, with some having no statute or case law related to the issue and others having very specific legal guidelines. This level of variability across time and jurisdictions makes it essential for clinicians to be well informed about their state or provincial obligations, especially because the professions' codes of ethics offer only general statements of permission to breach confidentiality in situations of danger to clients and/or third parties and admonitions to avoid harm to clients and others.

Still another reason for professionals to be better informed about dangerousness stems from some unique responsibilities with clients who make threats against public officials, are at risk of infecting others with HIV or other potentially deadly illnesses, or are perpetrators of domestic violence. Consider the following scenarios:

- After a recent election, a client expresses rage at the outcome of the congressional race, vowing to "do whatever is necessary to be sure that the winner does not get a chance to have that kind of power."
- A client discloses that she has broken her husband's nose and given him a black eye. The client suffers from paranoid schizophrenia, has become medication noncompliant, and believes that her husband may be trying to poison her. She has threat-

ened to kill him and kill herself before he can succeed in poisoning her.

- A young female graduate student enters therapy because she wants to get up the courage to get an HIV test after learning that someone with whom she had unprotected sex is HIV positive. She is unwilling to be abstinent currently or to inform her current partner of her history, but she has committed to try to use safer sex practices with the person she is now dating, if he is willing to do so.

As the chapters to follow illustrate, professionals may have specific (and sometimes conflicting) legal duties depending on the jurisdiction in which they practice. Moreover, several other complications related to the duty to protect loom on the horizon. The following scenarios hint at these complications:

- A client reveals that he smokes several marijuana cigarettes each day before going to work during the night shift. Because he operates heavy equipment in a steel-making plant, his intoxication in this setting could endanger other workers.
- A couple reveals to their therapist that they have decided not to disclose to their 18-year-old son his genetic risk of experiencing Huntington's disease. The therapist knows from the literature that most young adults at risk of Huntington's disease want to know their risk and make informed decisions about their own futures. The parents are adamant that disclosure not be made.
- A psychologist agrees to exchange e-mails with a 21-year-old client while the young woman is volunteering at a rural camp for youngsters. He has been seeing her for symptoms of depression and anxiety. During the e-mail exchanges, the client begins to reveal information that she never disclosed in their face-to-face sessions, which suggests that she has a history of self-mutilation and suicide attempts. The e-mails also indicate that she is experiencing high levels of distress at the camp and her self-destructive urges may be returning. Because he does not possess the client's current cell phone number, the psychologist has no other way to contact the client at this camp aside from e-mail, and he is very worried that she is a danger to herself.

This book clarifies the current legal and ethical obligations for professionals across North America and offers guidelines for best practice in these situations. Some consistent themes when providing clinical services with such clients are presented, and these are highlighted in the concluding chapter, including the need to know (and not assume) what the legal language is in the state(s) or province(s) in which one practices, the need to provide thorough informed consent to clients before evaluation and treatment begin, and the importance of a strong therapeutic alliance (when possible) to enable accurate assessment and intervention.

As editors, we believe the chapter authors have provided readers with succinct summaries of the large literature available that will be useful to practitioners in a variety of fields and settings. We hope that the book will help provide the best care possible to clients who may be dangerous to themselves or others. By becoming familiar with the content of this book, we believe that readers will realize that the concept and application of the duty to protect allow for significantly more possibilities for assessment and intervention than an overly narrow focus on a duty to warn.

REFERENCES

American Counseling Association. (2005). *ACA code of ethics*. Alexandria, VA: Author. Retrieved May 14, 2007, from http://www.counseling.org/Resources/CodeOfEthics/TP/Home/CT2.aspx

American Psychiatric Association. (2008). *The principles of medical ethics with annotations especially applicable to psychiatry*. Washington, DC: Author. Retrieved July 24, 2008, from http://www.psych.org/MainMenu/PsychiatricPractice/Ethics/ResourcesStandards/PrinciplesofMedicalEthics.aspx

American Psychological Association. (2002). Ethical principles of psychologists and code of conduct. *American Psychologist, 57*, 1060–1073. Retrieved from http://www.apa.org/ethics/code2002.html

Ewing v. Goldstein, 120 Cal. App. 4th 807 (2004).

Givelber, D. J., Bowers, W. J., & Blitch, C. L. (1984). *Tarasoff*, myth and reality: An empirical study of private law in action. *Wisconsin Law Review, 1984*, 443–497.

Haggard-Grann, U. (2007). Assessing violence risk: A review and clinical recommendations. *Journal of Counseling & Development, 85*, 294–302.

Kramer, L. (1997). A comparison study of the psychologist's duty to protect third parties from the potential violence of their patients. *Dissertation Abstracts International, 58*(7), 3927B.

Leedy, S. (1989). Psychologists' knowledge and application of *Tarasoff* in their decisions about dangerousness. *Dissertation Abstracts International, 50*(10), 4775B.

Lingefelter, C. O. (1997). Potentially dangerous clients: A study of Pennsylvania licensed psychologists' working knowledge of ethics and law. *Dissertation Abstracts International, 58*(6), 3320B.

Mossman, D. (1994). Assessing predictions of violence: Being accurate about accuracy. *Journal of Consulting and Clinical Psychology, 62*, 783–792.

National Association of Social Workers. (1999). *NASW code of ethics*. Washington, DC: Author. Retrieved May 14, 2007, from http://www.socialworkers.org/pubs/code/default.asp

Otto, R. (1992). The prediction of dangerous behavior: A review and analysis of "second generation" research. *Forensic Reports, 5*, 103–133.

Otto, R. K. (2000). Assessing and managing violence risk in outpatient settings. *Journal of Clinical Psychology, 56*, 1239–1262.

Pabian, Y. L., Welfel, E. R., & Beebe, R. (2007, August). *Psychologists' knowledge and application of state laws in* Tarasoff-*type situations*. Paper presented at the 115th Annual Convention of the American Psychological Association, San Francisco.

Scott, C. L., & Resnick, J. (2006). Violence risk assessment in persons with mental illness. *Aggression and Violent Behavior, 11*, 598–611.

Tarasoff v. Regents of the University of California, 131 Cal. Rptr. 14, 551 P.2d 334 (1976).

2

A REVIEW OF DUTY-TO-PROTECT STATUTES, CASES, AND PROCEDURES FOR POSITIVE PRACTICE

G. ANDREW H. BENJAMIN, LE'A KENT,
AND SKULTIP SIRIKANTRAPORN

In many states and provinces/territories, the duty to warn or protect is established by statutes or administrative rules.[1] Throughout this book, the authors discuss case examples in which extraordinary clinical circumstances have arisen in duty-to-warn or duty-to-protect contexts. The examples highlight circumstances that require mental health professionals (MHPs) to evaluate whether a duty-to-warn or duty-to-protect context has arisen and, in light of the evaluation, whether a particular intervention is necessary. This chapter articulates the steps MHPs should take when conflicting duties arise. Failure

---

[1]Statutes result from legislation enacted by the state or provincial legislatures. Rules or codes are created by state or provincial agencies operated under the authority delegated to them by the legislatures to perform specific administrative agency functions. Appellate judges must apply the statutes and rules or code when reviewing criminal or civil cases. When the law is ambiguous, judges may interpret the intent of the legislature or administrative agency within the jurisdiction or turn to other jurisdictional law for direction. The subsequent rulings create law and are referred to as *the common law*. When no statutory framework exists or the statutes are interpreted by the appellate judge, and the common law creates new duties, such behavior is referred to as *judicial activism* by some commentators of the courts.

to follow the duty of the jurisdiction can expose an MHP to malpractice liability or ethical violations when it conflicts with the duty of confidentiality. After reviewing the current statutes and case law on the duty to protect, we discuss five procedures that are key to meeting the legal and ethical obligations established by each jurisdiction's law while evaluating and intervening effectively: (a) disclosure and informed consent before evaluation and treatment begin, (b) therapeutic alliance, (c) assessment of the threat, (d) peer consultation, and (e) documentation. On the basis of actual clinical experiences, we believe this approach can reduce both the likelihood of injury to any person and the likelihood of the filing of a malpractice lawsuit or an ethical complaint.

METHOD FOR COLLECTING INFORMATION ON STATE AND PROVINCIAL/TERRITORIAL STATUTES

To determine whether the duty to warn or protect exists within a particular jurisdiction and to understand the exact contours of the duty, we reviewed all of the books in the American Psychological Association's *Law and Mental Health Professionals* series (this series is designed to provide a resource for both MHPs and attorneys regarding mental health law in each state). We also conducted searches using the Westlaw database for all 50 states, the District of Columbia, and the 13 Canadian provinces/territories. Our research attempted to answer the following questions for each jurisdiction: (a) Does a statute or an administrative rule create a duty to protect? (b) Have court rulings created a common-law duty or interpreted the statutes or administrative rules? (c) What is the specific duty in light of the law? (d) To which types of MHPs does the law apply? (e) How does the MHP discharge the duty? (f) Does the duty extend to assault against property, domestic violence, stalking, communicable diseases, driving, threats to public officials, or harm to self (e.g., suicidal ideation self-injury)? (g) Can the procedures for involuntary hospitalization be used as part of an evaluation and an intervention to meet the duty? (h) Do immunities from liability exist for the MHP who exercises the duty? The reader can find the narrative summaries answering these questions for each jurisdiction's law in an online appendix (see http://www.apa.org/books/resources/dutytoprotect; username: duty2protect; password: appendix).[2]

To confirm our research, we sent a summary of our results to the psychologist licensing board of each state and province/territory and requested that the board confirm the accuracy of our summary. Twenty-five of the

---

[2]Henceforth, duty to warn or protect is referred to as *duty to protect*. Most jurisdictions in which such a duty has been created have now constructed law that creates a duty to protect rather than a duty to warn.

jurisdictions (39%) agreed that the summaries of their law were accurate. Eleven of the jurisdictions (17%) indicated that they could issue no opinion for various reasons, the most common reason being that the board could not issue legal opinions. Twenty-eight of the jurisdictions (44%) failed to respond despite three written requests and two phone calls. Readers will be able to determine which of the boards responded by examining the online appendix (http://www.apa.org/books/resources/dutytoprotect). In addition, we requested that each licensing board provide any published ruling in regard to an ethics complaint regarding the duty to protect filed against an MHP within that jurisdiction. No jurisdiction forwarded published rulings.

DATA ON JURISDICTIONAL RESPONSES TO *TARASOFF*

The law regarding the duty to protect remains in transition throughout North America. Since the California Supreme Court ruling in *Tarasoff v. Regents of the University of California* (1976), a rapidly increasing number of jurisdictions have created a duty to protect. For example, in the first few years after *Tarasoff*, DeKraai and Sales (1982) reported that three states had implemented such a duty. Later, Glosoff, Herlihy, Herlihy, and Spence (1997) identified 20 states with such laws. Currently, a mandatory duty to protect has been created by statute or rule in 24 states, and 9 states operate under a common-law duty created by court decisions. Mandatory duty laws create a legal obligation for the MHP to take actions to protect third parties from a patient's threatened violence. Violating such a law exposes the MHP to lawsuits and ethics violations but not to criminal charges. In addition, 10 other states and 8 provinces/territories have statutes or rules giving MHPs a *permissive duty to protect*. A permissive duty to protect means that the law allows, but does not require, the MHP to breach patient confidentiality to protect third parties from a patient's threatened violence. MHPs are not subjected to liability for failing to protect third parties. Such a law provides more discretion to the MHP in defining how to act under the emerging circumstances of the case. The remaining 30 jurisdictions have not developed law about the duty to protect.

Although judicial activism first created the duty to warn,[3] many of the jurisdictions that started with common-law duty have modified the duty through the legislative process. The online appendix (http://www.apa.org/books/resources/dutytoprotect) to this volume provides a summary of how each jurisdiction has responded to the trend to establish and implement a duty to protect. Table 2.1 includes the following information for each juris-

---

[3]The original *Tarasoff* decision—which used the language *warn*—represents one of the most striking examples of judicial activism that has affected the regulation and practice of mental health evaluation and treatment.

TABLE 2.1
Overview of Duty-to-Protect Statutes in the United States and Canada

State	Mandatory or permissive duty by statute	Court-created duty exists	Courts have interpreted statute	Means of discharge specified	Duty explicitly extends to self-harm	Duty explicitly extends to harm to property	MHPs explicitly immune from civil liability for reasonable attempts to meet duty	Licensing board ratified summary
Alabama	N	N[a]	N	N	Y	N	N	Y
Alaska	P	N	N	N	N	N	N	Y
Arizona	M	Y	Y	Y	N	N	Y	D
Arkansas	N	N	N	N	N	N	N	
California	M	N	Y	Y	N	N	Y	D
Colorado	M	N	Y	Y	N	N	Y	Y
Connecticut	P	Y	N	N	N	N	N	D
Delaware	M	N	N	Y	N	Y	Y	Y
Florida	P	Y[b]	N	N	N	N	N	D
Georgia	N	N	N	N	N	N	Y	Y
Hawaii	P	N	N	N	N	N	N	
Idaho	M	N	Y	Y	N	N	N	D
Illinois	M	N	N	N	N	N	N	
Indiana	M	Y[c]	N	Y	N	N	N	
Iowa	N	Y[d]	Y[e]	N	N	N	N	Y
Kansas	N	N	Y	Y	N	N	Y	Y
Kentucky	M	N	Y	N	N	N	Y	
Louisiana	M	N	Y	Y	N	N	Y	Y
Maine	N	N	N	N	N	N	N	
Maryland	M	N	Y	Y	N	N	Y	Y
Massachusetts	M	N	N	Y	N	N	Y	Y
Michigan	M	N	Y	Y	N	N	Y	Y
Minnesota	M	N	Y	Y	N	N	Y	D

Mississippi	P	N	N	Y	N	N	N	Y
Missouri	N	Y	Y	Y[f]	N	N	N	
Montana	M	N	N	Y	N	N	N	Y
Nebraska	M	N	Y	Y	Y	N	Y	
Nevada	N	N	N	N	N	N	N	Y
New Hampshire	M	Y	Y	Y	N	Y	Y	D
New Jersey	M	N	Y	Y	Y	N	Y	D
New Mexico	N	Y[g]	N	N	N	N	N	Y
New York	P	N	Y	N	N	N	N	Y
North Carolina	P	Y[h]	N	N	N	N	N[i]	Y
North Dakota	M	N	N	Y	N	N	Y	
Ohio	M	N	Y	Y	N	N	Y	Y
Oklahoma	M	Y	N	Y	Y	N	N	
Oregon	P	Y[j]	N	Y	N	N	N	Y
Pennsylvania	P	Y	N	Y	N	N	N	D
Rhode Island	P	N	N	N	N	N	N	Y
South Carolina	P	Y	N	N	N	N	N	Y
South Dakota	P	N	N	N	N	Y	N	
Tennessee	M	Y[k]	N	Y	N	N	N	D
Texas	N	N	N	N	N	N	N	
Utah	M	N	Y	Y	N	N	Y	Y
Vermont	N	Y	Y	N	N	Y[l]	N	Y
Virginia	M	N	Y	Y	N	N	Y	D
Washington	M	N	Y	Y	N	N	Y	Y
West Virginia	P	N	N	N	N	N	N	Y
Wisconsin	N	Y[m]	Y[m]	Y[n]	N	N	N	
Wyoming	P	N	N	N	N	N	N	
District of Columbia	P	N	N	Y	N	N	N	

continued

TABLE 2.1
Continued

State	Mandatory or permissive duty by statute	Court-created duty exists	Courts have interpreted statute	Means of discharge specified	Duty explicitly extends to self-harm	Duty explicitly extends to harm to property	MHPs explicitly immune from civil liability for reasonable attempts to meet duty	Licensing board ratified summary
CANADA								
Alberta	P	N	N	Y	N	N	Y	Y
British Columbia°	P	N	N	Y	N	N	N	
Labrador and Newfoundland°	N	N	N	N	N	N	N	
Manitoba°	P	N	N	N	Y	N	Y	
New Brunswick°	N	N	N	N	N	N	N	
Northwest Territories°	N	N	N	N	N	N	N	
Nova Scotia°	P	N	N	Y	Y	N	N	
Nunavut°	N	N	N	Y	N	N	N	
Ontario°	P	N	N	N	N	N	Y	
Prince Edward Island°	N	N	N	N	N	N	N	
Quebec°	P	N	N	Y	Y	N	Y	
Saskatchewan°	P	N	N	N	N	N	Y	

Note. Y = Yes; N = No; M = A statute or administrative rule has created a mandatory duty; P = A statute or administrative rule has created a permissive duty; D = The licensing board of the jurisdiction declined to ratify the summary of its law or provide corrections.
a Opinions have some language favorable to duty.
b Limited duty for MHPs who have physical control over client.
c Duty found when MHP had explicitly promised third parties that they would be warned.
d Very limited duty to warn in inpatient context.

eStatute interpreted once by federal, not state, court.

fMeans of discharge are outlined in common law case.

gDuty owed to the driving public.

hDuty exists only when patient is involuntarily committed and harm is foreseeable.

iMHPs only are explicitly immune from liability for following accepted professional practice, judgment, and standards while attempting to involuntarily commit a patient.

jLimited duty for hospitalized patients.

kLimited duty for hospitalized patients.

lDuty extends only to property damage that presents a risk to life.

mVery broad duty to protect whenever harm is foreseeable.

nCommon law case specifies that warning, commitment, or detention may discharge duty.

oThe Association of Canadian Psychology Regulatory Organizations sent a letter on behalf of all Canadian regulatory Colleges/Boards. It stated that since the inquiry to the various provinces and territories regarded a legal concept requiring interpretation through provincial and/or federal legislation, the regulatory Colleges/Boards could not provide any legal opinions.

diction: Does a statute(s) or administrative rule(s) create a mandatory or permissive duty to protect within the jurisdiction? Have court rulings created a common-law duty or interpreted the statute or rules related to the duty subsequent to the statute or rule being created? Does the law specify how MHPs can discharge the duty (yes or no)? Does the duty to protect others also explicitly extend to harm to self, such as suicidal ideation and self-injury (yes or no)? Does the duty to protect others extend to assault against property (yes or no)? Is immunity from liability provided to the MHP who engages in reasonable evaluation and interventions to meet the duty to protect (yes or no)? Did the licensing board of the jurisdiction ratify the summary of its law or provide its own summary (yes or no)?

CASE EXAMPLES OF THE IMPACT OF THE EMERGING LAWS ON PRACTITIONERS

Early court cases offered MHPs little clarity about how to meet the duty. Typically, these cases resulted from judicial activism in response to egregious lapses of professional behavior within institutional contexts. For example, the Iowa Supreme Court, after earlier cases in which it refused to create a duty to protect on the basis of *Tarasoff* (e.g., *Matter of Votteler's Estate*, 1982), found a duty to protect existed under the circumstances of *Estate of Long* ex rel. *Smith v. Broadlawns Med. Ctr.* (2002). Although no statutory duty to protect exists within Iowa, the Iowa Supreme Court found that a common-law duty to protect existed when the staff of an inpatient facility, after promising to do so, failed to notify Ms. Long (the client's wife) that her violent husband was being discharged. Mr. Long killed Ms. Long the day he was released.

The inpatient facility was found liable for Ms. Long's wrongful death. According to the court record, she had endured acts of domestic violence that included being fired at with a gun 6 days before her murder. On the day of the first gun violence, Mr. Long sought voluntary psychiatric care at the Veterans Administration Hospital in Des Moines. He was transferred because of his health insurance policy to Broadlawns Medical Center. The attending physician, Dr. Shin, diagnosed him "as suffering from post-traumatic stress disorder versus dissociative disorder and dependencies on alcohol, marijuana, and methamphetamine" (*Estate of Long* ex rel. *Smith v. Broadlawns Med. Ctr.*, 2002, p. 78). Presumably, Dr. Shin also knew that the evaluation at the Veterans Administration Hospital earlier that day showed Mr. Long was "exhibiting homicidal and suicidal tendencies, was suffering from hallucinations and flashbacks, and stated that he was 'losing control'" (p. 78). The court record also showed that during that day, Ms. Long had a conversation with a Broadlawns social worker. Ms. Long had discussed her history of domestic violence, why her husband was voluntarily committed at that point, and the danger of his returning to their marital home if he was discharged. The social worker promised that she would call and warn Ms. Long of Mr. Long's discharge should it occur. Mr. Long was released 6 days later without escort to voluntarily enter a chemical dependency center. He did arrive at the center, but after taking part in initial assessment he returned to his home. He waited for Ms. Long to return later that evening and fatally shot her.

In this Iowa case, and several other similar cases in other jurisdictions, common-law duties were created from negligent acts in institutional settings. These judicially created standards are then generally thought to apply to all MHPs, although they provide little guidance to MHPs practicing in noninstitutional contexts. As a result, in many instances MHPs have turned to the legislative process to modify the judicially imposed duties. Developments in Washington State are typical of the process.

Washington's Supreme Court created a duty to protect in *Petersen v. State of Washington* (1983) and founded the duty on other jurisdictions' common law. *Petersen* involved a patient who had been stopped by hospital security for driving recklessly in the hospital's parking lot after returning from a day pass. Knowing this, the psychiatrist in *Petersen* nonetheless discharged the patient the next morning. The case record showed that the psychiatrist also knew the following data about the patient at the time of the discharge: The patient had an extensive history of drug abuse, the patient had partially castrated himself 16 days earlier while intoxicated on drugs, and the patient had entered the hospital after being adjudged gravely disabled (unable to take care of his basic life needs) and mentally ill—"schizophrenic reaction, paranoid type with depressive features" (*Petersen v. State of Washington*, 1983, p. 423). At the end of the 14-day involuntary hospitalization, despite his reckless driving of the night before, he was assessed on the day of release by the same psychiatrist to have recovered from the drug overdose and to have regained "full contact with reality" (*Petersen v. State of Washington*, 1983, p. 427). Five days later, under the influence of drugs, the patient ran a red light in his vehicle and hit Ms. Petersen's vehicle at 50 to 60 miles an hour. Ms. Peterson was someone unknown to the patient. The court held that the psychiatrist had "incurred a duty to take reasonable precautions to protect anyone who might be foreseeably endangered by . . . the [patient's] drug-related mental problems" (*Petersen v. State of Washington*, 1983, p. 428). The decision created great uncertainty within Washington because the court relied on two common-law cases from other jurisdictions to create the ruling, and both cases emphasized the foreseeability of the dangerousness in defining the MHPs' duty to exercise reasonable care, but neither case involved identifiable victims or those who could reasonably be identified.

DEVELOPMENT OF THE DUTY TO PROTECT

Petersen left Washington MHPs alarmed at their new common-law liability primarily because the case imposed a standard of foreseeability that was unsupported by any reasonable scientific basis. MHPs were uncertain about how to arrive at valid and reliable clinical judgments in light of the poor research evidence about predicting violent behavior. *Petersen* also offered little clarity about how to meet the new duty.

MHPs turned to the state legislature. During legislative hearings to enact a more reasonable duty, testimony cited the Monahan (1981) findings demonstrating that violent behavior is not consistently foreseeable. Other testimony documented an unintended consequence of creating such a liability: After the *Petersen* decision, MHPs, in increasing numbers, obtained involuntary commitment evaluations even for vague threats of violence uttered by their clients (*The Impact of the Uncertainty*, 1985). It was noted that MHPs sought evaluations at a significantly greater rate than before the common-law decision. The increase in evaluation requests overwhelmed the involuntary treatment systems of many counties in Washington and led to greater county expenditures for the involuntary treatment evaluations (*The Impact of the Uncertainty*, 1985). Washington psychologists mobilized with other MHPs to advocate for a statute that would define the duty specifically, and it was enacted to focus on actual threats of physical violence to reasonably identifiable third parties.

In the current review of the cases and laws, it appears that in many jurisdictions the duty to protect first emerged from the common law and was later clarified by statute. As a result, the laws across jurisdictions vary considerably. The laws vary not only as to the nature and scope of duty but also as to who must act when the duty arises. They also vary as to whom to protect, how the MHP can discharge the duty, and if the clinician meets the duty, whether immunity will exist for breaching confidentiality. Some jurisdictions appear to have enacted statutes in response to the development of common-law duties in other jurisdictions, hoping to head off the development of a broad common-law duty by passing the statute first. Judges have tended to expand the duty to protect more readily than have legislators. Legislators are accountable to constituents and generally engage in extensive fact finding before creating statutes. Almost without exception, common-law cases have focused on curbing the practices of MHPs within hospitals and other institutions that have greater control over their clients. Quite typically, the new common-law duty would not explicitly be limited to the institutional setting and would appear to MHPs to encompass outpatient practice.

The state of Washington has not been alone in enacting legal standards that are more reasonable to meet. The emerging laws provide clearer standards about assessing a client's risk of committing violence, the target(s) of the threatened violence, and how to meet the duty to protect. Nevertheless, a worrisome trend has occurred throughout the civil and criminal law of North America: MHPs are expected to provide evidence and predictions about the future violence of their clients (Monahan, 1996). In addition, it appears that fear of liability and a genuine desire to protect patients and potential victims from harm are inspiring MHPs and mental health researchers to develop better predictions of violence; certainly, they have driven the development of better methodology for making better predictions (Monahan, 1996). Responding to the threat of liability and to pressures from managed health care and public funding of state and provincial/territorial institutions, MHPs are also increasingly likely to provide community management of potentially violent clients (Mulvey & Lidz, 1998). The 1990s saw outpatient commitment options used much more frequently as a less restrictive alternative to involuntary hospitalizations. After reviewing the empirical research studies, Monahan (2006) concluded that "outpatient commitment, in combination with outpatient services, halve[d] the risk of patient violence . . . it improved medication adherence and it diminished substance abuse" (p. 517). Both licensing boards and courts will develop greater expectations about how MHPs should intervene to affect the conditions and changes in their clients' lives that may lead to violence.

PRACTITIONER APPROACH TO WORKING WITH THE DUTY TO PROTECT

Preparation for this type of context begins with knowing the law about the duty to protect and what constitutes the standard of care within the jurisdiction (Benjamin, Rosenwald, Overcast, & Feldman, 1995). Readers should view the information in the online appendix (http://www.apa.org/books/resources/dutytoprotect) and the narrative summary of their jurisdiction's law as a starting point for interpreting how the law within their own jurisdiction applies to their own cases. As discussed above, the rapid expansion of the duty to protect will lead to further development. Judicial activism will continue to affect the laws, and MHPs should expect further judicial interpretations of the legal vagaries.

Legal standards for negligence and ethical conduct require that MHPs conduct reasonably prudent assessment and interventions. Whether an MHP has acted reasonably under the circumstances of the case will be exposed through expert witness testimony about how an MHP "with comparable training and experience in the same community would have done when faced with a similar situation" (Mills, Sullivan, & Eth, 1987, p. 72). The results of the present survey suggest that many psychology licensing boards of the states and provinces/territories are unwilling to review the standards by which MHPs can best serve their clients and the public (only 25 boards were willing to review, for accuracy, the summary of their law found in the online appendix [http://www.apa.org/books/resources/dutytoprotect]; a note in the online appendix indicates the boards willing to conduct the review). MHPs can check with their state and provincial/territorial professional associations (SPAs) to see whether current recommendations for meeting the duty to protect may be developed. Many SPAs have ethics committees that can be consulted as part of the SPA benefits. In addition, SPAs can refer MHPs for individual consultation to lawyers specializing in legal practices focused on MHPs. Professional liability carriers also provide free legal and professional consultation. Finally, continuing education conducted under the auspices of the SPAs will update practitioners about how the duty to protect is changing within their jurisdiction. Once the legal and ethical standards in the MHP's jurisdiction are identified, the MHP can engage in the following practices to establish a reasonable course of action while meeting any duty to protect: (a) disclosure and informed consent before evaluation and treatment begins, (b) therapeutic alliance, (c) assessment of the threat, (d) peer consultation, and (e) documentation.

Disclosure and Informed Consent

A therapeutic alliance is founded on the informed consent process (Waitzkin, 1984). One of the linchpins of successful evaluation and intervention in a duty-to-protect context is full disclosure with the client about the limitations for protecting confidences before any dangerous ideation has been expressed (Glosoff et al., 1997). From the beginning of the professional relationship, to help the client make an informed decision about whether to pursue treatment, the MHP should let the client know that the MHP must disclose confidential information in certain defined legal contexts.[4] The laws related to all mandatory reporting duties and the duty to protect should be delineated clearly by the MHP to the client. In part, this process forewarns the client about issues that would require disclosure, and if the MHP must act on the duty, forewarning the client can avoid the client's feeling surprised and betrayed. Individuals seeking mental health services expect confidentiality (VandeCreek, Miars, & Herzog, 1987). The early transparency with clients encourages them to work with the MHP to remain within the confines of the law.

In addition, explicit dialogue about the disclosures leads to a more efficacious informed consent process (Pomerantz & Handelsman, 2004). Clients may not always read the informed consent document carefully and may skip the portion explaining when the law requires the MHP to breach confidentiality; they may also feel uncomfortable about seeking clarification with

---

[4]For example, all jurisdictions have enacted a mandatory reporting duty that MHPs must exercise whenever reasonable suspicion of child abuse, neglect, and exploitation emerges in their cases.

a MHP they have just met. Ideally, MHPs should delineate what legal and ethical disclosure duties exist within the jurisdiction. Later, if a threat of violence emerges, the MHP has a solid foundation on which to launch an active collaboration with the client to determine what precipitating and inhibiting factors exist.

Therapeutic Alliance

The development of a positive, cooperative relationship between the MHP and the client remains a significant factor in reducing the risk of a client's acting out in a violent manner (Pope, Simpson, & Weiner, 1978). Research has shown that the therapeutic alliance is one of the most critical factors in determining effective treatment outcome (Horvath & Bedi, 2002). As discussed earlier, the development of a positive, collaborative relationship between the MHP and the client begins with the informed consent process. Clients who have difficulty forming a therapeutic alliance are more likely to object to the cited limitations about protecting confidences during the informed consent process. This interaction can provide the MHP with data about whether a meaningful therapeutic alliance can be formed. If a healthy connection does not begin to emerge at this point of the relationship, and before any duty-to-protect context might arise, the MHP should consider the possibility of transferring the client to one of two or three other colleagues who may be better at forming an effective, working clinical relationship with that particular client. Without a therapeutic alliance, if a duty-to-protect situation emerges, the client will not provide sufficient information for the therapist to be able to make good clinical decisions. Certainly, without a therapeutic alliance it will be quite difficult to collaborate effectively with the client. For such a client, follow-through with various interventions on the basis of the assessment conclusions is likely to result in ill-informed interventions, a sense of abandonment or betrayal, and greater likelihood of ethics complaints or malpractice actions. (For more discussion of the role of the therapeutic alliance in protecting clients and third parties from harm, see chap. 5, this volume.)

In discussing risk variables believed to be related to violence perpetration, Monahan (1996) identified that communications about the risks of violence would become a significant factor in curbing violence. Although his focus was on communication with decision makers, such as judges or managed health care gatekeepers, interactions during the risk assessment process also can negatively affect the therapeutic alliance and impair the MHP's ability to work with the client on the violent ideation. The process of identifying and influencing the precipitating and inhibiting factors related to threats of violence will not work as well without the client's facilitative qualities contributing in an effective manner. If the therapeutic alliance is strong, when a client raises a threat of violence with the MHP, the client more easily accepts the risk assessment process, provides releases to obtain additional data, and collaboratively engages in the interventions.

Assessment of the Threat

The MHP engages in an assessment to determine whether a threat of violence is significant enough to warrant intervention. A general approach that has gained greater validation in the literature is to identify the risk factors and to orchestrate interventions that reduce the effects of possible precipitating factors and increase the power of inhibiting factors (Heilbrun, O'Neill, Strohman, Bowman, & Philipson, 2000). Decisions about evaluation can be approached in a standardized manner from one case to the next. Such a standardized approach, combined with an ongoing risk assessment of the particular case, leads to more efficacious clinical judgments (Monahan et al., 2001; Mulvey & Lidz, 1998).

Since *Tarasoff*, research studies have proliferated in an attempt to improve clinical judgment regarding the assessment of violence and to improve the validity of violence prediction. The seminal work by Monahan (1981) represented the first step in the development of psychological research to develop more accurate methods for predicting dangerousness. Since then, a myriad of biopsychosocial factors have been identified that can precipitate and inhibit the dangerous behavior (Scott & Resnick, 2006). After a thorough review of the literature, Scott and Resnick (2006, p. 608) concluded that the "inexact science" of predicting violence is best accomplished by considering the results of a risk assessment instrument combined with a detailed past history. Standardized risk assessment approaches have improved significantly (Harris, Rice, & Camilleri, 2004; Scott & Resnick, 2006).

Structured risk assessments (Monahan, 2006) are designed to obtain actuarial and clinical assessments that reduce clinical judgment errors and increase the accuracy of violence assessments. Recent studies on predictions of violence have shown that structured risk assessments that combined actuarial with clinical assessments resulted in the lowest rates of false-positive and false-negative errors (Harris et al., 2004; Scott & Resnick, 2006). Because of the variability of each client's disposition, history, contextual situation, and clinical issues, "only so much violence can ever be predicted using individually based characteristics, given the highly transactional nature of violence" (Mulvey & Lidz, 1998, p. 107). The research has also suggested that clinicians should examine the relevant changes in a client's life that may lead to violence (Mulvey & Lidz, 1998).

A very accessible actuarial instrument to evaluate a threat of violence against another person is the Iterative Classification Tree. It is viewed as the "instrument of choice for nonforensic" (i.e., noncriminal) clients (Harris et al., 2004, p. 1071). The MacArthur Violence Risk Assessment Study developed the Iterative Classification Tree on a large, multicultural community sample discharged from inpatient psychiatric facilities (Monahan et al., 2000, 2001; see the measure at http://bjp.rcpsych.org/cgi/reprint/176/4/312). Software (Classification of Violence Risk) is also available for processing a 10-minute structured interview and the data from a chart review (Monahan, 2006). Answers to both forms of the approach rely on a series of nested risk factors that lead to accurate classifications of low- to high-risk actuarial determinations about future violence. The Iterative Classification Tree and Classification of Violence Risk draw on easily obtained clinical information, including seriousness of prior arrests, motor impulsiveness, recent violent fantasies, diagnosis of any major mental disorder without any co-occurring substance abuse diagnosis, self-report of violence in the past 2 months, and anger reactions (see http://socialecology.uci.edu/faculty/rwnovaco).

During the session in which the threat emerges, the MHP collaborates with the client to begin to understand the possible impact of variables associated with violence The MHP engages in a structured risk assessment to determine the specific risks and how to mediate those risks. Corroboration of the findings of an actuarial assessment instrument and the clinical assessment about the various relevant precipitating and inhibiting factors can lead to effective interventions. Obtaining collateral information from key respondents or sources (e.g., spouses or partners, prior treatment professionals, hospital records) can also lead to better clinical judgments as multiple-measure corroboration about a pattern of behavior may be more likely to emerge from the evaluation. Recent literature has clustered the variables related to violence in four domains (Monahan et al., 2001):

- *Dispositional variables*, including age, age of first criminal conviction, sex, personality variables involving impulsivity or those involving long-range planning abilities, and neurological factors, such as closed-head injury;
- *Historical variables*, including educational level, childhood and adolescent antisocial behavior, prior convictions for violence, comparable circumstances of prior violence, pattern of unstable conflictual interpersonal relationships, substance abuse history, and history of mental hospitalization;
- *Contextual variables*, including family stability, dangerous or criminal social network, quality of social support, level of occupational responsibilities, financial resources, access and presence of weapons, and availability of victim(s); and
- *Clinical variables*, including types and symptoms of mental disorder, physical warning signs, level of functioning to cope with stressors, recent changes in mood states (anger, anxiety, and sadness), daydreams or thoughts about physically hurting or injuring someone, specificity of violent thoughts or plans, and level of intention to act on violent thoughts.

Scott and Resnick (2006) recommended detailing the likely impact of each known variable and the management or treatment strategy to implement the violence prevention plan. On the basis of corroboration of findings from the risk assessment, the MHP can explore a range of violence prevention interventions with the client as part of the assessment process. For example, if the client admits to owning guns, the client can ask an uninvolved family member to hold the guns and ammunition during the course of the treatment. This type of intervention is founded on the MHP's conclusions about how the precipitating and inhibiting factors are interacting. Each significant precipitating variable is linked to a specific intervention.

Ongoing assessment will also allow the MHP and client to refocus on how to ameliorate variables that may trigger future violence. On the one hand, if progress has not occurred in reducing the impact of a particular precipitating variable, a midcourse correction to the original plan can result in more efficacious treatment. For instance, if the client fails to remove the guns as agreed on, the MHP and the client can arrive at another approach to accomplish the task. Perhaps an effective midcourse intervention would be to call the client's favorite relative during the session and ask that relative to visit the client to pick up the guns. On the other hand, if a particular inhibiting variable seems to be working well, the MHP can focus on increasing its impact. For example, if the client reports that a definite reduction in anger and tension follows each psychotherapy session, then increasing the number of psychotherapeutic sessions per week would be a reasonable next step.

In some cases in which the therapeutic alliance is waning and the precipitating variables appear to be escalating, more intrusive interventions must occur. A useful approach in this context is for the MHP to suggest that an objective evaluation for an involuntary treatment occur. In some jurisdictions, such an evaluation will be conducted within the MHP's office. In other jurisdictions, a police officer can take both the MHP and the client to the facility where such evaluations are conducted. In both instances, no abandonment of the client occurs, and a new management and treatment plan can be developed. Such a formal approach can lead to involuntary outpatient treatment with allied intensive case management being ordered. For other cases, a period of voluntary admission to the hospital or even involuntary inpatient treatment might be ordered. Both types of interventions will lead to a treatment team and the client addressing whether continued treatment of the client by the MHP should occur subsequent to the hospitalization or commitment.

Peer Consultation

A fourth strategy involves seeking peer consultation whenever a doubt arises as to what would be a reasonable evaluation or treatment of the client, particularly if the client discloses material that may call for disclosure because of the law or if the client's condition is worsening despite the MHP's care (Gutheil & Appelbaum, 1982). The MHP conveys to the peer the salient facts about the case (facts that do not lead to the identification of the client) to corroborate whether sufficient assessment has occurred and whether the planned interventions are adequate. Once the peer consultation is obtained, the MHP sends a contemporaneous written communication to the peer that memorializes the facts relied on by the peer and the opinions provided by the peer (Benjamin et al., 1995). The peer consultation shows a transparent decision-making process that has taken into account the facts at hand while attempting to meet the standard of care. Such an action may decrease the risk of an ethics complaint or lawsuit and, if a complaint is filed or the MHP is sued, can help to bolster the MHP's contention that he or she acted reasonably at the time within the standards of care of the MHP's community of peers (Benjamin et al., 1995).

If the outpatient management plan appears not likely to work or if it has failed to reduce the risk of violence, in many jurisdictions an interdisciplinary approach will combine the realms of law and mental health through the strategic use of the law to serve the best interests of the client and the public. The structured risk assessment can lead to interventions that can use the law to protect the client, the public, and the MHP. Many jurisdictions provide a qualified immunity to an MHP for obtaining an involuntary treatment assessment of a client who is mentally ill and a danger to self or others. The client and the public may be best served when an independent evaluation by a specialist working within the involuntary mental health system provides direction about subsequent interventions. The use of such an evaluation can insulate the MHP from liability in many jurisdictions and end the need for the MHP to manage legal risk.

Documentation

Finally, a last recommendation involves documenting the rationale and procedures of the evaluation and treatment of the client. The extraordinary event of disclosing a threat of violence requires thorough documentation to establish what kind of threats prompted the MHP's disclosure, how those threats were assessed, and that the MHP acted reasonably under the circumstances (Benjamin et al., 1995). The documentation about the evaluation and intervention is strengthened by the inclusion of the peer consultation notes. Documentation could include direct quotes from the client about the threat, the results from the structured risk assessment, a listing of the precipitating and inhibiting factors about the threatened violence, and an analysis about how to manage the risk in light of those factors. Every subsequent action related to the management plan requires documentation. For example, documentation of the written releases to talk with collateral witnesses or supporters of the client, and their views about the context, can bolster the reliability of the data. Forwarding the brief written narratives to the collaterals and asking whether they have any other facts to add can also increase the reliability of the data. As the risk is lowered, the evidence establishing the diminution of the risk should also be documented. If the management plan appears not to have reduced the risk of violence, another evaluation and further peer consultation should occur and be documented.

CONCLUSION

Ambiguity about how to fulfill the duty to protect can arise because of a lack of clarity about the laws of many jurisdictions, the conflict between a duty to protect and the duty of confidentiality to the client, and the inexact science of predicting violence. The purpose of this chapter was to acquaint MHPs with the scope and impact of the issue, including the existing statutes, rules, and case law from different states and provinces/territories throughout North America and practical suggestions about how the MHP can meet the duty to protect.

Most jurisdictions have defined some type of standards for meeting the duty to protect, which have led to different implications for MHPs from jurisdiction to jurisdiction. Continued judicial activism in response to egregious fact patterns will lead to the development of further common law. SPAs must use the legislative process to delineate and refine the common law so that the legal and ethical obligations of MHPs are possible to carry out within the bounds of our inexact science. Reasonable approaches to discharging the duty to protect will lead to greater protection of the public while balancing the needs of confidentiality.

As a profession, the mental health field has attempted to increase an understanding of the duty to protect and its implications for MHPs. From a review of the statutes, a series of consultations with other MHPs, and several research studies, we found that a combination of five different practical approaches can enhance MHPs' ability to engage in efficacious behavioral, legal, and ethical actions. Such actions further the best interests of the client. Using the law of the jurisdiction, the MHP can conduct adequate disclosure during the informed consent process regarding confidentiality and its exceptions so that a collaborative relationship develops at the onset of the therapeutic relationship. While maintaining the therapeutic alliance, the MHP can conduct an assessment of the threat by using a combination of actuarial assessment and clinical judgments. Peer consultation can contemporaneously corroborate the reasonableness of the assessment and interventions. Finally, sufficient and timely documentation of incidents and actions taken by the MHP can show to anyone who gains access to the record later that the MHP conscientiously acted in the best interests of the client while meeting the duty to protect.

REFERENCES

Benjamin, G. A. H., Rosenwald, L., Overcast, T., & Feldman, S. B. (1995). *Law and mental health professionals: Washington*. Washington, DC: American Psychological Association.

DeKraai, M. B., & Sales, B. D. (1982). Privileged communications of psychologists. *Professional Psychology: Research and Practice, 13,* 372–388.

Estate of Long *ex rel.* Smith v. Broadlawns Med. Ctr., 656 N.W.2d 71 (Iowa 2002).

Glosoff, H. L., Herlihy, S. B., Herlihy, B., & Spence, E. B. (1997). Privileged communication in the psychologist–client relationship. *Professional Psychology: Research and Practice, 28,* 573–581.

Gutheil, T. G., & Appelbaum, P. S. (1982). *Clinical handbook of psychiatry and the law*. New York: McGraw-Hill.

Harris, G. T., Rice, M. E., & Camilleri, J. A. (2004). Applying a forensic actuarial assessment (the violence risk appraisal guide to nonforensic patients). *Journal of Interpersonal Violence, 19,* 1063–1074.

Heilbrun, K., O'Neill, M. L., Strohman, L. K., Bowman, Q., & Philipson, J. (2000). Expert approaches to communicating violence risk. *Law and Human Behavior, 24,* 137–148.

Horvath, A. O., & Bedi, R. P. (2002). The alliance. In J. C. Norcross (Ed.), *Psychotherapy relationships that work* (pp. 37–69). New York: Oxford University Press.

The impact of the uncertainty for mental health professionals created by Petersen v. State of Washington: Hearings before the House and Senate Judiciary Committees, 49th Leg. Wash. St. (1985).

Matter of Votteler's Estate, 327 N.W.2d 759 (Iowa 1982).

Mills, M. J., Sullivan, G., & Eth, S. (1987). Protecting third parties: A decade after *Tarasoff. American Journal of Psychiatry, 144,* 68–74.

Monahan, J. (1981). *The clinical prediction of violence*. Beverly Hills, CA: Sage.

Monahan, J. (1996). Violence prediction: The past twenty and the next twenty years. *Criminal Justice and Behavior, 23,* 107–120.

Monahan, J. (2006). Tarasoff at thirty: How developments in science and policy shape the common law. *University of Cincinnati Law Review, 75,* 497–521.

Monahan, J., Steadman, H., Appelbaum, P., Robbins, P., Mulvey, E., Silver, E., et al. (2000). Developing a clinically useful actuarial tool for assessing violence risk. *British Journal of Psychiatry, 176,* 312–319.

Monahan, J., Steadman, H., Silver, E., Appelbaum, P., Robbins, P., Mulvey, E., et al. (2001). *Rethinking risk assessment: The MacArthur study of mental disorder and violence*. New York: Oxford University Press.

Mulvey, E. P., & Lidz, C. W. (1998). Clinical prediction of violence as a conditional judgment. *Social Psychiatry and Psychiatric Epidemiology, 33,* 107–113.

Petersen v. State of Washington, 100 Wn.2d, 421, 671 P.2d 230 (1983).

Pomerantz, A. M., & Handelsman, M. M. (2004). Informed consent revisited: An updated written question format. *Professional Psychology: Research and Practice, 35,* 201–205.

Pope, K. S., Simpson, M. H., & Weiner, N. F. (1978). Malpractice in outpatient psychotherapy. *American Journal of Psychotherapy, 32,* 593–602.

Scott, C. L., & Resnick, P. J. (2006). Violence risk assessment in persons with mental illness. *Aggression and Violent Behavior, 11,* 598–611.

Tarasoff v. Regents of the University of California, 17 Cal. 3d 425, 551 P.2d 334 (1976).

VandeCreek, L., Miars, R., & Herzog, C. (1987). Client anticipations and preferences for confidentiality of records. *Journal of Counseling Psychology, 34,* 62–67.

Waitzkin, H. (1984, November 2). Doctor–patient communication: Clinical implications of social scientific research. *JAMA, 252,* 2441–2446.

3

THE DUTY TO PROTECT AND THE ETHICAL STANDARDS OF PROFESSIONAL ORGANIZATIONS

RITA SOMMERS-FLANAGAN, JOHN SOMMERS-FLANAGAN,
AND ELIZABETH REYNOLDS WELFEL

The duty to protect as discussed in the mental health literature, and probably as understood by most mental health professionals, is most strongly associated with the law—either as statutes passed by states and provinces/ territories or as holdings in court cases. The duty also has clear ethical dimensions, embedded in the responsibility of psychotherapists to promote the welfare of those they serve, respect their dignity, and work to help and avoid harm to their clients. Protecting client privacy is fundamental to these lofty ethical goals, and the ethics codes of the American Psychological Association (APA, 2002; http://www.apa.org/ethics/code2002.html), the American Counseling Association (ACA, 2005), and the National Association of Social Workers (NASW, 1999) fully endorse these values both through their aspirational statements and through their enforceable standards. None of these codes, however, sees the protection of client privacy as an absolute requirement, and all permit the breach of client privacy in some circumstances.

As the following sections of this chapter illustrate, each code endorses the responsibility of the professional to safeguard others when they are in danger. Moreover, each code clarifies the responsibility of professionals when their ethical duties appear to conflict with legal requirements. The wording in Standard 1.02 of the APA "Ethical Principles of Psychologists and Code of Conduct" is illustrative:

> If psychologists' ethical responsibilities conflict with law, regulations, or other governing legal authority, psychologists make known their commitment to the Ethics Code and take steps to resolve the conflict. If the conflict is unresolvable via such means, psychologists may adhere to the requirements of the law, regulations, or other governing authority. (p. 1063)

APA'S ETHICS CODE

The responsibility to maintain client privacy and keep others in society safe is expressed in the Introduction to APA's (2002) Ethics Code in the following aspirational (and therefore nonbinding) statements:

Principle A: Beneficence and Nonmaleficence
> Psychologists strive to benefit those with whom they work and take care to do no harm. In their professional actions, psychologists seek to safeguard the welfare and rights of those with whom they interact professionally and other affected persons, and the welfare of animal subjects of research. When conflicts occur among psychologists' obligations or concerns, they attempt to resolve these conflicts in a responsible fashion that avoids or minimizes harm. (p. 1062)

Principle E: Respect for People's Rights and Dignity
> Psychologists respect the dignity and worth of all people, and the rights of individuals to privacy, confidentiality, and self-determination. Psychologists are aware that special safeguards may be necessary to protect the rights and welfare of persons or communities whose vulnerabilities impair autonomous decision making. (p. 1063)

One fundamental component of respect for individual autonomy and dignity is the protection of clients' privacy, keeping both their contact with therapists and the content of their disclosures confidential. Indeed, every version of the seven revisions of the APA Ethics Code endorsed by the association after 1952 has identified the protection of client privacy as a central ethical responsibility of the psychologist and a central ethical value of the profession. Even the most famous court rulings in mental health law (e.g., *Jaffee v. Redmond*, 1996; *Tarasoff v. Regents of the University of California*, 1976) have affirmed the pivotal role of confidentiality of client communications in effective counseling and psychotherapy. The U.S. Supreme Court's statement in *Jaffee v. Redmond* (1996) is illustrative of court interpretations of the role of confidentiality in psychotherapy:

Effective psychotherapy [. . .] depends on an atmosphere of confidence and trust in which the patient is willing to make a frank and complete disclosure of facts, emotions, memories and fears. Because of the sensitive nature of the problems for which individuals consult psychotherapists, disclosure of confidential communications made in counseling sessions may cause embarrassment or disgrace. For this reason, the mere possibility of disclosure may impede development of the confidential relationship necessary for successful treatment. (Section III, para. 1)

Using this reasoning, APA's Ethics Code grants exceptions to confidentiality without client consent only in circumstances in which other ethical values carry greater weight and in jurisdictions in which the law permits or mandates such disclosure. The protection of vulnerable children and elders from abuse and neglect by caretakers is one instance in which another ethical value takes precedence over client privacy. Protecting the safety of third parties at risk of serious harm from clients is another ethical value of psychologists, so that if breaching confidentiality is the only feasible method to safeguard others, then that action is ethically permissible and advisable.

The APA Ethics Code first referred directly to the responsibilities of psychologists with clients whom they judge to be a danger to others in 1981. Earlier publications (APA, 1953, 1959, 1963, 1977) made no specific mention of this topic. The timing of the appearance of such language is not coincidental—the 1981 revision was the first version the association published after the impact of the 1976 *Tarasoff* decision was clear. Specifically, that code read as follows:

Principle 5: Confidentiality
    Psychologists have a primary obligation to respect the confidentiality of information obtained from persons in the course of their work as psychologists. They reveal such information to others only with the consent of the person or the person's legal representative except in those unusual circumstances in which not to do so would result in clear danger to the person or others. Where appropriate, psychologists inform their clients of the legal limits of confidentiality. (APA, 1981, pp. 635–636)

The 1981 Ethics Code is the only version in the history of these standards that refers directly to the issue of clients who are dangerous to self or others. The current revision of the Ethics Code (APA, 2002) uses language that is more general in scope and that more fully acknowledges the legal restraints on client–therapist confidentiality that exist in many jurisdictions.

4.05 Disclosures
    (a) Psychologists may disclose confidential information with the appropriate consent of the organizational client, the individual client/patient, or another legally authorized person on behalf of the client/patient unless prohibited by law.
    (b) Psychologists disclose confidential information without the consent of the individual only as mandated by law, or where permitted by

law for a valid purpose such as to (1) provide needed professional services; (2) obtain appropriate professional consultations; (3) protect the client/patient, psychologist, or others from harm; or (4) obtain payment for services from a client/patient, in which instance disclosure is limited to the minimum that is necessary to achieve the purpose. (p. 1066)

These sections of the 2002 Ethics Code highlight the psychologist's fundamental obligation to confidentiality. It is important to note that nothing in any version of the APA Ethics Code has *mandated* a breach of confidentiality in relation to the duty to protect in the absence of client consent. The language simply *permits* such actions under particular limited situations, expressing deference to legal mandates and regulations related to disclosure without client consent. In other words, in the absence of a legal requirement to break confidentiality (but in the presence of legal permission to breach) psychologists are allowed to use their professional judgment about the advisability of a breach of confidentiality even when clients represent a danger to themselves, to others, or even to the psychologist providing the service. Such a stance makes sense in light of the wide variability in state statutes regarding the duty to protect and the dynamic nature of case law rulings in civil cases against mental health professionals (see chap. 2, this volume). It also makes sense given the variety of circumstances under which a psychologist may be working with a potentially violent or self-destructive client. Unfortunately, both research findings (Givelber, Bowers, & Blitch, 1984; Pabian, Welfel, & Beebe, 2007) and our experience in teaching and consulting with psychologists suggest that at times professionals do not fully appreciate the distinction between the legal duty to protect and the ethical obligations as expressed in the APA Ethics Code. Often, they mistakenly believe that the ethical standards of the profession require a breach of confidentiality when they clearly do not. The permissive language in the professional ethical standards underscores the need for psychologists to understand and stay current with the court rulings and legislation in their jurisdictions. Unfortunately, misunderstandings of the legal duties of psychologists are as common as misunderstandings of the language in the APA Ethics Code (Givelber et al., 1984; Kramer, 1997; Leedy, 1989; Pabian et al., 2007).

It is important to note that even when disclosures are permitted and appropriate to prevent serious and foreseeable harm, the current code (APA, 2002) cautions psychologists to limit the extent of the disclosure as follows:

4.04 Minimizing Intrusions on Privacy
  (a) Psychologists include in written and oral reports and consultations, only information germane to the purpose for which the communication is made. (p. 1066)

In other words, psychologists have ethical responsibilities not only to judge whether a breach of confidentiality is warranted but also to determine what client information is truly essential to a necessary disclosure (p. 1066).

THE ACA *CODE OF ETHICS* AND THE DUTY TO PROTECT

The ACA (2005) *Code of Ethics* is distinct in the mental health professions for the extensive detail it provides regarding the ethical duties of counselors in relation to the protection of client confidentiality. The wording in the ACA *Code of Ethics* on confidentiality and its limits is as follows:

> Section B: Confidentiality, Privileged Communication, and Privacy
> B2 Exceptions
> a. The general requirement that counselors keep information confidential does not apply when disclosure is required to protect clients or identified others from serious and foreseeable harm or when legal requirements demand that confidential information must be revealed. Counselors consult with other professionals when in doubt as to the validity of an exception. Additional considerations apply when addressing end-of-life issues. (p. 7)

Counselors are allowed to break confidentiality to protect others from serious and foreseeable harm. Doing so is a choice, not a mandate, although states vary in their laws in this area (see chap. 2, this volume). The wording represents a significant change from ACA's (1995) *Code of Ethics and Standards of Practice*. Language from the 1995 version of that code included the phrase "The general requirement to keep information confidential does not apply when disclosure is required to prevent clear and imminent danger" (B.1.b). This language insinuated a kind of power to foresee the future that counselors simply do not possess. Disclosing a client's intentions to do harm will not necessarily prevent harm from occurring. Rather than an assumption that disclosure will "prevent clear and imminent danger," counselors are urged to disclose as an effort to protect others from "serious and foreseeable harm."

Although ACA's (2005) *Code of Ethics* does not seem to assume that helping professionals can prevent dangerous things from happening, it still sets the bar rather high. Confidentiality should be broken to try and protect clients or others from harm, but simply providing confidential information will not necessarily constitute protection. As many in the fields of child abuse and intimate partner violence know, disclosures can sometimes increase the possibility of harm, rather than serve as protection (Sundelson, 1999).

Adding to the complexity, the terms *serious* and *foreseeable* both have significant subjective latitude in interpretation. Who is to say what constitutes "serious" as opposed to "less-than-serious" harm? If a client is planning to engage in an affair, will this seriously harm his or her spouse or partner? If an adolescent client is determined to place an overdose of laxative in his or her parent's breakfast cereal to get even for a recent grounding, is this serious harm? What if the parent were diabetic and such dietary meddling could cause complications beyond indigestion?

Further confusion arises when considering the word *foreseeable*. Those of us without the ready use of a crystal ball have difficulty in accurately predicting the future. If an older person discloses that she is going to drive herself and her neighbor five blocks to see a movie, despite the fact that she no longer has a driver's license, is this foreseeable harm to the client or the neighbor? If a client is clearly angry at his boss, has a history of assault, drops hints that it would be quite gratifying to give his boss something to worry about, and then backs off when you query for specifics, how likely is the acting out?

These situations are fairly common in many counseling settings. The counseling relationship provides a safe haven where clients can let off steam, make bold claims, work out less-than-wise impulses, and face their losses and limits. Ethical counselors are clearly invested in the immediate and long-term welfare of their clients. They are also advocates for a better, safer, more just society (Toporek, Gerstein, Fouad, Roysircar-Sodowsky, & Israel, 2005). However, breaking confidentiality in an attempt to prevent harm to someone other than the client does not constitute such advocacy. Instead, in many cases, it is a step that feels like a betrayal of trust. Sometimes students who have little experience working with clients assume it is their duty to report every form of law breaking or threat they hear about. They have yet to experience the intense and focused loyalty and protectiveness that develop in the therapeutic relationship.

The necessarily subjective judgment calls faced by the mental health professional can be a significant source of worry and angst. Note that ACA's (2005) *Code of Ethics* urges the counselor to consult with others before taking steps that break trust and have such potentially serious repercussions. This gives us a chance to underscore advice we give our students and supervisees repeatedly: It is very wise to participate in an ongoing peer consultation group and to periodically get supervision from a more seasoned professional. There is both wisdom and safety in numbers (see Gottlieb, 2006, for an excellent model for peer consultation regarding ethical issues).

NASW'S *CODE OF ETHICS* AND THE DUTY TO PROTECT

The language in the NASW (1999) *Code of Ethics* also takes a permissive approach to the disclosure of confidential information with clients who appear dangerous to self or others, but it offers more specificity regarding the conditions under which a social worker is relieved of the obligation to maintain confidentiality. It identifies three conditions that must be met in this circumstance, paralleling the approach of the court in *Tarasoff* (1976):

Section 1.07 *Privacy and Confidentiality*
    (c) Social workers should protect the confidentiality of all information obtained in the course of professional service, except for compelling professional reasons. The general expectation that social workers will

keep information confidential does not apply when disclosure is necessary to prevent *serious*, *foreseeable*, and *imminent* harm to a client or other *identifiable person* [italics added]. In all instances, social workers should disclose the least amount of confidential information necessary to achieve the desired purpose; only information that is directly relevant to the purpose for which the disclosure is made should be revealed.

(d) Social workers should inform clients, to the extent possible, about the disclosure of confidential information and the potential consequences, when feasible, before the disclosure is made. This applies whether social workers disclose confidential information on the basis of a legal requirement or client consent.

The statement that when feasible, clients should be informed about the disclosure of confidentiality information even when such disclosure is legally mandated is not included in the APA (2002) Ethics Code, although it does appear in the ACA (2005) *Code of Ethics*. In other words, under this section, social workers are generally obligated to inform clients of disclosures made without client consent before the revelation whenever possible, although the code does offer them some latitude in situations in which it does not appear possible to follow this standard (Millstein, 2000; Strom-Gottfried, 2007). It differs from the ACA *Code of Ethics* insofar as it adds the criterion of imminent harm to the criteria of foreseeable and serious harm.

SPECIAL CIRCUMSTANCES: HIV DISEASE AND END-OF-LIFE ISSUES

There are two special situations related to confidentiality and the duty to protect that have received attention in the ACA (2005) *Code of Ethics* but not in either of the other codes (APA, 2002; NASW, 1999) that we highlight here to demonstrate the importance of being familiar with one's own code and with the codes of other professionals with whom one may be collaborating.

HIV Disease

The 1995 ACA *Code of Ethics* provided guidance that would allow counselors, under certain circumstances, to warn someone in danger of unknowingly being exposed to a deadly disease. Although HIV is not specifically mentioned, many professionals see HIV as the prototypical disease that would qualify under this standard, although other conditions (such as tuberculosis) would also be covered (see chap. 10, this volume). Quite similar to the 1995 version, the 2005 version reads as follows:

Section B: Confidentiality
B.2.b. Contagious, Life-Threatening Diseases

When clients disclose that they have a disease commonly known to be both communicable and life threatening, counselors may be justified in disclosing information to identifiable third parties, if they are known to be at demonstrable and high risk of contracting the disease. Prior to making a disclosure, counselors confirm that there is such a diagnosis and assess the intent of clients to inform the third parties about their disease or to engage in any behaviors that may be harmful to an identifiable third party. (p. 7)

Providing this possible justification is not without controversy. Neither the APA (2002) nor the NASW (1999) ethics code addresses this concern as specifically, and many would question such a disclosure (Melchert & Patterson, 1999). Because APA's Ethics Code does not include any specific language related to the ethics of breaching confidentiality in this circumstance, the broad statements in Section 4.05 Disclosures have the most applicability here. The APA Ethics Code permits but does not mandate disclosure to third parties without client consent on the basis of relevant laws and the judgment of the psychologist about the risk of harm to the client or others. In 1991, APA's Board of Directors and Council of Representatives issued further guidance on the profession's views of confidentiality related to client disclosures of HIV status. This resolution, titled *Legal Liability Related to Confidentiality and the Prevention of HIV Transmission,* affirmed the association's support for the confidentiality of client disclosures on this topic and formally expressed APA's opposition to the imposition of a legal duty to protect related to HIV transmission. It went on to state that if such legislation were to be enacted,

then it should permit disclosure only when (a) the provider knows of an identifiable third party who the provider has compelling reason to believe is at significant risk for infection; (b) the provider has a reasonable belief that the third party has no reason to suspect that he or she is at risk; and (c) the client/patient has been urged to inform the third party and has either refused or is considered unreliable in his/her willingness to notify the third party. (APA, 1991, para. 10)

Unfortunately, research in this area of decision making about disclosures of HIV status without client consent suggests that the therapist's views of homosexuality and the sexual orientation of the person at risk for infection influence professional decision making. For example, in responses to vignettes including a client with HIV, Palma and Iannelli (2002) found that counseling psychology students used different decision rules when deciding to breach confidentiality to warn unprotected sexual partners. Uninformed male partners of gay men were significantly less likely to be identified as parties to warn than were uninformed female partners of heterosexual men. In a study of the association between homophobia and a willingness to breach confidentiality about HIV status, McGuire, Nieri, Abbott, Sheridan, and

Fisher (1995) found that practicing psychotherapists who scored higher on a measure of homophobia were more likely to breach confidentiality.

Of course, breaking confidentiality regarding a client's HIV status is of great concern because of the likelihood of discrimination, job loss, and related risks (Breurer, 2005). It should never be done casually, without extensive consultation, or without comprehension of relevant legal requirements. However, the ACA (2005) *Code of Ethics*, in the spirit of protecting specific third parties, has created potential ethical justification for this kind of action. Please refer to chapter 10, this volume, for an extensive discussion of legal and ethical issues in working with clients with HIV spectrum disorders.

End-of-Life Issues

In its 2005 *Code of Ethics*, ACA again led the way in opening and examining an area directly relevant to the generally assumed counselor's duty to act always to protect and preserve life. This version includes discussion of considerations that may come into play with clients near the end of life. Similar to the unique stand taken on breaking confidentiality in certain situations with a client who has a communicable disease, this new standard opens the door for the counselor to take very particular aspects of a situation into account. In some ways, such permission places a significant burden on the counselor. Section A.9.c. of the 2005 ACA *Code of Ethics* states,

> Counselors who provide services to terminally ill individuals who are considering hastening their own deaths have the options of breaking or not breaking confidentiality, depending on applicable laws and the specific circumstances of the situation and after seeking consultation or supervision from appropriate professional and legal parties. (p. 6)

This statement provides counselors more latitude than previous ethical standards may have allowed. Although it is likely that some mental health professionals have chosen to keep confidential a terminally ill client's plans to hasten his or her own death, it has been an ethical issue about which mental health professionals disagree. Deeply held personal and professional values vary widely in this area (Byock, 1997; Koppel, 1999). This statement, new to the 2005 ACA *Code of Ethics* and still absent from the APA (2002) and NASW (1999) ethics codes, allows professional discretion in an area that could otherwise lead to a duty to protect requiring a break in confidentiality.

Psychologists must once again rely on Section 4.05 (APA, 2002), which allows a breach of confidentiality when clients are considering hastening their own deaths in jurisdictions in which laws permit such disclosures. The profession's stance on end-of-life issues is more fully stated in the reports of the APA Working Group on Assisted Suicide and End-of-Life Decisions (2000) and in the resolutions passed by the Council of Representatives that do not mandate prevention when an individual at the end of life is considering hastening his or her death (see http://www.apa.org/pi/eol; Farberman, 1997).

Practitioners and policymakers are continuing to grapple with the factors that would come into play on either side of this decision (Werth & Rogers, 2005). This topic is covered in greater depth in chapter 13 of this volume.

CONCLUSION

In summary, the ethics codes of ACA (2005) and NASW (1999) place the ultimate responsibility for making the determination to disclose confidential information about dangerousness without client consent on the professional. The APA (2002) Ethics Code highlights legal considerations more prominently in this judgment, allowing the psychologist this latitude when legal considerations permit such disclosures. In addition, the APA Ethics Code does not qualify the level or foreseeability of harm in its comments on disclosure of confidential information, in contrast to the other professions, both of which use the qualifiers of *serious and foreseeable* harm. NASW adds a third qualifier, *imminent*, to its language. These additions make sense because these codes do not explicitly limit breaches of confidentiality without client permission to circumstances in which there are legal mandates or legal permission.

Only the ACA (2005) *Code of Ethics* offers specific enforceable provisions regarding the breach of confidentiality for end-of-life situations and situations in which a client is placing another at risk for a life-threatening communicable disease. The discretion offered to the professional is fitting in light of the complex and confusing circumstances professionals typically face when attempting to sort out whether a client is at risk of harming someone and which therapeutic intervention is best suited to deescalate the risk and protect the safety and privacy of all involved.

Each code of ethics encourages clinicians not to make ethical judgments in isolation and to consult with other professionals when in doubt about the ethics of an action or when an action is likely to have serious consequences for a client or therapist (APA, 2002, Preamble; ACA, 2005, Section C.2.e.; NASW, 1999, Section 2.05[a]). Or as Steven Behnke, director of the APA Ethics Office, commented in a workshop sponsored by the Ohio Psychological Association in 2004, "Never worry alone."

REFERENCES

American Counseling Association. (1995). *Code of ethics and standards of practice.* Alexandria, VA: Author.

American Counseling Association. (2005). *ACA code of ethics.* Alexandria, VA: Author. Retrieved July 1, 2006, from http://www.counseling.org/Resources/ CodeOfEthics/TP/Home/CT2.aspx

American Psychological Association. (1953). *Ethical standards of psychologists.* Washington, DC: Author.

American Psychological Association. (1959). Ethical standards of psychologists. *American Psychologist, 14,* 279–282.

American Psychological Association. (1963). Ethical standards of psychologists. *American Psychologist, 18,* 56–60.

American Psychological Association. (1977, March). Ethical standards of psychologists. *APA Monitor,* pp. 22–23.

American Psychological Association. (1981). Ethical principles of psychologists. *American Psychologist, 36,* 633–638.

American Psychological Association. (1991). *Legal liability related to confidentiality and the prevention of HIV transmission.* Retrieved June 28, 2007, from http:// www.apa.org/pi/hivres.html#confihiv

American Psychological Association. (2002). Ethical principles of psychologists and code of conduct. *American Psychologist, 57,* 1060–1073.

APA Working Group on Assisted Suicide and End-of-Life Decisions. (2000). *Report to the Board of Directors of the American Psychological Association.* Retrieved November 1, 2005, from http://www.apa.org/pi/aseolf.html

Breurer, N. L. (2005). Teaching the HIV-positive client how to manage the workplace. *Journal of Vocational Rehabilitation, 22,* 163–169.

Byock, I. (1997). *Dying well: The prospect for growth at the end of life.* New York: Riverhead.

Farberman, R. K. (1997). Terminal illness and hastened death requests: The important role of the mental health professional. *Professional Psychology: Research and Practice, 28,* 544–547.

Givelber, D. J., Bowers, W. J., & Blitch, C. L. (1984). *Tarasoff,* myth and reality: An empirical study of private law in action. *Wisconsin Law Review, 1984,* 443–497.

Gottlieb, M. C. (2006). A template for peer ethics consultation. *Ethics & Behavior, 16,* 151–162.

Jaffee v. Redmond, 518 U.S. 1, 116 S. Ct. 1923 (1996).

Koppel, M. S. (1999). A Jungian perspective on therapy at the end of life. *Pastoral Psychology, 48,* 45–56.

Kramer, L. (1997). A comparison study of the psychologists' duty to protect third parties from the potential violence of their patients. *Dissertation Abstracts International, 58*(7), 3927B.

Leedy, S. (1989). Psychologists' knowledge and application of *Tarasoff* in their decision about dangerousness. *Dissertation Abstracts International, 50*(10), 4775B.

McGuire, J., Nieri, D., Abbott, D., Sheridan, K., & Fisher, R. (1995). Do *Tarasoff* principles apply in AIDS-related psychotherapy? Ethical decision making and the role of therapist homophobia and perceived client dangerousness. *Professional Psychology: Research and Practice, 26,* 608–611.

Melchert, T. P., & Patterson, M. M. (1999). Duty to warn and interventions with HIV-positive clients. *Professional Psychology: Research and Practice, 30,* 180–186.

Millstein, K. (2000). Confidentiality in direct social work practice: Inevitable challenges and ethical dilemmas. *Families in Society, 81,* 270–282.

National Association of Social Workers. (1999). *NASW code of ethics.* Washington, DC: Author. Retrieved June 28, 2007, from http://www.socialworkers.org/pubs/code/default.asp

Pabian, Y. L., Welfel, E. R., & Beebe, R. (2007, August). *Psychologists' knowledge and application of state laws in Tarasoff-type situations.* Paper presented at the 115th Annual Convention of the American Psychological Association, San Francisco.

Palma, T., & Iannelli, R. (2002). Therapeutic reactivity to confidentiality with HIV positive clients: Bias or epidemiology? *Ethics & Behavior, 12,* 353–370.

Strom-Gottfried, K. (2007). *Straight talk about professional ethics.* Chicago: Lyceum.

Sundelson, D. (1999). Restoring the confessional: Reporting laws and the destruction of confidentiality. In H. Kaley, M. N. Eagle, & D. L. Wolitzky (Eds.), *Psychoanalytic therapy as health care: Effectiveness and economics in the 21st century* (pp. 89–102). Hillsdale, NJ: Analytic Press.

Tarasoff v. Regents of the University of California, 17 Cal. 3d 425, 551 P.2d 334 (1976).

Toporek, R. L., Gerstein, L. H., Fouad, N. A., Roysircar-Sodowsky, G., & Israel, T. (Eds.). (2005). *Handbook for social justice in counseling psychology: Leadership, vision, and action.* Thousand Oaks, CA: Sage.

Werth, J. L., Jr., & Rogers, J. R. (2005). Assessing for impaired judgment as a means of meeting the "duty to protect" when a client is a potential harm-to-self: Implications for clients making end-of-life decisions. *Mortality, 10,* 7–21.

4

INTERNATIONAL ETHICS CODES AND THE DUTY TO PROTECT

MARK M. LEACH

Carrying out a duty to protect, especially when it involves a breach of confidentiality in the absence of client consent, becomes more complex when discussing international ethics issues because ethical and legal decisions surrounding confidentiality and duty to protect tend to be culture specific, given cultural and legal variations across countries. The purpose of this chapter is threefold: (a) to discuss the relationship between ethics guidelines and duty-to-protect issues from a cross-cultural perspective; (b) to determine the extent to which an ethical duty to protect, through confidentiality and disclosure, is found in ethics codes internationally and to discuss implications; and (c) to offer a glimpse into the variations involved in confidentiality and disclosure standards as presented in international ethics codes.

ETHICS CODES

Ethics and ethics codes are designed to protect the public and guide practice, although codes differ internationally in their breadth, depth, structure, and relationships with legal statutes and standards (Leach & Harbin,

1997; see also chap. 3, this volume). Codes consist of two types of guidelines, principles and standards. Principles make up the foundation for critical appraisal of ethical reasoning and are associated with philosophies that guide good practice. Originally discussed by Aristotle, principles emphasize overarching guidelines, higher level norms, and ambitious goals. They are nonenforceable rules to assist in decision making (Kitchener, 1984). For example, beneficence (do good and promote growth) and nonmaleficence (do no harm), fidelity and responsibility (create loyalty and trust), integrity (honesty), justice (fairness), and respect for individual rights and dignity (autonomy) are all highlighted in the American Psychological Association's (APA's; 2002) "Ethical Principles of Psychologists and Code of Conduct" and in numerous other codes in a variety of professions. Principled ethics such as beneficence and autonomy can become competing values, especially when considering disclosures surrounding duty-to-protect issues. The competition stems from valuing a client's decision-making abilities but also needing to disclose previously confidential information to protect the client and others. Though some ethics codes are comprised solely of principles, the majority consists of combinations of principles and standards.

Standards are the specified guidelines that practitioners often consult during their daily ethical decision making. They are "legalistic" and enforceable rules that guide practice and can be met with some disagreement about and variation in interpretation among psychologists because no ethics code can cover all possible ethical scenarios. Although psychological organizations internationally may have ethics codes that share similar standards, they can be interpreted differently on the basis of national culture, individual morality, and local legal standards. Regardless of interpretation, standards are associated with good professional ethical behaviors and are a reason why some ethics codes are called "codes of conduct."

INTERNATIONAL ETHICS CODES

Gauthier (2005), in conjunction with the International Union of Psychological Sciences, the International Association of Applied Psychology, and the International Association for Cross-Cultural Psychology, has been developing a document titled the *Universal Declaration of Ethical Principles for Psychologists*, designed to act as a common set of principles from which ethics codes internationally can be developed or modified. It is a means through which to find common psychological values, regardless of country and culture, and is highly likely to be ratified in 2008. Related to this chapter, it has the potential to offer an ethical foundation from which psychologists can construct the conditions under which disclosure of previously held confidential information can occur when clients may be dangerous to third parties.

The level to which the declaration eventually interfaces with the legal duty to protect will be associated with individual national laws.

Many psychological organizations internationally have developed ethics codes, some receiving initial direction by relying on already established codes from other countries, and others creating their codes with little external guidance. For example, the authors of the *Turkish Psychological Association Ethics Code* (Turkish Psychological Association, 2004) reviewed several countries' codes of ethics across multiple cultures, resulting in a code that reflects Turkish professional psychology culture (Yeşim Korkut, personal communication, October 21, 2006). Although most codes of ethics contain both principles and standards, they typically emphasize one over the other in terms of code content, language, and format. For example, the APA (2002) Ethics Code begins with a preamble and principles, but the majority of the content, language, structure, and form of the code lends itself to legalistic, enforceable standards (Leach & Harbin, 1997). Conversely, the Maltese *Charter of Professional Ethics* (Malta Union of Professional Psychologists, n.d.) is shorter and incorporates aspirational language, and the content focuses on principles.

Ethics codes standards are culture centered insofar as they are developed within a particular culture and reflect the values of that culture (see Leach, Glosoff, & Overmier, 2001). By virtue of sharing the same profession, though, psychologists internationally also share certain values that the field of psychology has deemed important. It would be expected that these common values, with consequent ethical principles and standards, would also be reflected in and consistent among many countries' ethics codes. In fact, some countries within the European Federation of Psychologists' Associations are assessing psychologists' practice mobility across European countries because of common educational and training backgrounds. This assessment includes discussion of common and disparate ethical principles and standards among ethics codes (Peiro & Lunt, 2002). However, little research guides the comparison of international ethics codes and their similarities and differences among principles and standards. Comparisons of ethics codes help determine ethics consistency internationally, including consistency in the duty-to-protect and risk management issues. By comparing codes, one can begin to illuminate common principles and standards and to examine common values across countries and cultures, as well as highlight principles and standards that are culture specific.

Few studies comparing psychological ethics codes internationally have been conducted. Leach and Harbin (1997) compared all principles and standards of codes from 24 countries and concluded that 10 individual standards approached universal agreement, especially the standards titled "Disclosures" and "Maintaining Confidentiality," found in 100% and 95% of codes, respectively. In essence, general ethical confidentiality statements are clearly universal, and confidentiality is a cornerstone from which psychological practice is grounded internationally. The broad standards related to maintaining and breaching confidentiality and to disclosures found in Leach and Harbin offer a glimpse into the importance of clinical guidance on duty-to-protect concerns, although these authors did not specifically review this concept.

A follow-up study (Leach et al., 2001) determined unique features of the codes, attesting to the cultural specificity of some of the standards. More broadly, within the international psychological ethics research field, a number of studies have been conducted in multiple countries comparing ethical dilemmas that psychologists face to determine ethically distressing incidents confronted regardless of country and culture (e.g., Pettifor & Sawchuk, 2006; Pope & Vetter, 1992; Slack & Wassenaar, 1999). In the most recent study assessing psychologists in nine primarily Western countries, Pettifor and Sawchuk (2006) reported that confidentiality issues created the greatest number of dilemmas that psychologists encountered internationally. It is unfortunate that they did not request information highlighting resolutions to the specific dilemmas, an important next step in this research area. As the daily practices and dilemmas faced by psychologists internationally begin to be understood, ethics codes will undergo further refinement leading to better ethical decision making (Lindsay & Clarkson, 1999).

DUTY TO PROTECT AND DISCLOSURE

Clinicians often immediately think of the potential for client suicide and homicide when considering imminent danger and disclosure, although additional issues are included in this text. Legal and ethical guidance for clinical decision making regarding potential client suicide and homicide is often less specific than, for example, such guidance regarding child abuse and elder abuse, which are often defined pretty clearly legally. With suicide and homicide ideation or threats, there may be some initial latitude for the psychologist legally, ethically, or morally as to whether disclosure is necessary. For example, a client recently fantasized about killing her partner for his infidelity and said that she would "probably use his gun . . . . I know where he keeps it." The extent of intent was unknown at that time, and a full homicide assessment was conducted to determine the degree of intent to which the client was a danger to her partner. Even after conducting an assessment, ultimate ethical decision making regarding disclosure statements rests with the judgment of the clinician. Strict legal guidance is not always available to clinicians. Not all states adhere to the *Tarasoff* (1976) holding (e.g., Texas) because of more recent case or statutory law, which can be confusing to psychologists, therefore requiring them to understand specific state statutes (see chap. 2, this volume). Regardless of specific case law or statutes, good, ethical clinical practice indicates that potential disclosure without the client's consent should be discussed in both oral and written formats for clients at the outset of therapy (APA, 2002). As Koocher and Keith-Spiegel (1998) indicated, a failure to tell clients of this limitation is not necessarily unethical, but informing clients of limits can help the wise therapist avoid concerns later in treatment. The extent to which other countries include disclosure statements in their ethics codes is unclear.

DISCLOSURE IN ETHICS CODES INTERNATIONALLY

Within ethics codes internationally, the duty to protect self and others often falls under ethics headings of Confidentiality or Informed Consent, with the overarching goal of protecting individuals from unjustifiable disclosures. To determine the extent to which duty-to-protect issues are included in psychology ethics codes internationally, 34 national codes were reviewed. Codes were assembled in a variety of ways, initially from mailings to all psychological organizations listed in the International Union of Psychological Sciences directory (see Leach & Harbin, 1997) and subsequently by downloading them from organization Web sites and through personal contacts. They have been updated when code revisions have become available. A number of codes were translated by native speakers, or if the full text could not be translated, international colleagues were contacted and asked whether a particular standard or principle was included in their respective code. For this chapter, a total of 34 codes were examined, representing 38 countries (5 countries—Denmark, Finland, Iceland, Norway, and Sweden—are under the purview of the Scandinavian code and therefore counted as a single code).

To establish the number of countries that include specific ethical disclosure statements (standards are assessed specifically, although some may fall under principled headings, e.g., Italy) in their code explicitly related to harming self or others (essentially, imminent danger), broadly defined, determinations based on five criteria were devised. First, inclusion of higher level aspirational principles such as autonomy and beneficence were not sufficient because they may be related to confidentiality broadly construed but not to disclosure and duty-to-protect standards specifically. Second, it was insufficient for codes to include only general confidentiality standards that did not specifically mention duty-to-protect issues. For example, the Filipino code (Psychological Association of the Philippines, n.d.) states, "The very nature of his [sic] work which touches the inner lives of his subjects, students and clients, the Clinical Psychologist is duty-bound to withhold information about any individual" (B. Confidentiality). Third, statements regarding disclosure with the client's consent, under court mandate, or under a third-party agreement were not included because they are related to disclosure but not specifically to the duty to protect. For example, the code from the Netherlands (Netherlands Institute of Psychologists, 1998) states,

If the contract includes the drafting of reports for an external principal or a third party, then there is no confidentiality. . . . The psychologist is obliged to treat as confidential any additional information that may have been revealed to them, but is not relevant to the report and to third parties. (III.2.4.2)

Fourth, general statements about informing the client of the limits of confidentiality were not specific enough to meet the criterion. Numerous countries' codes had statements similar to one found in the New Zealand code (New Zealand Psychological Society, 2002): "Psychologists discuss with persons and organizations with whom they establish a research or professional relationship (a) the limits of confidentiality" (1.6.3). Finally, the codes had to include specific duty-to-protect statements regarding disclosure of confidential information. For example, the Turkish code (Turkish Psychological Association, 2004), one of the more comprehensive in this area, explicitly states that psychologists may disclose confidential information "if the person being served has already harmed and or will harm himself, the psychologist or a third party" and "all harassment situations involving a child or an adolescent who is under the age of 18, an elderly or a person with a mental impairment who is legally incapable" (3.3d).

It should be noted that some codes included ethics statements that may have been implicitly related to duty to protect through reference to the law (e.g., Germany, Israel, Malta). Therefore, clinicians may have disclosure guidelines embedded within law but not explicitly stated in their respective ethics code. For example, Malta's code (Malta Union of Professional Psychologists, n.d.) states,

> Psychologists respect, and strive to promote, the fundamental rights, freedom, dignity, confidentiality, autonomy, and the psychological well-being of the individual. They can only accomplish this with the consent of the individual concerned except in cases where otherwise sanctioned by law. (Respect and Development of the Rights and Dignity of Persons)

Similarly, Israel (Israel Psychological Association, 2005) has a standard stating, "Psychologists will keep materials concerning their clients obtained during their professional work confidentially, unless the law permits" (2.5, Professional Confidentiality).

The German code (German Psychological Society & Association of German Professional Psychologists, 1999) is unique in that it explicitly provides the applicable legal statute:

> Pursuant to §203 of the German Criminal Code (StGB), psychologists are required to protect the confidentiality of all information confided to them in the course of exercising their professional activities except in those exceptional instances defined by law or in the event that other higher-ranking legal interests are in jeopardy. (Standard B.III.1.1)

International ethics codes offer unique ethical perspectives on duty-to-protect issues, and at least two areas can be considered: (a) general disclosure statements surrounding the limits of confidentiality and (b) specific duty-to-protect statements within the limits of confidentiality. In this study, 97% of the 34 codes (representing 38 countries) included at least a general statement regarding the possibility of disclosing confidential information. This finding is consistent with Leach and Harbin (1997), who found disclosure statements contained within 100% of the codes. Only the Estonian code (Union of Estonian Psychologists, 1990) did not include a disclosure statement, a finding that was expected given the aspirational language of the code, consisting of only 10 briefly stated principles.

The ethics codes were also evaluated for specific ethical standard examples related to the duty to protect. Results indicated that approximately 70% of countries' codes included specific information regarding disclosing confidential information to protect clients or others from harm, although countries define their ethical standards in multiple ways (see Exhibit 4.1). Thus, the duty to protect was explicitly contained in the majority of the codes available.

DISCUSSION

The purpose of this chapter is to determine the extent to which ethics standards related to duty-to-protect issues are included in international psychological ethics codes. As indicated earlier, the intent is to determine the inclusion of enforceable standards. Consistent with Leach and Harbin (1997), almost 100% of the codes included general disclosure statements. Approximately 70% of the codes included specific reference to duty-to-protect concerns, suggesting that it, too, is approaching a universal psychological standard.

Specifics of the International Codes

Certain sections of the codes are noteworthy, and four are briefly mentioned because this study is the first to review duty-to-protect issues internationally. First, nearly all of the codes that mentioned limits of confidentiality also indicated that psychologists should strive to arrive at a working agreement with the client before taking further steps. For example, the Netherlands code (Netherlands Institute of Psychologists, 1998) states that the

> psychologist is not obliged to observe confidentiality if [she or he] has legitimate reason to believe that a breach of confidence is the sole remaining measure that can prevent clear and imminent danger to any individual, or if they are required by law to disclose confidential information. (Standard III.2.4.3)

EXHIBIT 4.1
Principles and Standards Within Ethics Codes Internationally
Specifically Related to Duty-to-Protect Issues

Australia

Section B: Relationships With Clients

6. Must not disclose criminal acts of a client unless there is an overriding legal obligation to do so or when failure to disclose may result in clear risk to themselves or others.

Canada

Principle I: Respect for the Dignity of Persons

Confidentiality

I.45 [Psychologists should] share confidential information with others only with the informed consent of those involved, or in a manner that the persons involved cannot be identified, except as required or justified by law, or in circumstances of actual or possible serious physical harm or death.

Principle II: Responsible Caring

Offset/Correct Harm

II.39 [Psychologists should] do everything reasonably possible to stop or offset the consequences of actions by others when these actions are likely to cause serious physical harm or death. This may include reporting to appropriate authorities (e.g., the police), an intended victim, or a family member or other support person who can intervene, and would be done even when a confidential relationship is involved.

Chile

None specifically stated.

China

Health System

IV. Other

3. Crisis Intervention: In the process of counseling or doing psychotherapy, if you discover that a patient or visitor could harm themselves or the safety of the society, the psychologist of counseling or psychotherapy should immediately take the necessary steps to prevent an accident from happening.

Costa Rica

Responsibilities of Practicing Professionals

Article 15b. Information which is under professional secrecy can only be transmitted in order to avoid grave harm to which the attendant person or third parties could be exposed.

Croatia

None specifically stated.

Czech-Moravia

1. Competence, Responsibility

2.1 Psychologists uphold the principle of working with clients with their consent unless the law expressly states otherwise, or with the exception of pressing situations demanding action for the benefit of the client.

Dominican Republic

Confidentiality

Article 3.02 Psychologists may present confidential information to professionals or authorities when there exists a real and imminent danger for the individual or society.

Estonia[a]

None specifically stated.

France

Chapter 2: Conditions of Professional Practice

Article 13 In accordance with the provisions of the criminal law as regards non-assistance to someone in danger, s/he is obligated to notify, to the judicial authorities in charge of the law's application, any situation which can endanger the integrity of the people. In the particular case where it is confidential information . . . the psychologist evaluates in good conscience the action to be taken, by considering the legal regulations regarding professional secrecy and assistance to anyone in danger. The psychologist can clarify his decision by consulting with colleagues.

Germany

None specifically stated.

Great Britain

Principle: Respect

1.2 Standard of Privacy and Confidentiality

(vi) Restrict breaches of confidentiality to those exceptional circumstances under which there appears sufficient evidence to raise serious concern about: (a) the safety of clients; (b) the safety of other persons who may be endangered by the client's behavior; or (c) the health, welfare, or safety of children or vulnerable adults.

Hong Kong

Confidentiality

2.4 In exceptional circumstances, where there is sufficient evidence to raise serious concern about the safety or interests of clients, or about others who may be threatened by the client's behavior, Members shall take such steps as are judged necessary to inform appropriate third parties even without the prior consent of the clients. Whenever possible, Members shall consult an experienced and independent colleague beforehand.

Ireland

1.0 Respect for the Rights and Dignity of the Person

1.2 Privacy and Confidentiality

1.2.5 [Psychologists] share confidential information with others only with the informed consent (see Section 1.3) of those involved, or in a manner that the individu-

continues

EXHIBIT 4.1
Continued

als involved cannot be identified, except as required or justified by law, or in circumstances of actual or possible serious physical harm or death.

1.3 Informed Consent and Freedom of Consent

1.3.6 [Psychologists] act in emergencies (for example, where a client threatens suicide) on the basis of their professional judgment, if necessary without consent, but if possible obtain fully informed consent at a later stage.

Israel

None specifically stated.

Italy

General principles

Article 14 In other cases he [*sic*] shall carefully evaluate the need to make a total or partial exception to the confidentiality he is bounded by, when serious dangers for the life or psychological well-being of the patient and others arise.

Latvia

1. Professional Responsibilities and Obligations

1.4 Psychologists obtain appropriate informed consent from their adult clients regarding psychological services. Exceptions are made only in working with clients who do not have the capacity to give consent, in which case an effort is made to obtain informed permission from a legally authorized person. Psychologists obtain appropriate informed consent from the parents of minors regarding psychological services, except in crisis situations where the minor is dangerous to him- or herself or to others.

1.5 Psychologists must report to child protection authorities any suspected incidents of sexual, physical, or psychological abuse.

3. Confidentiality

3.4 When working with children or youth, psychologists obtain consent from parents before releasing confidential information to professionals in other agencies. An exception to the policy exists when the psychologist believes the student is in immediate danger to him- or herself or to others.

Lithuania

None specifically stated.

Malta[a]

None specifically stated.

Netherlands

Autonomy and Self-Determination

III2.4.3 Psychologist is not obliged to observe confidentiality if he [*sic*] has legitimate reason to believe that a breach of confidence is the sole remaining measure that can prevent clear and imminent danger to any individual, or if they are required by law to disclose confidential information.

New Zealand

1.6 Privacy and Confidentiality

Psychologists recognize and promote persons' and people's [*sic*] rights to privacy. They also recognise that there is a duty to disclose to appropriate people real threats to the safety of individuals and the public.

1.6.10 Psychologists recognize that there are certain exceptions and/or limitations to non-disclosure of personal information, and particular circumstances where there is a duty to disclose. These include[b,c] . . . (c) Urgent need: Where a situation arises when it is impossible or impracticable to seek consent to disclosure in time to prevent harm or injury to the person, persons, family, whanau, or community group; In these circumstances psychologists should report to the person, persons, or the person authorized to represent his/her interests, as soon as practicable, any information disclosed to a third party . . . (e) Client or public safety: Where a psychologist believes that non-disclosure may endanger a client, research participant or another person but is denied permission to disclose, the psychologist exercises professional judgment in deciding whether to breach confidentiality or not.

Peru

None specifically stated.

Philippines

B. Confidentiality

3. He [*sic*] releases information to appropriate individual/authorities only after careful deliberation or when there is imminent danger to the individual and the community.

Poland

The Practicing Psychologist

21. Information covered by professional secrecy may only be divulged when the safety of the client or other persons are seriously at risk. Whenever possible, decisions in such cases should be carefully discussed with an experienced and unbiased colleague.

24. The psychologist will advise assistants (or other professionals) of the obligation of absolute observance of professional secrecy, with the exception of risks to the safety of other persons, while reports and documents passed on for elaboration must be protected as far as possible to preserve the anonymity of the person concerned.

Puerto Rico

Confidentiality

3. The confidential information received is revealed only to professional and/or pertinent public authorities when the client threatens or infers hopeless damage to himherself and/or to third parties.

Russia[d]

Article 5: . . . if there are medical indications for controlling the patient's behaviors, the interference should be confined to clinical necessity; in such cases the psychiatrist should inform the patient about the nature of the measures taken and the reasons for them.

continues

EXHIBIT 4.1
Continued

In caring of his patients, the psychiatrist should follow the principle of minimal constraint of freedom and should help develop the patient's responsibility for his actions. In case of conflicting interests, the psychiatrist must give preference to the interests of the patient, unless their realization could cause serious damage to the patient and threaten the rights of other persons.

Article 7: Intervention cannot be used against or irrespective of the patient's own will, except where, because of severe mental disorder, the patient is incapable of forming a judgment as to what is beneficial to him [*sic*] and when lack of such interference might cause serious damage to the patient or to other people. Application of involuntary measure is necessary in such cases and is morally justified, though it is acceptable only within the limits defined by such necessity.

Article 8: The psychiatrist is permitted to disclose confidential information without the patient's consent only in cases specified by law or when the psychiatrist has no other means to prevent serious harm to the patient or to other persons. In these cases the patient should be informed of the disclosure whenever possible.

According to the Russian Federation "On Protection of Health of Citizens" (Article 61), "medical disclosure is necessary regardless of the patient's desires . . . [under the following conditions]: (a) the examination and treatment of a citizen incapable of expressing his will because of his condition; (b) the threat of the spread of infectious disease, mass poisonings, or strikes; (c) inquiry by authorities in connection with an investigation, inquest, or trial; (d) provision of information to the parents or legal guardians of a minor under 15 years of age who requires care; or (e) evidence that a citizen's health was harmed as a result of illegal actions" (p. 165; Polubinskaya & Bonnie, 1996).

Scandinavia

IV Confidentiality

A.1 Psychologists do not maintain confidentiality if they thereby risk harming the client. Exceptions from the requirements of confidentiality shall be made if there is obvious danger for the client or others, but information must be passed on to those who can initiate adequate actions in the situation at hand.

Serbia

None specifically stated.

Singapore

Principle 6: Confidentiality

Safeguarding information . . . is a primary obligation of the psychologist. Such information is not communicated to others unless certain conditions are met: Information received in confidence is revealed only after most careful deliberation and when there is clear and imminent danger to an individual or to society, and then only to appropriate professional workers or public authorities. [Note: Other conditions not related to this chapter are included in the code.]

Slovenia[a]

Confidentiality

(6) Psychologists may renounce this obligation only in cases when this is necessary for the benefit of the client or society, and shall be personally and morally responsible for making judgments in this case.

South Africa

3 Privacy, Confidentiality, and Records

3.4 Disclosures

3.4.1 Psychologists may disclose confidential information only with the permission of the individual or mandated by law, or when permitted by law for a valid purpose, such as to provide needed professional services to the client, to obtain appropriate professional consultations, to protect the client or others from harm, or to obtain payment for services, in which instance disclosure is limited to the minimum necessary to achieve that purpose.

3.8 Reporting of Abuse of Children and Vulnerable Adults

Psychologist shall report the abuse of children and vulnerable adults in terms of relevant law and professional responsibility.

Spain

None specifically stated.

Switzerland

None specifically stated.

Turkey

3.3 Maintaining Confidentiality of the Records

Conditions under which confidentiality may not be maintained: If the party being served has already harmed and/or will harm himself (*sic*), psychologist, or a third party; All harassment situations involving a child or an adolescent who is under the age of 18, an elderly or a person with a mental impairment who are (*sic*) legally incapable.

---

aDenotes use of more abstract and aspirational language in the ethics code. bDenotes that other concerns are listed but only this one pertains to this chapter. cDenotes that an Urgent Need category is also included in standard 1.7.9 relating to informed consent. dDenotes a psychiatric code.

The "sole remaining measure" implies that other avenues were exhausted before disclosure.

Second, the language used within the codes sets the tone and intent of specific standards. More than 90% of codes with specific limits of confidentiality statements allowed for psychologist judgment and used language that allowed for that judgment. Many codes use the terms *may, should,* or *strives,* reflecting respect for individual clinical determinations. This type of language reinforces "the advisory nature of the Code as a framework in support of professional judgement" (British Psychological Society [2006] *Code of Ethics and Conduct,* p. 6). The flexibility and professional judgment reflected in these statements is typical of the majority of codes. A minority of countries' codes contain more stringent language. For example, the French code (Société Française de Psychologie, 1996) indicates that "s/he is *obligated* [italics added] to notify" (Article 13). As this type of statement indicates, differences in meaning may signal the degree to which psychological organizations are willing to dictate behaviors. It should be noted, though, that ultimately psychologists use their judgment with individual clients, and regardless of ethics code language, individual ethical decisions must be made at particular clinical points in time.

Third, the category heading of Confidentiality appeared in more than half of the countries' codes with duty-to-protect standards. Others primarily included headings such as Professional Practice, Competence and Responsibility, and Autonomy and Self-Determination. The message is consistent with Woody (2001), who reiterated that confidentiality is the cornerstone of good professional psychological practice. Fourth, it is interesting to note that the Chinese code (Chinese Psychological Society, 1992) uses the term *accident* when discussing disclosure. Specifically, it reads, "If you discover that a patient . . . could harm themselves or the safety of the society, the psychologist . . . should immediately take the necessary steps to prevent an accident from happening." Although there may be translational issues with phrasing, when the English translation of the standard was sent to a Chinese colleague, she indicated that during the Cultural Revolution of Mao Zedong (1966–1976) there was no acceptance of mental illness, and all harmful events were explained politically. The formal field of psychology has only recently developed in China (Houcan Zhang, personal communication, October 16, 2006).

Duty to Protect and Community Resources in International Settings

Practical considerations faced daily by clinicians cannot be overlooked when examining ethics codes from an international, cultural perspective. When considering confidentiality and disclosure issues within an international cultural context, one must consider the relationships between professional obligations and resources. In the United States, most psychologists have access to nearby hospitals, generally trust the police, and can refer if necessary to a psychiatrist or at least a general, primary care physician. Let us assume that a psychologist has a suicidal client requiring inpatient care. In some countries (e.g., Peru), there are very few comprehensive mental health service options for individuals seeking treatment because most psychologists work in private or small group practices. As a clinician, if a suicidal client arrives at your private practice office and you are ill equipped to handle the case, there are extremely few alternatives. The duty to protect that might result in having the client committed to an inpatient unit or other treatment alternative becomes almost a moot point. Commitment proceedings are nonexistent in Peru, and individual clinicians are generally on their own (Isabel Nino deGuzman, personal communication, October 10, 2006), so it would be expected that the Peruvian code of ethics would not include specific confidentiality and disclosure ethical standards surrounding duty to protect. It does not.

Similarly, cultural issues should be considered with clients who may hurt others. Because of political and economic strife in many countries, the police are often not trusted. In the United States, mental health practitioners often must contact law enforcement if imminent danger to others exists. In other countries, police reporting may not be a reasonable option.

In addition, psychiatrists and the number of primary care physicians in the United States are a luxury when compared with other countries with fewer resources, especially when psychotropic medications are needed to diminish psychotic and other behaviors that can lead to harming self or others. Although the number of psychiatrists is decreasing in the United States, primary care physicians are generally readily available, constitute 80% of all psychotropic medication prescribers, and can assist with hospital admittance (Lavoie & Barone, 2006). Many countries have psychiatrists, although most do not, and primary care physicians may not be readily available. In countries in which psychotropic medications are cost prohibitive and family members are not available or unwilling to help intervene with treatment, the protection issue for the clinician becomes more convoluted.

CONCLUSION

As the results indicate, ethical standards related to the duty to protect are included in the majority of psychological organizations' codes and are not generally dependent on cultural influences. Of course, individual issues surrounding the duty to protect may be interpreted by psychologists on the basis of cultural attitudes and expectations, but the inclusion of the statements themselves in the codes is near universal. Ethical standards consistent with the duty to protect were found in more than 70% of the ethics codes internationally. Many ethics codes were initially developed in individual countries after reviewing the APA and other Western codes, borrowing many of the ethical guidelines. Therefore, some overlap among codes was expected. Although Leach and Harbin (1997) found that confidentiality and disclosure standards were universal among codes, this is the first study to evaluate specific duty to protect from an international ethical guidelines perspective. In the approximately 30% of codes without direct ethics statements, it is quite likely that some of the psychologists in those countries are still bound by duty-to-protect legal standards, although this was difficult to determine. For example, some national ethics codes are more intimately tied to legal statutes and laws than others, suggesting that the inclusion of duty-to-protect ethical standards may not be viewed as necessary because of their close connection to the law. To obtain a more robust picture of duty to protect, contact should be made with psychologists in those countries asking not only whether they are bound legally, but the origins of particular ethics standards. Consistent with Gauthier's (2005) *Universal Declaration of Ethical Principles for Psychologists* demonstrating common ethical principles across countries, further research may help define specific common standards that psychologists share, regardless of country and culture.

REFERENCES

American Psychological Association. (2002). Ethical principles of psychologists and code of conduct. *American Psychologist, 57,* 1060–1073.

Asamblea General del Colegio Profesional de Psicólogos de Costa Rica. (n.d.). *Código de ética professional.* San Jose, Costa Rica: Author.

Asociación de Psicologia de Puerto Rico. (2007). *Código de ética.* San Juan, Puerto Rico: Author.

Australian Psychological Society. (2007). *Code of ethics.* Victoria, Australia: Author.

British Psychological Society. (2006). *Code of ethics and conduct.* Leicester, England: Author.

Canadian Psychological Association. (2000). *Canadian code of ethics for psychologists.* Ottawa, Canada: Author.

Chinese Psychological Society. (1992). *Ethical code for psychologists of mental tests.* Beijing, China: Author.

Czech-Moravian Psychological Society. (1998). *Code of ethics.* Prague, Czech Republic: Author.

Dominican Psychological Association. (1980). *Code of ethics for psychology.* Santo Domingo, Dominican Republic: Author.

European Federation of Psychologists' Associations. (1998). *Ethical principles for Scandinavian psychologists.* Brussels, Belgium: Author.

Gauthier, J. (2005). *Moving closer to a Universal Declaration of Ethical Principles for Psychologists: Progress report and draft.* Retrieved October 27, 2006, from http://www.am.org/iupsys/ethprog2.pdf

German Psychological Society & Association of German Professional Psychologists. (1999). *Ethical principles of the German Psychological Society and code of conduct of the Association of German Professional Psychologists.* Berlin, Germany: Author.

The Hong Kong Psychological Society. (1998). *Professional code of practice.* Retrieved September 6, 2006, from http://www.hkps.org.hk/www/code.htm

Israel Psychological Association. (2005). *Code of ethics.* Haifa, Israel: Author.

Kitchener, K. S. (1984). Intuition, critical evaluation, and ethical principles: The foundation for ethical decisions in counseling psychology. *Counseling Psychologist, 12,* 43–55.

Koocher, G. P., & Keith-Spiegel, P. (1998). *Ethics in psychology: Professional standards and cases.* New York: Oxford University Press.

Latvian Association of Professional Psychologists. (2004). *Code of ethics.* Retrieved September 21, 2004, from: http://www.psy.it.normativa_ue/latvian_code_of_ethics.htm

Lavoie, K. L., & Barone, S. (2006). Prescriptions privileges for psychologists: A comprehensive review and critical analysis of current issues and controversies. *CNS Drugs, 20,* 1–66.

Leach, M. M., Glosoff, H., & Overmier, J. B. (2001). International ethics codes: A follow-up study of previously unmatched standards and principles. In J. B.

Overmier & J. A. Overmier (Eds.), *Psychology: IUPsyS Global Resource* [CD-ROM]. Florence, KY: Taylor & Francis.

Leach, M. M., & Harbin, J. J. (1997). Psychological ethics codes: A comparison of twenty-four countries. *International Journal of Psychology, 32,* 181–192.

Lindsay, G., & Clarkson, P. (1999). Ethical dilemmas of psychotherapists. *The Psychologist, 12,* 182–185.

Malta Union of Professional Psychologists. (n.d.). *Charter of professional ethics.* Valletta, Malta: Author.

Netherlands Institute of Psychologists. (1998). *Code of ethics for psychologists.* Amsterdam: Author.

New Zealand Psychological Society. (2002). *Code of ethics.* Wellington, New Zealand: Author.

Peiro, J. M., & Lunt, I. (2002). The context for a European framework for psychologists' training. *European Psychologist, 7,* 169–179.

Pettifor, J. L., & Sawchuk, T. R. (2006). Psychologists' perceptions of ethically troubling incidents across international borders. *International Journal of Psychology, 41,* 216–225.

Polish Psychological Association. (n.d.). *Code of professional ethics for the psychologist.* Retrieved September 21, 2004, from: http://www.psy.it.normativa_ue/polish_code_of_ethics.htm

Polubinskaya, S.V., & Bonnie, R.J. (1996). The code of professional ethics of the Russian Society of Psychiatrists: Text and commentary. *International Journal of Psychiatry and Law, 19,* 143–172.

Pope, K. S., & Vetter, V. A. (1992). Ethical dilemmas encountered by members of the American Psychological Association: A national survey. *American Psychologist, 47,* 397–411.

The Professional Board for Psychology Health Professions Council of South Africa. (2002). *Ethical code of professional conduct.* Killarny, South Africa: Author.

Psychological Association of the Philippines. (n.d.). *Code of ethics for psychologists.* Quezon City, Philippines: Author.

The Psychological Society of Ireland. (2003). *Code of professional ethics.* Dublin, Ireland: Author.

Russian Society of Psychiatrists. (1994). *The code of professional ethics of the psychiatrist:* Moscow: Author.

Singapore Psychological Society. (2000). *Code of professional ethics.* Singapore: Author.

Slack, C. M., & Wassenaar, D. R. (1999). Ethical dilemmas of South African clinical psychologists: International comparisons. *European Psychologist, 4,* 179–186.

Société Française de Psychologie. (1996). *Code de déontologie des psychologues praticiens.* Retrieved October 18, 2007, from http://www.sfpsy.org/Code-de-deontolgie-des.html

The Slovene Psychological Association. (2002). *The code of professional ethics of the Slovene psychologist.* Ljubljana, Slovenia: Author.

Società Italiana di Psicologia. (2006). *Codice deontological.* Retrieved January 28, 2008, from http://www.psy.it/codice_deontologico_inferiore.html

Tarasoff v. Board of Regents of the University of California, 551 P.2d 334 (1976).

Turkish Psychological Association. (2004). *Turkish Psychological Association ethics code.* Kizilay-Ankara, Turkey: Author.

Union of Estonian Psychologists. (1990). *Ethical principles.* Tallinn, Estonia: Author.

Woody, R. H. (2001). *Psychological information: Protecting the right to privacy: A guidebook for mental health practitioners and their clients.* Madison, CT: Psychosocial Press.

II

HARM TO OTHERS

5

PROTECTING OTHERS FROM HOMICIDE AND SERIOUS HARM

DEREK TRUSCOTT AND JIM EVANS

Consider the following situation:

George[1] was an ironworker who specialized in working on structural steel at very great heights. He took immense pride in his work, his unique and valued skills, his place in the family as a third-generation ironworker, and his membership in a peer group revered for their ability to walk the high steel. As a result of the demand for his particular combination of attributes, he was also able to earn a considerable wage and be a good provider for his family. In short, for George his work was his life.

George had severely injured his knee in an accident on the job and had undergone surgery on it, but efforts at rehabilitation were not having the desired effect. He was receiving treatment at a physical rehabilitation center from a team of health care professionals that included a physician, physical therapist, exercise therapist, occupational therapist, psychologist, and rehabilitation coordinator. It seemed almost certain that he would never again be able to work as an ironworker because the

---

[1]For the purposes of protecting the client's confidentiality, a pseudonym is used and all personal material has been significantly disguised.

instability of his knee posed too much of a risk to him and his coworkers when working at the perilous heights of his trade. He was extremely frustrated with his situation and was seeing the team psychologist for regular psychotherapy sessions.

One of the rehabilitation coordinator's roles on the treatment team was to keep George informed as to the team's assessment of his progress and the status of his workers' compensation claim. As it became increasingly likely that he would not be able to return to his job as an ironworker, the rehabilitation coordinator had to tell George that because he had few employment skills that he could use in a line of work commensurate with his new physical limitations, it was pretty certain that he was going to have to find a different line of work. The nature of workers' compensation insurance was such that he could not be compensated at a rate that would bring his income up to his preinjury level. Also, because workers' compensation is a no-fault insurance, he was not allowed to sue his employer and was thereby unable to regain any of his lost income in this way.

George told his therapist about the meeting with the rehabilitation coordinator in which the bad news was delivered and how he felt it was "just not fair." This theme had been raised by George many times during therapy, and he had expressed anger and made threats toward a number of people involved in his rehabilitation. As he talked on this occasion, he became extremely angry and agitated, jumped up out of his chair, and with startling strength punched the corner of the therapist's metal filing cabinet. This act caused his hand to bleed profusely, and it looked to the therapist as though he had broken some knuckles. George's response to seeing his damaged and bloodied hand was to say, "Boy . . . does this feel good!" He then stated that he wanted to find the rehabilitation coordinator—who was in the same building—and "give him a taste" of what he (George) was going through. The therapist feared greatly for the rehabilitation coordinator's life.

DUTY TO PROTECT

What tends to be particularly troubling about the idea of protecting others from homicide and serious harm is that the influence therapists have on our clients' lives is limited—it occurs largely within our therapy sessions. We work very hard to help those seeking our services and to assist them in applying the lessons learned, behaviors mastered, or insights gained to diminish their troubling symptoms or improve the quality of their lives. We feel responsible if they do not implement this learning or if they apply strategies without success. We then consider ways to assist them further, if they return, or to be more effective with other clients in similar circumstances. We also attempt to respond immediately if a client is in crisis. That our client may kill or seriously harm someone else seems quite obviously to be the result of the client's choice or of forces outside of our control, however, and therefore not our fault. Therefore, unless we have acted with gross incompetence, it seems unreasonable to place the blame on us if our client seriously harms another.

This, however, is not how society tends to see us. We have a legal obligation to exercise a degree of care and skill expected of a typical practitioner, and if we fail to do so and our client is harmed (or others are harmed), we can be sued for malpractice. In particular, society, as reflected in court decisions, sees the typical therapist as having unique skills beyond the average person for predicting and influencing how others will act. Arising out of this skill is an obligation to protect others from homicide and serious harm—a duty to protect. Largely as a result of legal decisions involving the duty to protect, professional associations and regulators have adopted standards of professional conduct that codify this obligation such that we can also face disciplinary action for lack of attention to the welfare of third parties (Truscott & Crook, 1993; see also chap. 3, this volume).

The duty to protect is generally triggered in Canada and the United States when a client has been (or reasonably should have been) assessed to be a serious threat to the life or physical integrity of a reasonably identifiable victim or victims and the therapist has an opportunity to act diligently to attempt to prevent the violent act from occurring (Truscott & Crook, 1993). Note that the duty consists of two parts: risk assessment and violence prevention.

RISK ASSESSMENT

It is the standard of foreseeability that presents the most serious ethical, legal, and practical dilemma for therapists. Although it is well established that even experts using actuarial methods do a pretty poor job of predicting violence (McGuire, 2004; Norko & Baranoski, 2005; Rice, Harris, & Quinsey, 2002), the legal standard is "reasonable foreseeability," not "certainty." In other words, we are held to the standard of whether a reasonable therapist would have foreseen violence on the part of the client. This standard is legally troubling for therapists because any judgment of liability brought against us will be made in hindsight, and thus the violence will tend to appear more foreseeable than it actually was.

The aims of risk assessment appear in principle to be perfectly straightforward: the identification of persons who pose a threat of violence to others. If we know who will commit a violent act, against whom they will commit it, and when they will commit it, effective preventive action can be taken. However, because our ability to predict violence is far from completely accurate, the ethical and practical aims of risk assessment become that of achieving a balance between the right of others to be protected from those likely to cause them harm and the rights and interests of the individual being assessed (McGuire, 2004).

Our ability to make accurate long-term predictions of any human behavior, particularly relatively rare behavior such as violence, is poor. This is because human behavior is rarely, if ever, predominantly the result of stable individual characteristics or consistent situational influences. Rather, the best understanding that we have is that violence (and indeed most human behavior) results from the interaction of individual traits and states with situational influences, and a healthy proportion of unexplained variance (Mischel, 2004).

Virtually anyone is capable of violent behavior in extreme violence-inducing situations (e.g., defending one's life) despite possessing few violent traits, whereas even the most violent individual will restrain him- or herself in certain situations (e.g., in church). Stated differently, individual characteristics are neither necessary nor sufficient causes of violent behavior, whereas situational influences can be. However, individual characteristics can alter the threshold at which situational influences precipitate violence: An individual who possesses more violent traits would be more likely to commit a violent act given relatively lesser situational influences than someone who possesses fewer violent traits. This is all well and good in theory; how does it translate to practice?

The practical difficulty with any risk assessment arises out of the rarity of the act. In fact, anyone whom we would call violent spends an infinitesimal proportion of time in any given day, week, month, or year actually harming someone. If you wanted to be correct in your assessment of risk more often than incorrect, you would always predict that any person will not commit a violent act over the short term of a few days or weeks. Even using the best techniques currently available to predict recidivism among people who have previously committed violent offenses results in a 24% false-positive rate (Banks et al., 2004). Rare events like violence will always be more difficult to predict than common ones because as the likelihood of the behavior being predicted lessens, the ratio of incorrect to correct predictions increases (Ægisdottir et al., 2006).

To make matters even more difficult for the practitioner, the information available for risk assessment is often fragmentary and unreliable. The therapist has to be concerned with many different possible outcomes, the risk of each of which can vary independently. When a wife and a depressed and jealous husband are no longer living together, for instance, the risk he poses to her may decrease while the risk he poses to others or to himself (Hillbrand, 2001) may increase (Bornstein, 2006; Buchanan, 1999). It is impossible to develop prediction rules that take into account the range of circumstances in which predictions are required (Ægisdottir et al., 2006; Davison, 1997). And then we have the challenge of how to respond appropriately to probability predictions applied to a particular case. Imagine that we have gone through a valid and reliable assessment of violence risk with a client before us, and the risk of violence is assessed as being low. Do we carry on as usual and not respond to the risk? Or do we respond to the low level of risk with some low level of intervention? And what if risk is assessed as being high? Do we go to exceptional lengths to prevent a violent act that statistically is very unlikely to occur?

The philosopher David Hume argued that there are two types of prediction, one founded on chance and the other founded on causes (Buchanan, 1999). When we respond to protect the potential victims of a person who is wielding a knife and angrily threatening violence, for example, we do so not because a high percentage of such people have gone on to attack someone in the past. We respond because this person has a weapon and is expressing a desire to harm someone in a manner that appears to be genuine. We base our judgment to some extent on that form of prediction that is founded on probability—angry people with weapons are likely to harm someone—and to a greater extent on a chain of causation—*this* person in *this* situation is expressing an intention to harm someone and has the means and opportunity to do so.

This type of prediction is familiar to therapists. It is what we rely on in most of our therapeutic work. Although we are knowledgeable of probabilities—for example, women who are in a violent relationship are at high risk immediately after they try to leave the relationship (Babcock, Jacobson, Gottman, & Yerington, 2000)—our particular skill is in understanding human situations—for example, when Stan becomes intoxicated from alcohol, he becomes angry and abusive toward his wife because deep down he is terrified that she will leave him. That is, we attempt to understand the particular circumstances and meanings that individuals make of their lives (Borum & Reddy, 2001). We know that it is these circumstances and meanings that shape how we act on the world and the people in it.

With someone who has acted violently before, we can examine the patterning of individual meanings and situational influences that have been associated with violent actions in the past. For example, under what conditions does the client become angry, abuse substances, isolate him- or herself, or act on strongly held beliefs? How have these patterns emerged before, how are they interrelated, and what combination of circumstances is likely to recur? When a client has never seriously harmed someone before, even though we know that the probability he or she will harm someone now is practically zero, we can strive to understand his or her personal sense of the current circumstances. Why is this particular situation so upsetting? To what extent does the client feel his or her life, livelihood, future, and intimate relationship needs are threatened? What options does he or she see as being available?

The Case of George Continued

The pattern of violence in George's life began with being exposed to a great deal of physical abuse as a child. Apparently, in his childhood home physical punishment and strapping were commonplace and accepted responses to his digressions from rules. Also, his father apparently had no qualms about punching and beating his son whenever he was angry with him. To George, his father was cruel and had to be endured and also respected because he was the head of the house and an ironworker. George's subsequent life was certainly more violent than the norm and his beating someone severely, while not exactly commonplace, was not out of character.

George described the childhood abuses he endured and the violence he inflicted on others in a matter-of-fact manner and did not attribute his violent behavior to his violent past. In fact, he did not see the difficulties in his life as arising out of interpersonal traits established in his past, from orderly sequences of objective cause and effect, or from dysfunctional interpersonal relationships. Rather, he saw life as a quest in which everyone has the choice to be a hero—or a villain—and to choose good versus evil, virtue over vice (Gold, 2006). For George, life was to be experienced fully in the moment, and opportunities for heroism were to be seized with a passion. Logic had its place, but it usually led to stifling, impassioned conclusions that deny the true nature of the human spirit. He saw people not as defined by their circumstances or problems, but as active agents in their lives. As such, they should be held responsible for their actions. And if anyone threatened or harmed him, his family, or his livelihood, he would dish out the vengeance they deserved.

In his sessions with the therapist, George expressed a great deal of anger toward the rehabilitation coordinator. It was as though all of his frustration with his situation was being channeled toward the rehabilitation coordinator—the bearer of bad news. This seemed to be exacerbated by a particularly bad fit between the worldview of the rehabilitation coordinator, who was trained in a very logical–analytical discipline, and that of George, who was very emotional and experiential in his approach to life. In moments of intense anger, George had made threats to harm the rehabilitation coordinator and "make him pay for what I have lost." He felt that if the rehabilitation coordinator could experience what he had, then he would understand. On the basis of the therapist's appreciation of George's past behavior and how he felt about his current circumstances, these were not idle threats.

VIOLENCE PREVENTION

It is commonly the case that therapists think we are legally obligated to *warn* the potential victims of our clients' violent behavior. This is not universally true—in only a few states in the United States is the duty worded such that warning is the only legal means to protect. The majority of courts in Canada and the United States have stated that therapists are expected to do whatever is reasonable under the circumstances to protect others from clients' violence, including warning the intended victim if this is the best available course of action. The intention of most of the courts is to *permit* therapists to break confidentiality if necessary, not to *require* therapists to do so. This is not true of all jurisdictions, however, and some states do expect therapists to both warn and prevent. Therapists are expected under normal circumstances to maintain clients' privacy and indeed can be found liable for damages resulting from harm caused by violating confidences, even if we are trying to prevent a violent act (*Garner v. Stone*, 1999; *Young v. Bella*, 2006). See chapter 2 for a comprehensive discussion of duty-to-protect statutes and case law.

> In the case of George, the therapist was concerned that if he warned the rehabilitation coordinator about the threat to his life, George would be discharged from the rehabilitation center, thereby terminating his access to treatment and probably resulting in his compensation benefits being cut off for noncompliance with treatment. This possibility would obviously exacerbate George's stress and make him more angry and may have increased the risk that he would engage in a violent act. He could also be deterred from seeking counseling for dealing with any future violent impulses because of feeling betrayed by the therapist. None of these outcomes would be good for George. Plus, the therapist knew that like most intended victims of violence (Binder & McNiel, 1999), the rehabilitation coordinator was probably aware that he was a target of George's anger and just accepted it as an aspect of his job. And yet the therapist felt he had to do something. Indeed, society (as reflected in professional standards of practice) expected the therapist to influence George to prevent him from harming the rehabilitation coordinator.

Although society's belief in therapists' ability to influence the lives of our clients via psychotherapy is well founded (Lambert & Ogles, 2004), when a client threatens the life or physical integrity of someone else, it *feels* different than therapy as usual. Even therapists experienced in dealing with clients who have a history of harming others feel anxious under these circumstances (Buckner & Firestone, 2000). Surely, the only similar circumstance is when a client threatens to take his or her own life (Truscott, Evans, & Knish, 1999). So, at the very least, therapists want to provide the best therapy possible. In fact, most therapists believe they should do something different, something exceptional, as befits the exceptional nature of the situation.

The body of research on the efficacy of psychotherapy, however, provides overwhelming support for one very important conclusion: There are no significant differences in the effectiveness of any system of psychotherapy or any psychotherapeutic technique over another (Ahn & Wampold, 2001; Chambless & Ollendick, 2001; Lambert & Ogles, 2004; Wampold et al.,

1997). Although there are some well-conducted studies that have shown some differences between therapies (e.g., Dimidjian et al., 2006), the number of studies that have shown significant differences are what would be expected by chance given the total number of studies that have been conducted (Wampold et al., 1997). Practitioners' belief in one theory over another, adherence to a particular therapeutic system, or application of a specific treatment technique has no consistent impact on whether they are more or less successful in relieving psychological distress, promoting mental health, or remediating particular problems such as violence (Wampold, 2007).

Most important from the point of view of trying to protect others from homicide and serious harm, therapists are not able to do anything to anyone to make them not harm someone. What therapists are able to do is facilitate a process in which problem solving, insight attainment, personal growth, and interpersonal harmony are far more likely to occur than in the circumstance of most people's lives. If providing therapy will result in a client's no longer being a threat to someone, then therapists should focus our efforts on doing so as best we can. If a therapist is unable to facilitate an effective therapeutic process, or if in his or her best judgment doing so would not significantly reduce the risk of harm, only then should he or she undertake nonprofessional actions that require no special expertise, such as warning the potential victim or alerting the police (Quattrocchi & Schopp, 2005; Truscott & Evans, 2001; Truscott et al., 1999; Truscott, Evans, & Mansell, 1995).

Effective psychotherapy is characterized by three conditions (Frank & Frank, 1991; Wampold, 2001). First, the client must seek help from a practitioner whom he or she believes to be helpful. Second, the client must experience a collaborative relationship with the therapist. Third, the therapy must have a rationale that is believable to the client and therapist and involve activities consistent with the rationale. If therapists want to be maximally effective, therefore, we need to maximize these conditions. Therapists should thus strive to collaborate with clients by understanding their personal worldview as a means to establish a common understanding of the nature of their problem. Each person's worldview serves as a filter by which he or she selectively attends to the vast amount of potential data that he or she experiences and enables people to make sense of their lives (Lyddon, 1989b; Unger, Draper, & Pendergrass, 1986). What is viewed as a "problem" from one worldview, therefore, may not be seen as one from another. It follows that the means by which to bring about problem remediation will vary by worldview. Duncan, Miller, and Sparks (2004) called this finding the client's "theory of change." By finding a theory of change that is acceptable and believable for the client and the therapist, both can work collaboratively toward shared goals via agreed-on tasks (Horvath & Greenberg, 1994).

Sometimes a client will present with an explicit theory of change, such as "I want to learn to control my anger." More often it is implicit, such as "If I could just figure out what is wrong with me I wouldn't get so frustrated all the time." In either case, it is not the ultimate "truth" of the theory that is predictive of success in therapy, it is the individual's belief in it (Lyddon, 1989b). If the therapist takes an experiential, emotion-focused approach and the client has a logical, action-oriented approach to life, for example, therapy is not expected to be successful (Lyddon, 1989a; Lyddon & Adamson, 1992). It would be similarly as unlikely if the therapist was systems oriented and the client was predisposed toward seeking personal insight. Although it may be possible to convince clients that their understanding of their problem and its solution is incorrect and they should adopt the therapist's, considerable time and effort will have to be devoted to the task in proportion to the degree of dissimilarity, with no guarantee of success. Indeed, it is much more likely that the client will not return, and each will experience the other as difficult or nonresponsive.

> In George's case, the therapist decided not to warn the rehabilitation coordinator of the threat to his life that this frustrated, angry, and violent man represented. What he did instead was to do everything he could to protect the rehabilitation coordinator; warning him of the threat to his life was still an option that could be exercised if all therapeutic efforts failed. Immediately after the angry, fist-injuring outburst, the psychologist gave the client tissues to clean the blood from his hand. He then suggested that they go for a walk in a nearby forested area. George agreed. As strange as it may seem, the fact that George's knuckles may have been broken was not attended to. The therapist thought that even mentioning the possibility at that moment would have strained the therapeutic alliance. They went out a back door of the center to avoid meeting anyone else and especially to prevent passing the rehabilitation coordinator's office on the way to the front door.
>
> On the basis of their work together and his efforts to understand George's worldview, the therapist felt confident that George would welcome a therapeutic relationship of unwavering acceptance and empathic contact—not of action or explanation—and that doing so would foster self-acceptance and self-understanding and thereby reduce his likelihood of harming the rehabilitation coordinator. Rather than being viewed as deficits to be remedied, George's frustrations were seen as powerful opportunities for the emergence of a more fully integrated self. In George's and the therapist's shared worldview, emotional expression had a functional role in unlocking his inherent self-organizing capacities and was thus encouraged. Feelings were understood as warranting being fully experienced, even when painful, to bring rich meaning to his life. Full focus on the present was valued as promoting personal growth. With this increased awareness and self-knowledge, George could achieve unique creative solutions. His strengths and talents were discussed as gifts to be appreciated and used in the service of others, especially his family.
>
> So, as they walked the therapist listened to George, facilitated emotional expression and deep, personal disclosure, and tried very hard to relate to him with unconditional positive regard (Rogers, 1957) while

not judging, evaluating, or presuming to know what was best for him. Note that this approach to helping George is not the only way to influence someone to not harm another. Its effectiveness arose out of the shared belief between George and the therapist that people are best understood from what would be called a humanistic worldview. If George had held a more empirical worldview, for example, the therapist would have taken a more active, directive stance and deliberately selected activities that promoted rational thinking or adaptive behaviors intended to address specific problems and achieve pragmatic, measurable outcomes. Similarly, if George had held more of a rationalist worldview, the therapist would have adopted an introspective, skeptical stance and encouraged a detailed description of events to foster honest self-perception so that patterns of personal experiences and old meanings could be discovered and understood and new, more realistic decisions made in light of these personal insights.

DIVERSITY CONSIDERATIONS

One of the most powerful influences on worldview is culture: the set of shared meanings about the nature of the world that inform the structure of social interactions by providing members a set of norms for acceptable behavior and lifestyle (Fowers & Richardson, 1996). These norms provide information about how to think, feel, and behave to remain a member of the group and also about who is not a member of the group. Cultural status is often inaccurately assigned by way of visible physical characteristics—such as skin color—commonly associated in some vague way with geographical ancestry. The imprecision of doing so is usually further compounded by the use of the term *race* to loosely imply some sort of genetic lineage that does not exist (Helms & Talleyrand, 1997). The degree to which one's worldview is shaped by cultural norms is highly individual, however. Some people are unaware of the extent to which they live by cultural norms, others consciously choose to belong and behave in accordance with the norms of certain groups, and most are influenced by some combination of nonconscious and conscious norms. This means that assignment to a particular cultural group cannot be made without knowledge of the individual's subjective experience. Although nationality and religious affiliation, for example, typically influence people's worldview via cultural norms, there are many other characteristics by which people can identify themselves as belonging to a normative group, such as age, gender, sexual orientation, occupation, and physical abilities.

The therapist's cultural norms can interfere with attending to the client's individual worldview in a number of ways (American Psychological Association, 2002). For example, psychotherapists are particularly prone to assume that our theories and therapies are equally applicable to anyone—regardless of cultural worldview—because we tend to believe that they are morally, ethically, and politically neutral (Ibrahim, 1996). Therapists therefore tend to assume that others, whether from the same cultural group or not, share our worldview. This mistaken assumption has been termed *cultural encapsulation* (Wrenn, 1962) and can prevent therapists from seeing the world as our clients see it.

Another possibility is that if therapists see the client as not of our cultural group, we tend to assume that they do not share our worldview and may then turn to whatever knowledge they possess (sometimes accurate, sometimes not) about the cultural group into which they have categorized them. Thus, one might expect that all individuals of a culture different than one's own are all different in the same way than individuals of one's own cultural group. Sometimes people expect that persons of a particular cultural heritage are inferior—the more common usage of the concept of discrimination—and sometimes they may idealize cultural stereotypes (e.g., the "noble savage"). In either case, therapists miss the opportunity to collaborate with the client from within their unique worldview.

With respect to the client's cultural norms, the importance of working collaboratively from within a shared worldview is highlighted when the client is a member of a cultural minority. The foci of most psychotherapies very much reflect the European–North American (Western) worldview in which they were developed. In particular, the focus of problems and their solution is typically the individual (Triandis, 1995). Many non-Western cultures, however, hold a collectivist worldview in which social context gives life meaning and purpose and is the source of personal difficulties (Hofstede, 1980; Kim, Triandis, Kaitçibasi, Choi, & Yoon, 1994). Personal problems and their solution are understood differently (Oyserman, Coon, & Kemmelmeier, 2002). Problems are seen as arising out of social pressures, interpersonal conflicts, or unhealthy role expectations and are best solved by involving others in the solution. Symptom relief and personal growth are sought by changing the nature of relationships with significant people within one's social system, not at their expense. Unhealthy social relationships or expectations are to be replaced with strong interpersonal ties and many-sided, nurturing relationships. Communion—contact, openness, and noncontractual cooperation between persons—is seen as the ideal human state, not individual freedom. Particularly different for many therapists of European–North American heritage is that someone with a collectivist worldview will tend to expect the therapist to be an ally and advocate. When a client who is of a minority heritage seeks therapy, therefore, there is a greater risk of a mismatch between the worldview of the client and that of the therapist as reflected in the therapy.

The process of acculturation, in which the norms of one culture (often that in which one is raised) are in conflict with those of another (often a group to which one chooses or aspires to belong), has a particularly important influence on the provision of psychotherapy (Merali, 1999). In George's case, he experienced a conflict between the expectations of his normative group that feelings are not to be shared in a heartfelt, intimate way with another person—especially another man—and those of his personal worldview, shared by his therapist, that emotional expression is healthy and healing. His therapist thus was very careful to honor both of these expectations and the conflict George was experiencing. They discussed how important belonging to his normative group was for him and how he did not completely accept all of the expectations of the group. Together they came to an understanding that psychotherapy was a special circumstance in which he could share his feelings in an open, honest way while at the same time not violate prohibitions against such behavior because he would never do so in "normal" circumstances.

> Once George had walked, talked, and worked through his emotionality to a degree that he and the therapist felt he was safe to be around other people, a taxi was called and the therapist made sure George got into it and left the center where the rehabilitation coordinator was still in his office working. The plan was to collaboratively determine how to continue with rehabilitation without having the rehabilitation coordinator's life threatened in any way. George had emergency contact numbers that he could use if he felt the need. They agreed to meet at the front door of the rehabilitation center on his return the next day.

SUPERVISION AND CONSULTATION

After George's therapist returned to his office, he contacted a trusted colleague to discuss, debrief, and consult about the situation, making sure to protect his client's identity. He stated that he wanted to speak with someone who would "not overreact" and would help him work through his thoughts and feelings about his work with George and the threat that he posed. Such consultation with another professional in difficult cases is both ethically and legally appropriate. Although from a legal perspective having a colleague concur with one's actions is not necessarily evidence that there is no negligence, it does speak to the reasonableness of one's conduct—an important component of any defense against malpractice. The legal value of such a consultation, however, will be diminished unless the therapist keeps a note of the meeting or, ideally, one is prepared by the consulted professional. Having a record may also reduce lawyers' interest in pursuing litigation unless the therapist has failed to follow the suggestions of the consultation. And, although it is prudent to consult with others, ultimately therapists are ethically and legally responsible for our professional actions.

From the supervisor's or consultant's perspective, the degree of responsibility assumed is inversely proportional to the therapist's degree of skill and experience. If the therapist is not a licensed professional or is a professional in training, then the supervisor is responsible for the well-being of the client and any harm to a third party arising out of a duty to protect. The only circumstance in which the supervisee ought to be held accountable for harm would be if the supervisor's input was knowingly not sought or if the supervisee willfully failed to follow the supervisor's direction. At the other end of the continuum, if the therapist is an experienced, licensed professional, the consultant would have very little responsibility for the therapist's action. It might, however, make for a rather interesting legal defense if a therapist were to claim that an expert consultant's improper advice was followed.

For the therapist trying to help George and protect the rehabilitation coordinator, risk had already been assessed as being present—a typical situation when consultation is sought regarding protecting others from homicide and serious harm. So a brief review of how the therapist came to the conclusion that there was a threat to a third party was undertaken. The consultant agreed that some professional action was indicated. Although it is certainly possible that the therapist might be worried for no good reason, unfounded worry is rare, and it is best to err on the side of caution. If one imagined oneself as a defendant on a witness stand, most would find it very uncomfortable saying, "I was worried that my client would harm someone and decided not to do anything about it." In addition, an accounting of the objective facts of a situation often fails to capture the subjective experience of being with the client. One person saying "I wish my mother was dead!" may be expressing feelings of frustration with no desire to actually harm anyone, whereas another person—or even the same person under different circumstances—may be expressing murderous intent. Only the therapist present when the utterance was made (and the client) has access to that information. So the consultant was wise to treat the therapist's worries seriously.

They talked about how the therapist felt about what had happened and what he did and about his fear that he may have done the wrong thing or not done enough. The consultant listened, asked questions to facilitate the therapist's thorough exploration of the situation, and reviewed with him the relevant professional and legal standards. Together, they concluded that he was right to take the threat seriously and that given the information available, the rehabilitation coordinator was best protected by the therapist providing the best psychotherapy he could, rather than by a warning.

CONCLUSION

The Case of George: The Next Day

The next day George did not return. The therapist attempted to contact him and learned from his wife that during the previous evening, George once again became very upset and agitated. His wife said that she felt she needed help because of his extreme anger. She then went with her husband to the psychiatric walk-in clinic of the local hospital. There, after an interview, George was admitted to the psychiatric ward. At the hospital, he made many of the same remarks in regard to the rehabilitation coordinator that he had made to the therapist.

The psychiatrist who interviewed George phoned the rehabilitation coordinator, told him about the threats George was making toward him, and advised him to take steps to protect himself. Security services at the rehabilitation center were notified, and they stationed a guard at the front door to prevent George's entry should he return. Later in the day, the rehabilitation coordinator informed the therapist of the psychiatrist's call and the steps taken in response. He asked the therapist if he knew of the threats. Knowing looks were exchanged, and nothing was said.

George never did return, and the therapist never saw him again. His physical rehabilitation ended that day, and he eventually undertook a less physically demanding, less dangerous line of work. Some years later, one of the other therapists from the rehabilitation team met George on the street, and they stopped to talk. George said he was doing well, mentioned the psychotherapist by name, and said to thank him for all the help and support he had given him during his time of need.

In preparing this chapter for publication, the rehabilitation coordinator was asked whether he would be interested in reading the case to see whether he could add to it on the basis of his memory of the situation. It was then about 10 years since the incident had occurred, and the authors thought that it was acceptable to share the details with him because George had long since left the rehabilitation center and was no longer on compensation. The rehabilitation coordinator said that he had suspected that the therapist had known about the threat and had acted to protect him. He (the rehabilitation coordinator) said that he understood why confidentiality was maintained and was thankful for the therapist's work.

In this chapter, we have attempted to highlight the central importance of doing good therapy when working with someone threatening to kill or seriously harm another. In George's case, this was exemplified by the therapist working intensely and collaboratively with him, maintaining confidentiality, and thereby protecting the rehabilitation coordinator. Psychotherapy with George worked out well for all concerned. Of course, sometimes things do not work out well. If George had returned and killed or seriously injured the rehabilitation coordinator, the therapist would have been in serious legal difficulty. Given the nature of the threat, there could be a strong legal argument for breach of duty to protect. We encourage therapists to consider this possibility very seriously, familiarize themselves with their jurisdiction's relevant laws, carry comprehensive liability insurance, and be prepared to defend themselves in court with a thoughtful, articulate rationale for their actions.

REFERENCES

Ægisdottir, S., White, M. J., Spengler, P. M., Maugherman, A. S., Anderson, L. A., Cook, R. S., et al. (2006). The meta-analysis of clinical judgment project: Fifty-six years of accumulated research on clinical versus statistical prediction. *Counseling Psychologist, 34,* 341–382.

Ahn, H., & Wampold, B. E. (2001). Where oh where are the specific ingredients? A meta-analysis of component studies in counseling and psychotherapy. *Journal of Counseling Psychology, 48,* 251–257.

American Psychological Association. (2002). *Guidelines on multicultural education, training, research, practice, and organizational change for psychologists.* Washington, DC: Author.

Babcock, J. C., Jacobson, N. S., Gottman, J. M., & Yerington, T. P. (2000). Attachment, emotional regulation, and the function of marital violence: Differences between secure, preoccupied and dismissing violent and nonviolent husbands. *Journal of Family Violence, 15,* 391–409.

Banks, S., Robbins, P. C., Silver, E., Vesselinov, R., Steadman, H. J., Monahan, J., et al. (2004). A multiple-models approach to violence risk assessment among people with mental disorder. *Criminal Justice and Behavior, 31,* 324–340.

Binder, R. L., & McNiel, D. E. (1999). Application of the *Tarasoff* ruling and its effect on the victim and the therapeutic relationship. *Psychiatric Services, 47,* 1212–1215.

Bornstein, R. F. (2006). The complex relationship between dependency and domestic violence. *American Psychologist, 61,* 595–606.

Borum, R., & Reddy, M. (2001). Assessing violence risk in *Tarasoff* situations: A fact-based model of inquiry. *Behavioral Sciences & the Law, 19,* 375–385.

Buchanan, A. (1999). Risk and dangerousness. *Psychological Medicine, 29,* 465–473.

Buckner, F., & Firestone, M. (2000). "Where the public peril begins": 25 years after *Tarasoff. Journal of Legal Medicine, 21,* 187–222.

Chambless, D. L., & Ollendick, T. H. (2001). Empirically supported psychological interventions: Controversies and evidence. *Annual Review of Psychology, 52,* 685–716.

Davison, S. (1997). Risk assessment and management: A busy practitioner's perspective. *International Review of Psychiatry, 9,* 201–206.

Dimidjian, S., Hollon, S. D., Dobson, K. S., Schmaling, K. B., Kohlenberg, R. J., Addis, M. E., et al. (2006). Randomized trial of behavioral activation, cognitive therapy, and antidepressant medication in the acute treatment of adults with major depression. *Journal of Consulting and Clinical Psychology, 74,* 658–670.

Duncan, B. L., Miller, S. D., & Sparks, J. A. (2004). *The heroic client: A revolutionary way to improve effectiveness through client-directed, outcome-informed therapy.* San Francisco: Jossey-Bass.

Fowers, B. J., & Richardson, F. C. (1996). Why is multiculturalism good? *American Psychologist, 51,* 609–621.

Frank, J. D., & Frank, J. B. (1991). *Persuasion and healing: A comparative study of psychotherapy*. Baltimore: Johns Hopkins University Press.

Garner v. Stone, No. 97A-30250-1 (Ga., Dekalb County Super. Ct. Dec. 16, 1999).

Gold, J. (2006). Patient-initiated integration. In G. Stricker & J. Gold (Eds.), *A casebook of psychotherapy integration* (pp. 253–260). Washington, DC: American Psychological Association.

Helms, J. E., & Talleyrand, R. M. (1997). Race is not ethnicity. *American Psychologist, 52*, 1246–1247.

Hillbrand, M. (2001). Homicide–suicide and other forms of co-occurring aggression against self and against others. *Professional Psychology: Research and Practice, 32*, 626–635.

Hofstede, G. (1980). *Culture's consequences*. Beverly Hills, CA: Sage.

Horvath, A. O., & Greenberg, L. S. (1994). *The working alliance: Theory, research, and practice*. New York: Wiley.

Ibrahim, F. A. (1996). A multicultural perspective on principle and virtue ethics. *Counseling Psychologist, 24*, 78–85.

Kim, U., Triandis, C., Kagitçibasi, Ç., Choi, S., & Yoon, G. (1994). *Individualism and collectivism: Theory, method, and applications*. Thousand Oaks, CA: Sage.

Lambert, M. J., & Ogles, B. M. (2004). The efficacy and effectiveness of psychotherapy. In M. J. Lambert (Ed.), *Bergin and Garfield's handbook of psychotherapy and behavior change* (5th ed., pp. 139–192). New York: Wiley.

Lyddon, W.J. (1989a). Personal epistemology and preference for counseling. *Journal of Counseling Psychology, 36*, 423–429.

Lyddon, W. J. (1989b). Root metaphor theory: A philosophical framework for counseling and psychotherapy. *Journal of Counseling & Development, 67*, 442–448.

Lyddon, W. J., & Adamson, L. E. (1992). Worldview and counseling preference: An analogue study. *Journal of Counseling & Development, 71*, 41–47.

McGuire, J. (2004). Minimising harm in violence risk assessment: Practical solutions to ethical problems? *Health, Risk & Society, 6*, 327–345.

Merali, N. (1999). Resolution of value conflicts in multicultural counselling. *Canadian Journal of Counselling, 33*, 28–36.

Mischel, W. (2004) Toward an integrative science of the person. *Annual Review of Psychology, 55*, 1–22.

Norko, M. A., & Baranoski, M. V. (2005). The state of contemporary risk assessment research. *Canadian Journal of Psychiatry/Revue Canadienne de Psychiatrie, 50*, 18–26.

Oyserman, D., Coon, H. M., & Kemmelmeier, M. (2002). Individualism and collectivism: Evaluation of theoretical assumptions and meta-analyses. *Psychological Bulletin, 128*, 3–72.

Quattrocchi, M. R., & Schopp, R. F. (2005). Tarasaurus rex: A standard of care that could not adapt. *Psychology, Public Policy, and Law, 11*, 109–137.

Rice, M. E., Harris, G. T., & Quinsey, V. L. (2002). The appraisal of violence risk. *Current Opinion in Psychiatry, 15*, 589–593.

Rogers, C. R. (1957). The necessary and sufficient conditions of therapeutic personality change. *Journal of Consulting Psychology, 21*, 95–103.

Triandis, H. C. (1995). *Individualism and collectivism*. Boulder, CO: Westview Press.

Truscott, D., & Crook, K. H. (1993). *Tarasoff* in the Canadian context: *Wenden* and the duty to protect. *Canadian Journal of Psychiatry/Revue Canadienne de Psychiatrie, 38*, 84–89.

Truscott, D., & Evans, J. (2001). Responding to dangerous clients. In E. R. Welfel & R. E. Ingersoll (Eds.), *The mental health desk reference: A sourcebook for counselors and therapists* (pp. 271–276). New York: Wiley.

Truscott, D., Evans, J., & Knish, S. (1999). A process model for clinical decision making in high risk outpatient situations: The therapeutic alliance and suicide. *Canadian Journal of Counselling, 33*, 307–316.

Truscott, D., Evans, J., & Mansell, S. (1995). Outpatient psychotherapy with dangerous clients: A model for clinical decision making. *Professional Psychology: Research and Practice, 26*, 484–490.

Unger, R. K., Draper, R. D., & Pendergrass, M. L. (1986). Personal epistemology and personal experience. *Journal of Social Issues, 42*, 67–79.

Wampold, B. E. (2001). *The great psychotherapy debate: Models, methods, and findings*. Hillsdale, NJ: Erlbaum.

Wampold, B. E. (2007). Psychotherapy: The humanistic (and effective) treatment. *American Psychologist, 62*, 857–873.

Wampold, B. E., Mondin, G. W., Moody, M., Stich, F., Benson, K., & Ahn, H. (1997). A meta-analysis of outcome studies comparing bona fide psychotherapies: Empirically, "All must have prizes." *Psychological Bulletin, 122*, 203–215.

Wrenn, C. G. (1962). The culturally encapsulated counselor. *Harvard Educational Review, 32*, 444–449.

Young v. Bella, 1 S.C.R. 108, 2006 SCC 3 (2006).

6

RISK ASSESSMENT AND THE DUTY TO PROTECT IN CASES INVOLVING INTIMATE PARTNER VIOLENCE

ALAN ROSENBAUM AND LYNN S. DOWD

The duty imposed on psychotherapists to take whatever steps are reasonably necessary to protect potential victims of their clients' violent acts is predicated on the special relationship presumed to exist between psychotherapist and client, wherein the therapist has access to information that should enable him or her to predict such violence. Although the empirical evidence supporting psychotherapist prescience may be lacking (Monahan, 1981), less clairvoyance may be necessary if the client is already known to be violent. Therapists working with aggressive populations may therefore need to be especially vigilant regarding the potential for violence and mindful of their duty to protect.

A recent survey of women in the United States revealed that one in five had been a victim of intimate partner assault (Tjaden & Thoennes, 2000). Victims often come into contact with the mental health system because of the emotional consequences of intimate partner violence (IPV), which include increased risk for depression, substance use, posttraumatic stress disorder symptoms, and chronic mental illness (Coker et al., 2002). Perpetrators are also likely to use mental health services, often in the context of batterer intervention programs, which are commonly mandated by courts and proba-tion departments and many of which are conducted by psychologists, social workers, or other professional counselors. This chapter addresses the most salient legal, ethical, and moral considerations that arise in the course of dealing with IPV.

PREVALENCE AND RELATED ISSUES

Our discussion focuses on aggression in adult intimate relationships. To identify the presence of IPV, clinicians must have some basic knowledge and include screening questions in the assessment process. All clinicians should be aware that partner violence is common, often bidirectional, and can vary from mild to severe. Representative studies have found that ap-proximately 12% of couples experience partner violence and that women may be aggressive as frequently as men (Straus, 1997). Although most would agree that male aggression results in significantly more negative physical and emotional consequences (Archer, 2000; Holtzworth-Munroe, 2005), Dutton and Corvo (2006) suggested that the consequences may be similar. Aggres-sion may serve a different function for men than for women. Johnson (2000) argued that when violence is used to exert power over, and to control, the partner, the perpetrator is almost always male. If the distinction between aggression and battering is based on the intent and effect of the violence (i.e., battering involves fear and coerced behavioral changes), then women may be aggressive, but they are rarely considered to be batterers.

Although bidirectional IPV is the most prevalent form (Dutton & Corvo, 2006), we primarily focus on male perpetrators. Many of the issues and recommendations, however, apply equally to female perpetrators. Simi-larly, despite the prevalent ideology that conceptualizes IPV as gendered, there is strong evidence that partner aggression occurs at least as frequently between same-sex couples as between heterosexual couples (Elliot, 1996; Lie, Schilit, Bush, Montagne, & Reyes, 1991). Although the treatment of IPV in homosexual couples entails unique dynamics and issues, space limits compel us to restrict our discussion to heterosexual couples. Nonetheless, many of the recommendations regarding the duty to protect will apply in either case.

TREATMENT CONSIDERATIONS

Most states have developed standards for the treatment of IPV perpe-trators, and those standards usually dictate time-limited, psychoeducational group intervention using a format such as the Duluth model (Pence & Paymar, 1993), with its focus on power and control issues and a coordinated commu-nity response that involves cooperation and communication among the police, courts, shelters, and intervention programs. Batterer intervention programs move in two broad directions: those viewing themselves as an extension of the legal system (management and control programs) and those using a therapeutic approach. Therapeutic programs evolved within the mental health professions, view victim protection as a by-product of successful intervention, consider the batterer to be the primary client, and in most cases observe the rules of confidentiality as articulated by the ethical principles of the mental health professions. Management and control programs are more likely to have originated within the battered women's movement, view victim protection as their primary responsibility, see the victim as their client, and conceptualize confidentiality for the batterer as an impediment to those objectives. Both types of programs typically focus on helping the batterer accept responsibility for his aggression, develop empathy with the victim, and recognize the many forms of coercive control. Many programs add modules on alcohol and substance use, positive parenting, and anger management. Several states prohibit the use of couples counseling, at least as a primary intervention, and some eschew the use of anger management, asserting that violence is more a manipulative strategy than an expression of angry emotions. The specifics of batterer intervention are well articulated elsewhere, such as in Aldarondo and Mederos (2002), and an in-depth discussion of state standards can be found in Geffner and Rosenbaum (2001).

Whether batterer intervention strategies are effective is a matter of contentious debate. Several recent meta-analytic studies have concluded that effect sizes are small to, at best, moderate (Babcock, Green, & Robie, 2004). However, others have noted that the Duluth model is overrepresented in these studies, and it may be that it is the Duluth model, with its nontherapeutic philosophy, that accounts for the apparent ineffectiveness of batterer intervention (Dutton & Corvo, 2006). Comparative studies using a broader range of approaches are warranted before firm conclusions can be drawn.

Case Example

In the course of discussion, we use the following clinical scenario for purposes of illustration. To protect client confidentiality, the case is a composite of several cases, but it illustrates a number of issues and patterns that are frequently seen in violent domestic relationships.

> David and Michelle have had an intermittent relationship for more than 10 years. David has been mandated by the local district court to attend domestic violence treatment after being arrested for domestic assault and battery. Michelle has two children from a previous relationship, and the couple has two children together. David also has a grown daughter in another state with whom he has had no contact for many years. He does not know her whereabouts. The family has an open case with the Department of Social Services because of sexual abuse of one child, and the

other three children are in foster care. David and Michelle are permitted only supervised visits because one of the protective issues has been their verbal and physical altercations in the children's presence. Both deny physical aggression toward the children. The couple has a history of mutual aggression during episodes of substance abuse. These occurred every weekend for the past several years, with David typically drinking a case of beer plus hard liquor, until his recent arrest. Michelle also acknowledged drinking heavily and smoking marijuana. Their fights have usually consisted of pushing, slapping, and grabbing. However, on at least one occasion, David admits to choking Michelle, and he has given her several black eyes and frequent bruises. Michelle has attacked David with a knife and once threw her cell phone at him, hitting him in the face. Several years ago, Michelle took out a restraining order on David, which he violated. He was incarcerated for 6 months, during which time Michelle began seeing another man. Since that time, they have gotten into frequent fights over Michelle's behavior toward other men, which David sees as flirtatious. Michelle denies any current infidelity. David has done factory work in the past, but is currently unemployed. Michelle works as a home health care provider and supports David. She resents that he is not working and that he spends money impulsively. The couple plans to move in with Michelle's stepmother to save money. David grew up in a housing project where he was exposed to a high degree of street violence. His father died when he was 12 of an alcohol-related illness, and his mother still drinks heavily. He is estranged from his own family of origin. "Michelle and the kids are my family," he stated. He indicated a much higher degree of relationship satisfaction than she did. Michelle has never used any battered women's services.

Preliminary Considerations for the Nondomestic Violence Specialist

Most states with standards also have policies that allow judges to mandate participation in batterer intervention programs, either as a diversion in lieu of prosecution or as a term of probation. Because most batterer intervention is initiated via this mechanism, most is also conducted by therapists having expertise in treating interpartner aggression. Although perpetrators rarely enter treatment voluntarily, they could come into therapy in a variety of ways, possibly becoming the responsibility of a clinician lacking specialized training in IPV. For example, IPV often occurs in the context of marital discord, and violence may be occurring even if this has not been identified as part of the presenting problem. Similarly, batterers are often depressed (Hamberger & Hastings, 1986) and/or have alcohol and substance abuse issues (Tolman & Bennett, 1990). Thus, even therapists who do not routinely accept domestic violence cases might find themselves having to assess risk and deal with questions regarding their duty to protect in the context of IPV.

Any risk assessment is dependent on the identification of violence. Often the information is not spontaneously offered, or the severity and frequency is minimized, by both perpetrators and victims. Compounding the problem is the failure by many mental health professionals to include inquiries about violence in their evaluations (Hamberger & Phelan, 2004). Structured screening procedures, which include rapport building and very specific questioning, are most likely to promote disclosure (see Hamberger & Phelan, 2004, for guidance in the screening process).

A client who initially denies domestic violence may later acknowledge its occurrence once a secure treatment alliance is in place. If the disclosing client is a victim, the clinician's focus must turn to safety planning, in which specific courses of action are formulated for implementation when the client feels endangered (see Davies, Lyon, & Monti-Catania, 1998, for an in-depth examination of these issues). The "Ethical Principles of Psychologists and Code of Conduct" (American Psychological Association, 2002) discourages clinicians lacking specialized training in an area from treating clients with those specific problems without appropriate supervision. Absent the availability of a knowledgeable consultant, referral to a therapist with the requisite expertise might be advisable. In such cases, both victims and perpetrators would benefit from referral to domestic violence services for further specialized assessment and intervention. Clinicians should also keep in mind that partner violence and child abuse are often co-occurring behaviors (Jaffe, Lemon, & Poisson, 2003; Smith Slep & O'Leary, 2005), and the necessity of reporting to child protective services may arise. In this regard, they should also be aware that the child abuse perpetrator might be the woman, and, in fact, Dutton and Corvo (2006) noted that perpetration by the mother might be more probable.

RISK ASSESSMENT PROCESSES AND MEASURES

It has long been recognized that batterers are a heterogeneous group, varying on a host of dimensions including severity and frequency of aggression, historical factors, alcohol use, generality of aggression, and level of psychopathy. These differences have been reflected in the development of typologies, such as the tripartite one developed by Holtzworth-Munroe and Stuart (1994), which includes the family only, the borderline–dysphoric, and the generally violent–antisocial subtypes. Johnson (2000) offered a dyadic typology in which he distinguished the more severe violence pattern, termed *patriarchal terrorism,* from the more common, less severe mutually violent pattern, termed *common couple violence.* Although physical and emotional injury can occur in either type, patriarchal terrorism represents the more serious threat. Distinguishing between the types and relative levels of risk can be difficult, creating problems for both treatment providers and the courts.

Although it is essential for the courts to have evaluative data with which to make informed decisions about the disposition of batterer cases and to assist with victim safety planning, predicting dangerousness is an inexact science, and the consequences of false positives (predicting reoffending when none, in fact, occurs) and false negatives (failing to predict reoffense when it does) are significant and potentially dire. Despite this dilemma, or perhaps because of it, many risk, or danger, assessments have been developed and evaluated to varying degrees. Recently, the National Institute of Justice released its Intimate Partner Violence Risk Assessment Validation Study (Roehl, O'Sullivan, Webster, & Campbell, 2005). This 5-year multisite field test compared four commonly used risk assessment instruments with victim report. Most of these measures were primarily designed to assess the risk of reassault, rather than the dangerousness of an individual who has not yet perpetrated an assault. Only one measure, the Danger Assessment (Campbell, 2004), was specifically constructed to assess lethality. It obtains information exclusively from the victim and can be used to assess danger in a relationship in which aggression has not yet occurred.

Choosing a risk assessment instrument depends on the type of information available to the assessor. The Domestic Violence Screening Inventory (Williams & Houghton, 2004), the Kingston Screening Instrument for Domestic Violence (Lyon, 1998), and the DV-MOSAIC (de Becker & Associates, 2005) all require information derived from criminal justice records (e.g., police reports). The Domestic Violence Screening Inventory and the Kingston Screening Instrument for Domestic Violence include information obtained from the offender. The Danger Assessment, Kingston Screening Instrument for Domestic Violence, and the DV-MOSAIC also include victim report. The Spousal Assault Risk Assessment (Kropp, Hart, Webster, & Eaves, 1995) is a clinical measure that was intended to assess reoffending in a criminal justice system context and requires a psychological assessment and clinical judgment. Despite its name, the authors intended the Spousal Assault Risk Assessment to be a guide as part of an in-depth assessment rather than an actuarial instrument (Kropp et al., 1995). Structured clinical methods of risk assessment, such as the Spousal Assault Risk Assessment, may reduce the degree of inconsistency in information (Kropp, 2004). It should be noted that assessment methods that rely on psychological evaluation as a primary source of data can only be used by trained mental health professionals.

Actuarial methods use variables that have been empirically demonstrated to predict aggression. Examples are the Violence Risk Appraisal Guide (Harris, Rice, & Camilleri, 2004; Quinsey, Harris, Rice, & Cormier, 1998) and the Ontario Domestic Assault Risk Assessment (Hilton et al., 2004). These measures use a parsimonious list of factors that have reliably predicted violent behavior, such as younger age, lower socioeconomic status, prior conflict and abuse in the relationship, antisocial behavior and personality traits, substance abuse, and possibly psychopathy (Hilton & Harris, 2005). Proponents of actuarial measures (e.g., Hilton & Harris, 2005) have pointed to their accuracy and focus on advantages in clinical use and their ability to compare a given individual's score with norms to produce a probability of reoffense. Although the Violence Risk Assessment Guide requires considerable time and information that may not be easily accessible, the Ontario Domestic Assault Risk Assessment is described as being shorter and easier to use. The Ontario Domestic Assault Risk Assessment may also be used in interviewing female victims (Hilton & Harris, 2005).

Many of the risk assessments (especially those in Roehl et al., 2005) were developed to aid the courts in making dispositional decisions, either with regard to trial versus diversion or in sentencing. For example, the purpose of the Domestic Violence Screening Inventory was to help determine the level of community supervision and the terms of probation or parole. The Kingston Screening Instrument for Domestic Violence provides data for decisions regarding probation release, and the DV-MOSAIC was intended to help determine the criminal justice response in cases of domestic assault. The Spousal Assault Risk Assessment is widely used in "Canada and Vermont for probation supervision and treatment decisions" (Roehl et al., 2005, p. 18). Significant decisions regarding an individual's life are made on the basis of the risk assessment measures. Consequently, the validity and sensitivity and specificity of these measures are of utmost importance. In the National Institute of Justice study (Roehl et al., 2005), all five measures had acceptable levels of sensitivity, meaning that women who were reassaulted were correctly classified as being at elevated risk of reassault. The Danger Assessment and the DV-MOSAIC were the most sensitive. Thus, these measures may be useful for safety planning with victims of IPV. It must be borne in mind, however, that although these are encouraging results, the false-negative rates (women predicted to be at low risk who were subsequently reassaulted) were between 16% and 33% for these measures. Therefore, although they may function well as aggregate measures, their utility for making decisions on an individual basis clearly requires caution.

In the Roehl et al. (2005) study, the above measures did less well in terms of specificity (predicting reassault when none subsequently occurred), which, as Roehl et al. pointed out, is "more of a concern for offender rights than victim safety" (p. 82). Given the commitment to protect the rights of the accused in the U.S. criminal justice system, a high rate of false positives is not acceptable. The conclusion of the authors of the National Institute of Justice study seems apropos: "Risk assessment instruments or methods should not be the only factors considered in making decisions about victim safety or offender sanctions. . . . Rather, they are meant to be one source of information among many others" (p. 82). The best practice is to gather information with multiple methods (e.g., interview, checklist, and record review, if available) and from multiple sources. Ideally, the perpetrator and victim would be interviewed separately and information from collateral sources, such as a protective services worker, victim advocate, or police reports, would be integrated into a comprehensive assessment.

The National Institute of Justice study concluded that the victim's perception of risk provided the best balance between sensitivity and specificity and that simply asking the victim whether she feels she is in danger may be the most economical and valid assessment strategy. As Roehl et al. (2005) stated, victims were "impressive predictors of their own risk" (p. 77). Women who are consulted about their perceptions of risk of reassault as part of the overall risk assessment process may be able to more accurately judge their level of risk and engage in appropriate safety planning as a result. Campbell (2004), for example, noted that the act of completing the danger assessment frequently raised the consciousness of women regarding their peril and prompted them to take action to promote their own safety.

Apart from the use of the above measures, clinicians should be familiar with the most salient risk factors in domestically violent couples. Regarding specific factors associated with lethality, Campbell et al. (2003) conducted an 11-city study of the Danger Assessment and identified several factors to be associated with lethality. Specifically, perpetrator access to a gun and prior threats to use it predicted lethality (but not reassault). Severe depression and suicidality in the perpetrator were also associated with the risk of a lethal outcome (especially murder–suicide), but again were not predictive of reassault. Elevated risk for lethal outcomes was associated with perpetrator unemployment, the victim leaving the perpetrator after having lived together during the past year, perpetrator avoidance of arrests for past offenses, the victim having a child that the perpetrator knew was not his (e.g., from a previous relationship), and forced sexual activities. In our case example, David is currently unemployed and has a history of separations from his partner (although they are now together, that status could change quickly), and his partner has two children by another man. Should he resume his former substance abuse pattern, this would add to the level of risk. Campbell (2004) also noted that because many of the risk factors are dynamic, treatment providers need to be continuously alert to changes in the relationship that could alter the risk profiles and therefore affect the duty to protect.

CHALLENGES ARISING IN TREATMENT

Historically, there has been intense debate regarding whether the treatment of IPV should even be the domain of the mental health professions. Straus (1972) minimized the importance of individual psychopathology. Twenty-two years later, the commission in Massachusetts charged with revising the batterer treatment standards took pains to change the wording from *treatment* to *intervention* to further depathologize the problem and distance it from the mental health professions.

This exemplifies a serious problem for mental health professionals working in this area, namely the significant impact of sociopolitical influences.

The aforementioned guidelines and standards for batterer intervention may have the force of law if they are established by agencies with authority derived from powers legislated to them by their state lawmakers. In many cases, these standards were developed absent the input of mental health professionals and, in some cases (e.g., Massachusetts) include requirements that may be at odds with the professional ethics of psychologists or other mental health practitioners. Thus, if state standards require notification of potential victims, or the authorities, for behaviors that would ordinarily not trigger protective actions by the treatment provider, the state standards might take precedence over the ethical standards of the professions. "Generally, state standards of batterer treatment require that programs severely limit client confidentiality and prescribe that programs inform courts about repeat acts of violence, alcohol or drug use, [program] attendance, and overall progress" (Adams, 1994, p. 9). We recently reviewed the standards from the states for which we could find standards. Of those states having standards, 64% specifically required routine victim contact. Although there was substantial variability, all standards that required victim contact specified that the contact be made at the point of entry into the intervention. Eleven required contact at termination, and 14 specified that victims be contacted regarding any change in perpetrator status or if a threat were made. Thirteen specifically permitted routine violation of confidentiality. The fact that confidentiality is generally viewed as essential to the effectiveness of psychotherapy was one of the bases for the U.S. Supreme Court ruling in the case of *Jaffee v. Redmond* (1996), which affirmed that therapist–client communications were privileged. The absence of confidentiality in many batterer intervention programs is a potential explanation for the mediocre effect sizes that have been attributed to these interventions (Babcock et al., 2004).

Regarding the treatment of IPV, various states not only require diluted confidentiality protections but also regulate the length, format, and content of the intervention. A question that arises is whether these state standards, given their lack of empirical support in the treatment literature, can be used by courts to define the standard of care for batterer intervention.

Standard of Care

Standard of care refers to the level of treatment that the reasonably prudent professional would provide under similar circumstances. The opinion of expert witnesses is necessary to define standard of care, at least in part, because the standard of care is rarely, if ever, codified, especially in the mental health professions. Although we are not aware of any malpractice cases in which state standards for batterer intervention were invoked to establish the standard of care, the possibility (and threat) remains. In an earlier work, Rosenbaum, Warnken, and Grudzinskas (2003) opined that "a psychologist who does not comply with certification standards because they are inconsistent with the ethical practice of psychologists should be held to the standard of care practiced by other psychologists and not those defined by the state standards" (p. 299). States (e.g., Utah) in which all persons treating batterers are required to conform to state treatment standards, irrespective of whether they are certified or working in a certified program, might be an exception. Practitioners are warned that the foregoing is our opinion and is offered in the absence of any legal test or statute.

Duty to Protect

It is our assessment that treatment providers who uncover IPV in the course of routine psychotherapy incur the same duties and responsibilities that would attach to the disclosure of threat or violent intent in any therapy situation. However, several issues unique to IPV may require action on the part of the practitioner. For example, in many states, exposing a child to interparental aggression is reportable to child protective authorities as neglect (or emotional abuse). This is clearly the case in California, Florida, Georgia, and Utah (personal communication with their respective child protective authorities, January 2008). In other states (e.g., Illinois, Minnesota, North Carolina), the reportability of exposure to IPV is less clear. Making a child maltreatment report, however, could lead to serious consequences for the batterer, such as revocation of probation. Our case includes just such a situation. Although David and Michelle deny physical aggression toward their children, the child protective agency in their state recognizes the harmful effect on children of exposure to domestic violence.

Defining exposure of a child to IPV as maltreatment has also led to dire consequences for victims. For example, the term *failure to protect* has been applied to battered mothers who remain in abusive relationships, thus exposing their children to the harmful effects of witnessing IPV, and children have been separated from their mothers as a result. In a well-known case in New York (*Nicholson v. Williams*, 2002), an injunction was issued against the state's children's services agencies, stating that said agencies "participated in widespread, unnecessary, and cruel practices [i.e. removing children from the mother predicated on the idea that exposing them to IPV constituted neglect] that punished abused mothers for their own victimization" (Fitzgerald, Richard, Torchia, & Allo, 2004, p. 12). In Minnesota, changes in the child maltreatment statute to include exposure to interparental violence as reportable maltreatment had to be repealed within a year because of the strain on the state's child protective agency produced by the large volume of reports.

In addition to whether the presenting problem automatically constitutes a reportable event, practitioners must also be concerned about the possibility of child maltreatment, not only by the batterer but also by the victim. Edleson (1999) summarized the findings of more than 30 studies examining the link between adult domestic violence and child maltreatment and found a median co-occurrence rate of 40% (i.e., if adult IPV is occurring, a child is also being maltreated in 40% of the cases). It must be noted, however, that in many of these cases, the maltreatment was classified as "failure to protect" and was thus a direct function of the IPV report. Also of concern is the possibility that the batterer may attempt to manipulate the treatment provider into colluding with him to make a report against his partner because a report of child maltreatment coming from a professional would be taken more seriously than one coming from a batterer, who might more likely be seen as retaliating against his partner. The potential for harm to all parties (child, victim, and perpetrator) would argue for careful consideration of the risks and benefits of each option on a case-by-case basis.

Many states require the reporting of injuries caused during the commission of a crime (including domestic violence), and a smaller number of states mandate the reporting of domestic violence if disclosed by a patient to a health care provider. Utah, for example, has an adult abuse statute that places providers under a legal obligation to report abuse to the authorities (Utah Statute 26-23a-2). Under this statute, health care professionals cannot be punished for making a report and, in fact, incur penalties (including being charged with a misdemeanor, jailed, and/or fined) for failing to report suspected or confirmed cases of abuse. It should be noted, however, that psychologists are not specifically included in the Utah definition of health care provider. Hamberger and Phelan (2004) reviewed the advantages and disadvantages of having such a law and concluded that overall there is ambivalence among the victims studied about whether such a law would be helpful or would place them at greater risk for harm and family disruption. In addition, clinicians may be placed in the difficult position of possibly breaching the confidentiality of a competent adult and the clinically unfeasible position of disempowering the victim by making the decision to share the information without the victim's consent (Glass & Campbell, 1998; Hamberger & Phelan, 2004). We strongly advise therapists to make sure that they are familiar with the specific requirements of the jurisdiction in which they practice and also to stay current regarding these requirements because, as exemplified by the Minnesota experience described above, the requirements are subject to revision.

On the one hand, one advantage for those working with a court-mandated population is that the primary potential victim (the female partner) of the batterer is already aware of the client's dangerousness, as is the legal system. Thus, the many negative sequelae of making the initial report (e.g., when a client's child abusive behavior is uncovered by a mandated reporter who must inform the appropriate agency) have already been experienced. On the other hand, because many court-mandated clients are already on probation, any report of potential violence could trigger a violation of probation and result in the client being incarcerated. The often competing elements of ethical reasoning—beneficence and nonmaleficence—necessitate that all of the potential consequences, to both perpetrator and victim, of any protective action be considered.

Discharging the Duty to Protect

The protective requirements imposed on therapists dealing with IPV are no different from those affecting any other case; however, the nature of the population increases the need for vigilance and complicates decision making. The usual responses to the threat posed by clients are to warn victims and notify the appropriate authorities (e.g., police, courts, child protective services), violating confidentiality, if necessary. Many batterer intervention programs, recognizing these responsibilities and the additional regulations that may be placed on them by state standards, require perpetrators to sign a statement releasing them from the obligations of confidentiality at the start of the intervention. They may also inform perpetrators that victims will be contacted, either regularly or as necessary, and obtain victim contact information from them at the same time.

A related concern is the possible assumption, particularly on the part of the victim, that the batterer's participation in treatment means that he can change and that the victim is now safer. This belief might increase the likelihood that the victim will stay in an abusive relationship, undermining the objective of many shelters and victim advocates who seek to empower victims to leave. Victim safety would require that victims be properly informed regarding the probability of success and also of the possibility that victims are not safer because the perpetrator is in a program. Many states require that programs make contact with victims and provide such information; however, we believe that it puts the clinician in the unfeasible position of delivering a pessimistic message about treatment effectiveness to the victim while communicating hope and expectation of change to the perpetrator. One possible solution is for programs to team with local shelters that would assume responsibility for educating victims while also informing them of any programs and services they offer. This is consistent with state standards in many states that require a collaborative relationship with the local battered women's shelter.

Finally, irrespective of whether a treatment provider (or program) views the victim or the perpetrator as his or her client, victim safety must be a priority. Historically, actions intended to help victims (such as mandatory arrest of batterers, characterizing exposure of children to interparental aggression as a form of child neglect, and even victim contact) have had unintended negative consequences for victims. Treatment providers must carefully consider the potential outcomes of all protective actions before proceeding and remain sensitive to the possibility that even the most well-meaning efforts to protect might inadvertently result in more harm than good.

Considerations Regarding the Therapeutic Alliance

Perpetrators who have been mandated to treatment often come in with a great deal of anger directed not only toward their female partners but also toward the courts and the program. Anger toward the courts frequently occurs because the batterer feels he was treated unfairly by the legal system. As noted above, violence often occurs in the context of a volatile dyad, is low level, and is mutual. Consequently, the man may not be the sole aggressor, yet he may feel that he alone is being sanctioned. In addition, to avoid the expense and risk of a trial, batterers often accept a plea when, in fact, they may not believe they are guilty or, at least, the only guilty party. It is important for therapists to acknowledge this anger rather than viewing it as the batterer's denial or failure to take responsibility for his or her behavior. It is equally important that therapists not be seduced into colluding with the batterer, viewing him, rather than his victim, as the injured party. Because therapists often see only one of the partners (the batterer), they are exposed to a biased perspective not only regarding what happened but also regarding the context in which it occurred. Invariably, a different picture emerges when other perspectives (e.g., victim report, police report) are included.

CONCLUSION

Intervening with partner-aggressive individuals entails many challenges. Thorough psychological evaluation and risk assessment are best done in an adequately structured manner by a trained mental health clinician to generate an understanding of the level of risk and the clinical needs of perpetrator, victim, and children. The victim's perceptions of risk must be included in this assessment, along with other sources of data, such as police reports and criminal and mental health histories. The clinician is advised to anticipate situations that may require a warning of imminent harm, as well as reportable protective issues. Although current risk assessments are flawed, and models of treatment are less effective than we would like, it is imperative to continue to intervene and protect to the best of our ability while striving to learn more effective ways to do so.

REFERENCES

Adams, D. (1994). Treatment standards for abuser programs. *Violence Update, 5(1),* 5–11.

Aldarondo, E., & Mederos, F. (2002). *Programs for men who batter: Intervention and prevention strategies in a diverse society.* Kingston, NJ: Civic Research Institute.

American Psychological Association. (2002). Ethical principles of psychologists and code of conduct. *American Psychologist, 57,* 1060–1073.

Archer, J. (2000). Sex differences in aggression between heterosexual partners: A meta-analytic review. *Psychological Bulletin, 126,* 651–680.

Babcock, J. C., Green, C. E., & Robie, C. (2004). Does batterers' treatment work? A meta-analytic review of domestic violence treatment. *Clinical Psychology Review, 23,* 1023–1053.

Campbell, J. C. (2004). Helping women understand their risk in situations of intimate partner violence. *Journal of Interpersonal Violence, 19,* 1464–1477.

Campbell, J. C., Webster, D., Koziol-McLain, J., Block, C., Campbell, D., Curry, M., et al. (2003). Risk factors for femicide in abusive relationships: Results from a multisite case control study. *American Journal of Public Health, 93,* 1089–1097.

Coker, A. L., Davis, K. E., Arias, I., Desai, S., Sanderson, M., Brandt, H. M., et al. (2002). Physical and mental health effects of intimate partner violence for men and women. *American Journal of Preventive Medicine, 23,* 260–268.

Davies, J., Lyon, E., & Monti-Catania, D. (1998). *Safety planning with battered women: Complex lives/difficult choices.* Thousand Oaks, CA: Sage.

de Becker & Associates. (2005). *Domestic violence method (DV-MOSAIC).* Retrieved June 20, 2007, from http://www.mosaicsystem.com/dv.htm

Dutton, D. G., & Corvo, K. (2006). Transforming a flawed policy: A call to revive psychology and science in domestic violence research and practice. *Aggression and Violent Behavior, 11,* 457–483.

Edleson, J. L. (1999). The overlap between child maltreatment and woman battering. *Violence Against Women, 5,* 134–154.

Elliot, P. (1996). Shattering illusions: Same sex domestic violence. In C. M. Renzetti & C. H. Miley (Eds.), *Violence in gay and lesbian partner relationships* (pp. 1–8). New York: Haworth Press.

Fitzgerald, A., Richard, J., Torchia, A., & Allo, J. (2004). *Civil and criminal responses to children and youth who experience domestic violence: A model policy response for Vermont.* (Available from the Vermont Network Against Domestic Violence and Sexual Assault, the Vermont Department for Children and Families, and the Vermont Center for Crime Victim Services)

Geffner, R. A., & Rosenbaum, A. (2001). *Domestic violence offenders: Current interventions, research, and implications for policies and standards.* New York: Haworth Maltreatment & Trauma Press.

Glass, N., & Campbell, J. C. (1998). Mandatory reporting of intimate partner violence by health care professionals: A policy review. *Nursing Outlook, 46,* 279–283.

Hamberger, L. K., & Hastings, J. E. (1986). Characteristics of spouse abusers: Predictors of treatment acceptance. *Journal of Interpersonal Violence, 1,* 363–373.

Hamberger, L. K., & Phelan, M. B. (2004). *Domestic violence screening and intervention in medical and mental healthcare settings.* New York: Springer.

Harris, G. T, Rice, M. E., & Camilleri, J. A. (2004). Applying a forensic actuarial assessment (the Violence Risk Appraisal Guide) to nonforensic patients. *Journal of Interpersonal Violence, 19,* 1063–1075.

Hilton, N. Z., & Harris, G. T. (2005). Predicting wife assault: A critical review and implications for policy and practice. *Trauma, Violence, & Abuse, 6*, 3–23.

Hilton, N. Z., Harris, G. T., Rice, M. E., Lang, C., Cormier, C. A., & Lines, K. (2004). A brief actuarial assessment for the prediction of wife assault recidivism: The Ontario Domestic Assault Risk Assessment. *Psychological Assessment, 16*, 267–275.

Holtzworth-Munroe, A. (2005). Male versus female intimate partner violence: Putting controversial findings into context. *Journal of Marriage and Family, 67*, 1120–1125.

Holtzworth-Munroe, A., & Stuart, G. L. (1994). Typologies of male batterers: Three subtypes and the differences among them. *Psychological Bulletin, 116*, 476–497.

Jaffee v. Redmond, 518 U.S. 1, 116 S. Ct. 1923 (1996).

Jaffe, P., Lemon, N., & Poisson, S. E. (2003). *Child custody and domestic violence: A call for safety and accountability*. Thousand Oaks, CA: Sage.

Johnson, M. P. (2000). Conflict and control: Images of symmetry and asymmetry in domestic violence. In A. Booth, A. C. Crouter, & M. Clements (Eds.), *Couples in conflict* (pp. 95–104). Hillsdale, NJ: Erlbaum.

Kropp, P. R. (2004). Some questions regarding spousal assault risk assessment. *Violence Against Women, 10*, 676–697.

Kropp, P. R., Hart, S. D., Webster, C. D., & Eaves, D. (1995). *Manual for the Spousal Assault Risk Assessment Guide* (2nd ed.). Vancouver: British Columbia Institute Against Family Violence.

Lie, G., Schilit, R., Bush, J., Montagne, M., & Reyes, L. (1991). Lesbians in currently aggressive relationships: How frequently do they report aggressive past relationships? *Violence and Victims, 6*, 121–135.

Lyon, E. (1998, May). *The Revised K-SID: Analysis of reliability and relationship to new arrests after one year (An interim report)*. Hartford: State of Connecticut, Office of Policy and Management.

Monahan, J. (1981). *The clinical prediction of violent behavior* (DHHS Pub. No. ADM 81-921). Washington, DC: U.S. Government Printing Office.

Nicholson v. Williams, 203 F. Supp. 2d 153 (E.D. N.Y. 2002).

Pence, E., & Paymar, M. (1993). *Education groups for men who batter: The Duluth model*. New York: Springer.

Quinsey, V. L., Harris, G. T., Rice, M. E., & Cormier, C. A. (1998). *Violent offenders: Appraising and managing risk*. Washington, DC: American Psychological Association.

Roehl, J., O'Sullivan, C., Webster, D., & Campbell, J. C. (2005, March). *Intimate partner violence risk assessment validation study: Practitioner summary and recommendations: Validation of tools for assessing risk from violent intimate partners* (NIJ No. 209732). Retrieved June 20, 2007, from http://www.ncjrs.gov/pdffiles1/nij/grants/209732.pdf

Rosenbaum, A., Warnken, W. J., & Grudzinskas, A. J. (2003). Legal and ethical issues in the court-mandated treatment of batterers. In D. G. Dutton & D. J.

Sonkin (Eds.), *Intimate violence: Contemporary treatment innovations* (pp. 279–303). New York: Haworth Trauma & Maltreatment Press.

Smith Slep, A. M., & O'Leary, S. G. (2005). Parent and partner violence in families with young children: Rates, patterns, and connections. *Journal of Consulting and Clinical Psychology, 73*, 435–444.

Straus, M. A. (1972). Foreword. In R. Gelles, *The violent home* (pp. 13–17). Beverly Hills, CA: Sage.

Straus, M. A. (1997). Physical assaults by women partners: A major social problem. In M. R. Walsh (Ed.), *Women, men, and gender: Ongoing debates* (pp. 210–221). New Haven, CT: Yale University Press.

Tjaden, P., & Thoennes, N. (2000). Prevalence and consequences of male-to-female and female-to-male intimate partner violence as measured by the national violence against women survey. *Violence Against Women, 6*, 142–161.

Tolman, R. M., & Bennett, L. W. (1990). A review of quantitative research on men who batter. *Journal of Interpersonal Violence, 5*, 87–118.

Williams, K. R., & Houghton, A. B. (2004). Assessing the risk of domestic violence reoffending: A validation study. *Law and Human Behavior, 28*, 437–455.

7

WORKING WITH THE STALKING OFFENDER: CONSIDERATIONS FOR RISK ASSESSMENT AND INTERVENTION

BARRY ROSENFELD, JOANNA FAVA, AND MICHELE GALIETTA

James, a 34-year-old financial planner, dated Suzanne for 3 months. The relationship was relatively superficial, seeing each other every week or two, and deteriorated when James began questioning Suzanne about her whereabouts during times they were apart. Suzanne eventually ended the relationship, although James continued to telephone her for several weeks after their breakup, at times becoming loud and angry with her on the telephone. After one particularly threatening voice message, Suzanne informed the police, and James was charged with stalking (a misdemeanor punishable by up to 6 months in prison). Because he had no prior criminal record, James was sentenced to a period of probation that included mandatory mental health treatment. However, his probation officer had difficulty finding an appropriate treatment setting. Several mental health clinics expressed concern that James might begin to harass their staff, and most stated that they did not have a treatment program appropriate to address James's behavior. A private psychologist, a specialist in domestic violence, accepted the referral and initiated weekly cognitive–

behavioral therapy with James. However, 3 weeks into treatment the patient revealed that he had been frequenting the bar across the street from Suzanne's apartment and was aware that she has been dating another man. During the very next session, James accidentally emptied out his backpack in the therapist's office, and a large knife and roll of duct tape fell out. James explained that he had planned to break into Suzanne's apartment with a knife and duct tape, tie up her boyfriend, and "scare him off." At this point, the therapist began to worry for Suzanne's safety and contemplated informing her of the possible risk.

THE PROBLEM OF STALKING

Stalking, also called obsessional harassment, involves repeatedly following, harassing, or attempting to contact another person in a manner that would cause a reasonable person fear or distress (Tjaden & Theonnes, 1998). Stalking can have serious repercussions on those who are harassed, including anxiety, sleep disturbance, and symptoms of posttraumatic stress disorder, as well as thoughts of suicide in extreme cases (Pathe & Mullen, 1997). In addition, being stalked often causes individuals to seek counseling, lose time at work, change jobs, or even relocate their home (Pathe & Mullen, 1997; Tjaden & Theonnes, 1998).

Although stalking has always existed, the 1989 killing of actress Rebecca Schaeffer by an obsessed fan propelled the issue into the nation's consciousness. In the 6 weeks after Rebecca Schaeffer's death, four other California women were killed by individuals who had been stalking them, leading the California legislature to write the first antistalking legislation. By 2000, similar legislation had been passed in all 50 states. Although the requirements vary by state, most statutes require three core elements (Beatty, 2003): (a) that a pattern of behavior be directed at a particular person (rather than a single threatening incident), (b) that the behavior be intentional, and (c) that the behavior actually cause the victim to fear for his or her safety.

Tjaden and Thoennes (1998) conducted a national survey of the prevalence of stalking in the general population. Defining stalking as

> a course of conduct directed at a specific person that involves repeated visual or physical proximity; nonconsensual communication; verbal, written, or implied threats; or a combination thereof that would cause fear in a reasonable person (with repeated meaning on two or more occasions) (p. 2),

they estimated that roughly 1 million women and 370,000 men are stalked annually. These figures correspond to a lifetime rate of 8% for women and 2% for men. The growing recognition of the problem of stalking, and of the potentially dangerous nature of this behavior, has spawned a burgeoning research literature focused on understanding who engages in stalking and why.

This literature has revealed a number of patterns, such as the high prevalence of psychological disorders in stalking offenders, including severe mental disorders (e.g., schizophrenia, delusional disorder), personality disorders (primarily borderline, antisocial, and narcissistic), and substance-related disorders (Rosenfeld, 2004). The rates of these disorders have varied across studies, but composite estimates indicate that roughly one third of stalkers suffer from a psychotic disorder, between 50% and 60% have a personality disorder, and roughly 30% to 50% abuse drugs or alcohol. Although early studies focused on identifying "types" of stalking offenders, subsequent studies have focused on risk factors for violence, often with surprising results (described later). For example, the presence of psychosis, a putative risk factor for violence, has been associated with lower rates of violence among stalking offenders (Rosenfeld, 2004). Instead, the most robust predictors of recidivism and violence include the presence of a prior intimate relationship, a history of overt threats, and the presence of substance abuse or a personality disorder diagnosis (Rosenfeld, 2004).

The literature has also demonstrated relatively high rates of violence among stalking offenders, with violence occurring in 30% to 40% of cases (Rosenfeld, 2004). Although relatively little of this violence is life threatening, serious incidents of violence, including homicide, have occasionally occurred and garnered significant media coverage. Accurately assessing risk for violence in stalking cases is crucial for appropriate legal decision making and for establishing treatment goals and procedures.

Although the literature on the treatment of individuals who exhibit stalking behaviors is limited, in this chapter we present guidelines for the assessment and treatment of stalking offenders. Some of the issues discussed pertain specifically to stalking, but many apply equally to any type of treatment in forensic settings and to community treatment of those at increased risk for violence. We address challenges associated with evaluating and treating individuals who engage in stalking behaviors, including how to develop a therapeutic alliance with individuals mandated to treatment, manage issues of confidentiality, and maintain awareness of one's personal limits. In addition, we address such clients' motivational deficits and how to overcome them. As noted previously, risk assessment is an essential component of treatment with this population. Thus, we provide detailed guidelines for conducting ongoing risk assessment, along with a discussion of the duty to protect in the context of stalking cases.

NEGOTIATING THE THERAPEUTIC RELATIONSHIP

Perhaps the most striking aspect of treating stalking offenders is the impact that this client population has on the therapeutic relationship. There is little dispute that the ability to develop a working relationship between the therapist and the client is one of the most (if not the most) critical elements in any mental health treatment setting. Numerous studies have demonstrated the importance of the therapeutic relationship to treatment outcome, finding that roughly 25% of the variance in treatment outcome is explained by therapist and process variables (e.g., therapists' personal style and clients' perception of an alliance; Lambert & Bergin, 1994; Matt & Navarro, 1997). Although this literature typically focuses on traditional psychotherapy settings, research with offender samples has similarly demonstrated the importance of therapist variables and the therapeutic relationship (e.g., Marshall, 2005).

Negotiating the therapeutic relationship with stalking offenders is fraught with difficulties that either do not apply or are greatly simplified in traditional mental health treatment settings. The first hurdle to overcome in most treatment cases involving stalking is the fact that many individuals are mandated by the court to attend treatment. This can create an environment of hostility even before treatment begins and should typically be addressed early on in the treatment. Acknowledging the compulsory nature of treatment and allowing clients to express their anger or resentment about this situation is often helpful. Motivation for treatment can often be increased when freedom and autonomy are maximized. This can be accomplished by highlighting the client's freedom to choose whether to meaningfully participate in treatment or to simply attend or feign active engagement in treatment. Ironically, patients who have developed a strong alliance with the therapist will often begin to disclose information that raises therapist concerns (e.g., thoughts and feelings about the target of their harassment), at times leading to heightened safety concerns (discussed further later).

A second hurdle that arises in treating stalking offenders involves demonstrating to the client (through speech and action) the therapist characteristics shown to be associated with successful treatment. Drapeau (2005), in a study of sex offenders referred for treatment, found that the offender's perception of the therapist's characteristics was the most important factor in treatment success. They characterized effective clinicians as being honest, caring, respectful, nonjudgmental, and noncritical. In sum, the basic Rogerian traits of warmth, authenticity, and positive regard that are important for all therapy are no less critical to developing a therapeutic alliance in forensic contexts. Yet, being authentic and having genuine regard for clients who have committed violent, threatening, or disturbing acts is often difficult and requires ongoing attention to one's own thoughts and feelings.

A third hurdle that should be addressed before initiating treatment pertains to the potential risk to the therapist. A number of studies have described the potential for clients to develop inappropriate attachments to their therapist, leading to a host of behaviors that may frighten or cause injury to the practitioner (e.g., Lion & Herschler, 1998). These problematic behaviors include, but are not limited to, stalking, harassing, threatening, and even attacking the therapist. Corder and Whiteside (1996) found that clients who are involved in the legal system (e.g., forensic clients) were more likely to exhibit threats, stalking, and physical violence than were clients with no history of legal system involvement. Although this study hardly provides conclusive support for clinician fears, there is little dispute that clinicians need to have a heightened level of concern and caution when working with clients known to have engaged in stalking. Moreover, risk to the therapist can be conceptualized in financial terms, not just physical terms, because the potential for litigation (e.g., for failure to warn or protect a victim) is not insignificant. As described below, these risks are best minimized through ethical and responsible practice (e.g., thorough risk assessment and, when appropriate, disclosures or intervention), but can never be eliminated altogether (although such risks exist to a greater or lesser extent in all treatment settings).

Addressing clinician concerns that may impair forming a therapeutic alliance remains complicated; however, a number of steps can help minimize the impact of these concerns on clinician behavior. To begin, acknowledgment of one's fears can help the clinician identify and address any obstacles that arise in the development of a therapeutic alliance. In particular, recognition and management of one's fears and distrust are critical to balancing the need to take appropriate precautions with the development of a genuine alliance. Development of an alliance is also facilitated by clinician behaviors within the therapy context, such as open acknowledgment of fears and concerns, integration of the client and his or her perspective into development of treatment goals, and the maintenance of a genuinely empathic relationship (without simply ignoring inappropriate behaviors; Marshall & Serran, 2004). Although the base rate for violence toward therapists in this context is low, taking reasonable precautions allows clinicians to feel safe so that they may concentrate on treatment issues.

When therapists initiate treatment with criminal offenders, another issue that arises early in the treatment process is negotiating the limits and boundaries of confidentiality. The complexities of confidentiality hinge, to some extent, on the nature of treatment because many individuals are court ordered to attend treatment and many treatment settings maintain collaborative relationships with court officers (e.g., probation or parole offices, mental health courts, diversion programs). Thus, although the specific issues that pertain to any individual setting may differ, the broader issues of confidentiality require clear and frank discussion with the prospective client as soon as treatment is initiated. Issues that should be outlined include the extent to which specific types of information will be disclosed to the justice system (e.g., only attendance or nonattendance, progress in treatment, specific topics discussed). Perhaps most important, procedures for dealing with perceived violence risk, continued criminal behavior, or other potential violations (e.g., alcohol use, drug use) require explicit discussion and agreement from the client in advance of any disclosures occurring. In particular, patients should be informed as to the duty to warn and/or protect identified victims. Such a course limits surprise and feelings of betrayal for the client when a reportable event emerges and reduces or avoids subsequent conflicts when such disclosures are warranted.

Although disclosures regarding the limits of confidentiality are often perceived by clinicians as hindering the development of a therapeutic alliance, such perceptions are often ill founded (Binder & McNiel, 1996). Most offenders, particularly when court ordered to attend treatment, perceive the therapy setting as simply an extension of probation or parole. Thus, offenders often minimize the amount of information they divulge or minimize and deny many of the behaviors and problems that are the focus of treatment. Hence, frank discussion of confidentiality issues at the outset of treatment can actually help build the therapeutic alliance because such conversations can serve to reassure the client as to the clinician's awareness of and vigilance to these issues. In addition, if a disclosure becomes necessary, informing the patient as to what information will be disclosed and the reason can reduce the likelihood of an adverse reaction to the disclosure. This type of therapist behavior models for the client honest and open communication even around difficult topics. It should be noted that although, in general, asking the client to make the disclosure of violence risk may be a good intervention, this is not true in the case of stalking. In fact, it is probably illegal in most instances (given the frequent existence of a no-contact order).

Another critical issue that warrants discussion immediately on initiating treatment is the nature of treatment itself (discussed in more detail later). Clients, whether court mandated or voluntary, must be informed as to the type and focus of treatment to develop realistic expectations. Particularly in offender treatment settings, in which the choice to attend treatment is not entirely the client's, clinicians should disclose any relevant information regarding the nature of treatment, the expectations of the clinician, the time commitment expected, and the indicators for determining treatment success or completion. Use of a formal written contract may even be beneficial in such settings to minimize subsequent allegations that disclosures were inappropriate or insufficient.

A special consideration in working with offender populations that is even more critical when treating stalking offenders involves the clinician's limits regarding self-disclosure. Clinicians should avoid providing any unnecessary information about themselves, their family, or their personal background. Avoiding displays of personal or family photographs and having an unlisted home phone number are advisable to minimize the client's access to the clinician outside of the treatment setting. Nevertheless, the Internet-savvy client can often locate considerable information about the clinician even when such precautions are taken, so monitoring of what information is accessible through the Internet is recommended. Despite precautions against disclosure of one's personal background, appropriate self-disclosures can be beneficial to treatment. Information about how one has handled strong emotions or frustrating experiences may be particularly useful, provided the disclosure does not violate the personal limits of the therapist or compromise his or her safety.

TREATMENT WITH STALKING OFFENDERS

Unfortunately, the choice of treatment approaches for stalking offenders is complicated by the lack of any interventions with demonstrated efficacy in reducing stalking per se. That said, many elements of treatment are well supported to target specific behaviors (e.g., the use of antipsychotic medications for psychotic symptoms or interventions for alcohol and substance abuse). Given the nature of forensic treatment settings, treatment should inevitably target the behaviors associated with either the criminal behavior or the violence risk. Treatment targets should be prioritized according to their importance and should be monitored throughout treatment.

Any treatment planning for stalking offenders, as with all treatment settings, requires a thorough assessment and determination of what, if any, diagnoses apply to the offender and how to operationalize the behaviors that must change to end the stalking behavior. Considerable research has focused on identifying the most common diagnoses among stalking offenders, with early studies emphasizing individuals with erotomanic delusions (typically, but not always, associated with a diagnosis of delusional disorder; e.g., Harmon, Rosner, & Owens, 1995; Meloy & Gothard, 1995). More recent research has identified high rates of personality disorder among stalking offenders (e.g., Rosenfeld & Harmon, 2002). In particular, Cluster B disorders, such as borderline, antisocial, and narcissistic personality disorders, alone or in combination with paranoid and dependent personality disorders or traits, account for roughly half of all stalking offenders and may be even more prevalent among the subset of individuals who are referred for outpatient mental health treatment (Rosenfeld, 2004). Other common diagnoses include mood disorders (depression and bipolar disorders) and substance abuse. Despite the seemingly "obsessive" behavior that characterizes stalking, obsessive–compulsive disorders are relatively uncommon. Instead, the seemingly obsessive preoccupation with another person is typically because of a delusional fixation on that individual (probably accounting for 20% of all stalking cases), intense anger and resentment related to feelings of rejection or unfair treatment (roughly 60% of cases), or other, more idiosyncratic reasons (described in more detail later; Rosenfeld, 2004).

The distinction between psychotic and nonpsychotic individuals is, of course, paramount because the former group almost invariably requires antipsychotic medication in addition to whatever other treatment approaches might be warranted. Although clinical lore suggests that antipsychotic medications are less effective in clients with encapsulated delusions (e.g., erotomania or other delusional disorders), pharmacological interventions are nevertheless warranted and have been increasingly supported for the treatment of delusional disorders (Kelly, 2005). In particular, older medications such as pimozide have been reported to be effective, as have some newer atypical antipsychotic agents such as risperidone and clozapine (Manschreck & Khan, 2006). Nonetheless, the response rate for clients with delusional disorders rarely exceeds 50%, and relatively little systematic research has focused specifically on this subgroup of individuals. Moreover, medication compliance is always a concern, and it is heightened when individuals are coerced (e.g., by the legal system) into treatment (described further later).

The list of psychotherapies with empirical support is growing, but evidence-based treatments for forensic populations and individuals at high risk for violence continue to lag behind. To date, few systematic mental health interventions exist for stalking offenders, and those that have been developed over the past few years still fall far short of being classified as evidence based. Two groups have described interventions specifically for stalking offenders, although neither has published data in support of effectiveness. Warren, MacKenzie, Mullen, and Ogloff (2005) described an intervention based on the problem behavior model that focuses on behavioral principles such as identifying the precipitants of stalking and harassment behaviors and developing alternative responses. In addition, our research group has used dialectical behavior therapy (Linehan, 1993) for stalking offenders. Although still under investigation, this application of dialectical behavior therapy has yielded encouraging pilot results (Rosenfeld et al., 2007).

These systematic interventions may show promise for helping guide the treatment of stalking offenders; however, at present most clinicians are forced to rely on eclectic or idiosyncratic approaches to dealing with this challenging population. Thus, clinicians may be wise to adapt existing techniques to the problems both unique to stalking (e.g., the obsessive fixation on another individual or attempts to initiate contact in response to feelings of inadequacy, rejection, or anger) and those that are common to many offender and nonoffender clients (e.g., substance abuse, depression). Many of these problems are well suited to cognitive–behavioral approaches, such as helping clients reassess distorted cognitions and develop alternative responses, but the effectiveness of any of these approaches is still largely unknown. One element of treatment that is essential, no matter what treatment approach one is using, is regular assessment of current level of risk.

RISK ASSESSMENT IN STALKING CASES

How a professional distinguishes genuine imminent risk from exaggerated fears is an important consideration for both treatment and evaluation settings. Using formal risk assessment procedures is helpful. In addition, seeking supervision or consultation from an experienced colleague (discussed below) can help the clinician maintain an accurate perception of the risk posed by his or her client. Although these steps will not eliminate all risk to clinicians (or others outside the treatment setting), they are likely to help the clinician develop and maintain a therapeutic alliance even with clients who engage in behaviors that are disconcerting.

Perhaps the most important aspect of treatment with stalking offenders is identifying when an individual presents a significant risk for violence. Not only is accurate risk assessment critical to managing the risks posed by one's client, but awareness of the risk factors for violence can help the clinician accurately appraise the risk posed to him- or herself. With accurate risk assessment, unnecessary precautions or restrictions can be minimized while simultaneously protecting those individuals who might be at risk. However, because few clients openly acknowledge their intent to engage in violent or high-risk behaviors, clinicians must be familiar with the risk factors for violence in stalking offenders and the formal methods available to conduct such assessments. In addition, integration of collateral data, from victims, probation or police officers, or medical or mental health records, is a critical element of a thorough risk assessment strategy. Such data can also be important in cases in which the clinician believes that a high risk of violence exists, particularly in helping provide the justification for a decision to intervene or warn the potential victim. Finally, collateral evidence can help the clinician to overcome the client's denial and minimization by providing additional examples of continued problem behaviors and can help identify the actions that must change for the stalking to end.

A growing literature has addressed the variables that correspond to an increased risk of violence in stalking offenders (see Rosenfeld, 2004, for review). A recent meta-analysis of the stalking violence literature identified several variables that have consistently, or sporadically, been associated with violence (Rosenfeld, 2004). One of the strongest predictors of violence observed in this review was the existence of prior threats. Although this variable was a robust predictor of violence in every study, it is also noteworthy that only a subset of those individuals who make explicit threats of harm actually engage in subsequent violence. In addition, a small but worrisome subset of violent individuals do not express their intentions in advance. Despite these *false positives* (threats that are not acted on) and *false negatives* (violence without a prior threat), the overall association between threats and subsequent violence is substantial and should raise concerns whenever a credible threat of violence (i.e., one that is not frankly implausible) is expressed, and such verbalizations must be thoroughly evaluated (see also Borum, Fein, Vossekuil, & Berglund, 1999).

Another strong predictor of stalking-related violence is the existence of a previous intimate relationship between the victim and the offender

(Rosenfeld, 2004). Across each study reviewed, individuals who harassed prior intimates were significantly more likely to be violent than were those who stalked or harassed strangers, family members, or acquaintances. Historical variables such as past violence unrelated to the stalking relationship and prior criminal history generated more equivocal findings, with significant associations observed in some but not all studies. Several clinical variables were also associated with violence, including the presence of a personality disorder (particularly Cluster B disorders such as narcissistic, antisocial, or borderline personality disorders), substance abuse, and the absence of psychosis (i.e., psychotic individuals were less often violent than were nonpsychotic individuals). Likewise, demographic variables such as age (younger adults are more often violent than older adults) and education (less educated individuals are typically more likely to be violent) that are often associated with violence in the general offender literature have also been supported in some stalking research (e.g., Rosenfeld & Harmon, 2002).

In addition to offender-related variables that have been the subject of systematic research, a number of situational or contextual risk factors have been identified but less often studied. Perhaps the most obvious of these context-related risk factors is the availability of the identified victim. Clearly, individuals who have access to the potential victim have far greater opportunity to act on violent impulses than do those whose potential victims are not easily approachable (e.g., individuals who target celebrities or other public figures). Likewise, the ready availability of weapons or a history of using weapons in the context of violence increases the likelihood that violent behaviors will have severe or life-threatening implications. Finally, an escalating pattern of stalking behaviors, whether in terms of frequency or severity (e.g., increasing level of risk or intrusiveness), can be an important cue to a heightened risk of violence.

Although traditional methods of risk assessment rely on clinicians to estimate violence risk on the basis of their own idiosyncratic methods, researchers have increasingly developed formal risk assessment techniques to guide the evaluation process. Two broad categories of risk assessment techniques have emerged in recent years: actuarial and structured professional judgment. Actuarial risk assessment relies on a statistically generated algorithm to generate a likelihood estimate, typically in the form of a probability of violence. Rosenfeld and Lewis (2005) described one such approach with stalking offenders, using a regression tree to distinguish stalking offenders with varying rates of violence. Structured professional judgment, however, involves identifying empirically supported risk factors, defining a method for determining their presence or absence, and relying on trained clinicians to integrate these risk factors into a summary judgment about violence risk (e.g., high risk, moderate risk, or low risk). Kropp, Hart, and Lyon (2008) developed one such measure specifically designed to assess risk in stalking cases, the Stalking Assessment and Management guide. The Stalking Assessment and Management guide elicits data regarding three different dimensions of violence risk: factors related to the stalking behaviors (e.g., threats, escalation), general psychological characteristics of the offender (e.g., anger, substance abuse, employment or relationship problems), and victim vulnerability factors (e.g., inconsistent behavior or attitudes toward the offender, unsafe living conditions). However, this measure, although promising, does not yet have any established validity to support its usefulness in differentiating highand lower risk stalking offenders.

The Duty to Protect

Once a significant risk of violence has been identified, clinicians are faced with an even more difficult challenge: determining when and how to intervene. Since the seminal case of *Tarasoff v. Regents of the University of California* (1976), in which the California Supreme Court ruled that a mental health professional can be held liable for failing to protect a potential victim when the client presents a serious risk of harm, clinicians have been increasingly cognizant of the limits of confidentiality and hospitalization requirements when a risk of serious violence exists. A comprehensive review of duty-to-protect requirements across all jurisdictions is beyond the scope of this chapter (see chap. 2, this volume), but the essential core of this requirement is similar in most jurisdictions. Clinicians are obligated to inform potential victims or take other necessary steps (e.g., notifying police, seeking hospitalization) to minimize the risk of violence that exists. Of course, the range of actions necessary varies tremendously across jurisdictions, and clinicians must familiarize themselves with the specific statutes and case law that apply to their jurisdiction. For example, some jurisdictions require taking steps to warn the victim, whereas others require interventions to prevent the violence from occurring. Still other states (e.g., Texas) have failed to follow the example set by *Tarasoff* at all and specifically prohibit civil lawsuits based on failure to warn or protect potential victims.

In addition to legal guidelines, the "Ethical Principles of Psychologists and Code of Conduct" promulgated by the American Psychological Association (2002) also addresses issues of confidentiality and when breaches are warranted. The American Psychological Association's (2002) Ethics Code asserts that "psychologists disclose confidential information without the consent of the individual only as mandated by law, or where permitted by law for a valid purpose" (Standard 4.05[b], p. 1066). Because of the adverse effect that breaches of confidentiality can have on the therapeutic relationship, clinicians must be vigilant of both the temptation to violate confidentiality unnecessarily and the opposite tension, to ignore risk factors and warning signs because of concern about jeopardizing the treatment relationship. Although little research has addressed the impact of confidentiality breaches on the therapeutic alliance, it is our experience that the impact is dramatically lessened when clients are informed about the steps that are to be taken.

Once the clinician determines that a serious risk of violence exists, the decision to break confidentiality and warn either the potential victim or the police becomes easier. In many treatment settings (particularly when working with stalking offenders), the clinician will not have direct contact with, or even access to, the identified victim. Thus, notification might take the form of informing the police, the offender's probation officer, or even the district attorney's office. Because time is often critical once the risk of violence seems imminent, clinicians are advised to identify potential contacts in advance and maintain a record of this information for all clients just in case the need to warn a victim arises. Identifying the most appropriate individual(s) to contact, and having contact information readily available, will be critical if a serious risk of imminent violence arises.

ISSUES FOR SUPERVISORS AND CONSULTANTS

Supervisors and consultants face a unique set of issues when the client presents a heightened risk of violence, whether that risk pertains to the clinician or to a third party. Trainees and supervisees inevitably look to the supervisor or consultant for guidance whenever difficult treatment dilemmas arise, many of which were described earlier. Thus, supervisors and consultants must first assess their own knowledge and comfort in overseeing the treatment of stalking offenders to ensure they possess adequate expertise to safely oversee the treatment or evaluation process.

Assuming adequate expertise, supervisors should consider their top priority the maintenance of a safe environment for their supervisee. This process involves both assessing the risk to the treating clinician or evaluator and monitoring the extent of risk posed to others (e.g., the target of harassment). Supervisors should be able to maintain greater objectivity than the treating clinician and therefore are better able to manage strong feelings that often arise in clinicians, particularly when the clinician has little or no experience working with stalking offenders. Also, naïve clinicians may overlook or fail to recognize warning signs that a more seasoned clinician or objective supervisor would readily identify. Thus, the supervisor can serve an important role by providing objective feedback regarding the accuracy of the clinician's perspective.

Because clinicians rely on a supervisor's expertise, supervisors and consultants must also maintain a heightened level of knowledge regarding treatment methods and risk assessment techniques, as well as legal guidelines for how and when to respond when an imminent risk of life-threatening violence exists. Although supervisors, like clinicians, will inevitably vary in their experience and knowledge, the minimum level of acceptable expertise is far higher for supervisors, and arguably higher still for consultants, than for treating clinicians. Particularly when supervision or consultation has been sought outside of a formal institutional setting (e.g., an independent practitioner seeking consultation on a difficult treatment or assessment case), the requirements for expertise are substantial, precisely because the clinician is likely to rely heavily on the opinions and guidance of a consultant.

Supervisors can also serve an invaluable role in monitoring the involvement of their supervisees to reduce burnout. Offender settings are particularly stressful both because of the resistance and denial that pervade offender evaluation and treatment relationships and because of the pervasive concern for oneself and others. Supervisors and consultants can help monitor and modulate these stressors to maintain a balanced therapeutic relationship that does not sacrifice either therapist safety or objectivity.

CONCLUSION

In recent years, antistalking legislation has led to an increase in the number of stalking offenders referred to the mental health system. Thus, there is greater need to improve risk assessment strategies and to develop appropriate interventions to target this particular population. Determining when stalking clients pose a serious risk of harm to others has clear and significant implications for offenders, potential victims, the therapist, and the legal system. The 1976 *Tarasoff* ruling, and the creation of the duty to protect in jurisdictions across North America, transcended the ethical duty to engage in accurate risk assessments and created a legal duty and responsibility. However, stalking research has not kept pace with the need for systematic intervention and assessment techniques. Without the benefit of empirically validated instruments, therapists must rely on clinical judgment and knowledge of the specific risk factors associated with violence in stalking offenders. In addition, no mental health interventions have been empirically validated for treating stalking behaviors. Because the underlying psychological features of stalking offenders vary tremendously, it is imperative that clinicians thoroughly evaluate their clients and develop a treatment approach that will best meet the needs of the individual. Supervision, ongoing inquiry regarding a client's violent or stalking-related impulses, and detailed documentation of all sessions should be considered standard practice for any therapist working with this population. With careful attention to all of these issues, decisions about when and how to warn or protect potential victims can be substantially enhanced.

REFERENCES

American Psychological Association. (2002). Ethical principles of psychologists and code of conduct. *American Psychologist, 57,* 1060–1073.

Beatty, D. (2003). Stalking legislation in the United States. In M. P. Brewster (Ed.), *Stalking: Psychology, risk factors, interventions, and law* (pp. 2-1–2-55). Kingston, NJ: Civic Research Institute.

Binder, R. L., & McNiel, D. (1996). Application of the Tarasoff ruling and its effect on the victim and the therapeutic relationship. *Psychiatric Services, 47*, 1212–1215.

Borum, R., Fein, R., Vossekuil, B., & Berglund, J. (1999). Threat assessment: Defining an approach for evaluating risk of targeted violence. *Behavioral Sciences & the Law, 17*, 323–337.

Corder, B. F., & Whiteside, R. (1996). A survey of psychologists' safety issues and concerns. *American Journal of Forensic Psychology, 14*, 65–72.

Drapeau, M. (2005). Research on the processes involved in treating sexual offenders. *Sexual Abuse: Journal of Research and Treatment, 17*, 117–125.

Harmon, R. B., Rosner, R., & Owens, H. (1995). Obsessional harassment and erotomania in a criminal court population. *Journal of Forensic Sciences, 40*, 188–196.

Kelly, B. D. (2005). Erotomania: Epidemiology and management. *CNS Drugs, 19*, 657–669.

Kropp, P. R., Hart, S. D., & Lyon, D. R. (2008). *Guidelines for stalking assessment and management.* Vancouver: Proactive Resolutions.

Lambert, M. J., & Bergin, A. E. (1994). The effectiveness of psychotherapy. In A. E. Bergin (Ed.), *Handbook of psychotherapy and behavior change* (4th ed., pp. 143–189). Oxford, England: Wiley.

Linehan, M. M. (1993). *Cognitive-behavioral treatment of borderline personality disorder.* New York: Guilford Press.

Lion, J. R., & Herschler, J. A. (1998). The stalking of clinicians by their parents. In J. R. Meloy (Ed.), *The psychology of stalking: Clinical and forensic perspectives* (pp. 163–173). San Diego, CA: Academic Press.

Manschreck, T. C., & Khan, N. L. (2006). Recent advances in the treatment of delusional disorder. *Canadian Journal of Psychiatry/Revue Canadienne de Psychiatrie, 51*, 114–119.

Marshall, W. L. (2005). Therapist style in sexual offender treatment: Influence on indices of change. *Sex Abuse, 17*, 109–116.

Marshall, W. L., & Serran, G.A. (2004). The role of the therapist in offender treatment. *Psychology, Crime & Law, 10*, 309–320.

Matt, G. E., & Navarro, A. M. (1997). What meta-analyses have and have not taught us about psychotherapy effects: A review and future directions. *Clinical Psychology Review, 17*, 1–32.

Meloy, J. R., & Gothard, S. (1995). Demographic and clinical comparison of obsessional followers and offenders with mental disorders. *American Journal of Psychiatry, 152*, 258–263.

Pathe, M., & Mullen, P. E. (1997). The impact of stalkers on their victims. *British Journal of Psychiatry, 170*, 12–17.

Rosenfeld, B. (2004). Violence risk factors in stalking and obsessional harassment: A review and preliminary meta-analysis. *Criminal Justice and Behavior, 31*, 9–36.

Rosenfeld, B., Galietta, M., Ivanoff, A., Garcia-Mansilla, A., Martinez, R., Fava, J., et al. (2007). Dialectical behavior therapy for the treatment of stalking offenders. *International Journal of Forensic Mental Health, 6,* 95–103.

Rosenfeld, B., & Harmon, R. (2002). Factors associated with violence in stalking and obsessional harassment cases. *Criminal Justice and Behavior, 29,* 671–691.

Rosenfeld, B., & Lewis, C. (2005). Assessing violence risk in stalking cases: A regression tree approach. *Law and Human Behavior, 29,* 343–357.

Tarasoff v. Regents of the University of California, 131 Cal. Rptr. 14, 551 P.2d 334 (1976).

Tjaden, P., & Thoennes, N. (1998). *Stalking in America: Findings from the National Violence Against Women Survey* (NCJ Report No. 169592). Washington, DC: U.S. Department of Justice.

Warren, L. J., MacKenzie, R., Mullen, P. E., & Ogloff, J. R. (2005). The problem behavior model: The development of a stalkers clinic and a threateners clinic. *Behavioral Sciences and the Law, 23,* 387–397.

8

THREATS AGAINST PUBLIC OFFICIALS: CONSIDERATIONS FOR RISK ASSESSMENT, REPORTING, AND INTERVENTION

MARISA REDDY RANDAZZO AND MICHELLE KEENEY

Someone threatens the life of a public official every day. The president of the United States, vice president, former presidents, and first families are the targets of several thousand threats per year (Coggins, Pynchon, & Dvoskin, 1998). Members of Congress have received as many as 1,500 threats in a year (e.g., Scalora et al., 2002). Other public officials, such as cabinet secretaries, governors, mayors, and judges, are threatened each year as well (Baumgartner, Scalora, & Plank, 2001; Calhoun, 1998; Vossekuil, Borum, Fein, & Reddy, 2001). Many of these officials are protected by federal, state, and local law enforcement agencies, such as the U.S. Secret Service, U.S. Capitol Police, U.S. Marshals Service, and respective state troopers.

The law enforcement agencies charged with protecting public officials accomplish their missions in part through the investigation of threats to their protectees. These protective investigations include a range of activities aimed at identifying, assessing, and managing individuals who may pose a risk of harm to a protectee. Collectively, these activities are referred to as *threat assessment* or *protective intelligence activities* (e.g., Borum, Fein, Vossekuil, & Berglund, 1999; Fein & Vossekuil, 1998; Scalora et al., 2002; Vossekuil et al., 2001).

This chapter describes the range of threats and other behavior directed toward public officials that may come to the attention of psychologists and other mental health professionals (MHPs) and that may prompt some concern or action regarding a duty to protect. The chapter includes legal, ethical, and professional considerations with respect to addressing a client-issued threat to a public official. Beginning with an overview of the range of threats that an MHP may encounter, we address conducting assessments of risk that a client may pose, reporting threats issued by a client, and partnering with law enforcement to create and implement case management plans to reduce violence risk as well as support the client. This chapter draws heavily on our experience as psychologists with the Secret Service and thus includes frequent references to threats against the president of the United States and other Secret Service protectees. However, the nature of the issues discussed here apply in a similar fashion to threats against other public officials, including members of Congress, governors, judicial officials, and others who may be targeted by virtue of their public status (Baumgartner et al., 2001; Fein & Vossekuil, 1999).

RANGE OF THREATS TO PUBLIC OFFICIALS

Those who threaten public officials communicate their intentions in a variety of ways: through written communications that are sent via post or e-mail, oral communications that are conveyed via telephone or in person, and gestures or behaviors that indicate some intent to harm. The threats themselves also take a range of forms. These include direct threats of harm, in which the threatener states clearly his or her intentions to kill, kidnap, or harm the public official; conditional threats of harm, in which the threatener conveys his or her intention to do harm if certain conditions are not met; and indirect or veiled threats of harm, in which the threatener indicates his or her desire that the public official die or otherwise suffer harm, but without a clear indication that the threatener is the one who will perpetrate the harm. In addition, individuals come to the attention of the agencies that protect public officials for what is characterized as "inappropriate interest" in a protectee. Such behavior does not include the conveyance of threats but does suggest some preoccupation with a public official that is coupled with some concerning behavior, such as efforts to approach, stalk, or harass the official. The agencies that protect public officials typically take all types of threats seriously, regardless of the directness of their nature or the manner in which they are conveyed (Baumgartner et al., 2001; Borum et al., 1999; Fein & Vossekuil, 1998; Scalora et al., 2002).

The U.S. criminal code (i.e., 18 U.S.C. § 871 and 18 U.S.C. § 879) treats all of these types of threats and inappropriate interest, when issued against the president or other Secret Service protectees, as federal violations and authorizes the Secret Service to investigate these cases (18 U.S.C. § 3056). In addition, individual states have passed legislation criminalizing certain types of threatening behavior toward public officials (e.g., in Virginia, threatening the governor or his or her immediate family is a felony; Va. Stat. § 18.2–60.1). Knowledge of such state and federal laws will assist clinicians who may be involved with the assessment or treatment of individuals who make or pose threats to public officials, particularly because these statutes often articulate the type of behavior (e.g., conveyance of an oral or written threat, more general behavior indicative of a risk of targeted violence) that is considered criminal and thus of interest to agencies charged with protective responsibilities. Such knowledge can help clinicians better understand the role of the law enforcement agencies involved and why they may ask for information from the clinician.

ASSESSING A CLIENT'S RISK OF TARGETED VIOLENCE AGAINST A PUBLIC OFFICIAL

Case Study 1: Outpatient Evaluation of a Presidential Threatener

Mr. S.,[1] a 51-year-old, separated White male who lived alone, was referred by his family for an outpatient evaluation after they had become increasingly concerned about his behavior, noting that he had not slept for several days and that he had become increasingly agitated. They were concerned about his well-being and worried that he might become violent. When Mr. S. presented for his intake appointment, he recounted an extensive history of mental health treatment that had begun several decades earlier following his emergency evacuation out of Vietnam, after, as he recounted, a "nervous breakdown." On his return to the United States, he was placed in a psychiatric hospital for the first time.

Mr. S. reported additional psychiatric hospitalizations, some of which followed his arrest for threatening various presidents. These included an arrest and hospitalization in 1970 after he threatened to kill President Nixon; an arrest in 1976 for threatening to kill President Ford; and an arrest in 1998 after threatening to blow up several buildings occupied by the federal government. He reported additional stays in psychiatric hospitals over the decades that were not tied to an arrest but were to help him "calm his nerves." He also reported taking psychotropic medication

---

[1]For purposes of confidentiality, all names in this case study are fictitious, and clinical material is significantly disguised.

at various times, and from his descriptions and the names of some of the medications it seemed that he had been prescribed antipsychotics and mood stabilizers.

Mr. S. also reported a significant history of impulsive and violent behavior directed toward those in his personal life. For example, he stated that his second wife left him 2 years earlier after he fired several shots in their house. Similarly, his most recent relationship ended after he reported firing "15 rounds over her head" inside his home.

When Mr. S. presented for his intake interview, his speech was fairly disorganized, and he tended to ramble, moving tangentially from one topic to another. He also made numerous statements referencing his status as the leader of several thousand warriors. When generally queried about his intentions to harm others or thoughts that he might have had about such action, he reported that he had wanted to telephone one of the Department of Defense installations to speak with the "highest ranking official" at the institution and threaten to blow up military bases and federal buildings. When asked why he would place such a call, Mr. S. shared several reasons. First, he wanted to ensure that the president could protect the United States against an attack by the warriors who were at the ready to attack if he directed them to do so. Mr. S. was concerned that the president did not have adequate defenses to protect the country should someone launch an attack on the homeland, and he wanted to ensure that in fact the country was well prepared. Second, he believed that placing such a call would show the allegations that he threatened Presidents Nixon and Ford to be false. He did not want his two sons to grow up believing that their father was a "presidential threatener."

In the course of their practice, clinicians may encounter a client similar to Mr. S. who threatens a public official or displays some inappropriate interest. A significant portion of those who threaten public officials have had contact with the mental health care system at some point in their lives or are actively symptomatic at the time they come to the attention of law enforcement. For example, approximately half of all those who threaten Secret Service protectees have at least one *Diagnostic and Statistical Manual of Mental Disorders* (4th ed.; American Psychiatric Association, 1994) diagnosis at the time they issue their threats or have had some contact with the mental health care system for evaluation or treatment (Fein & Vossekuil, 1999). Among those who are assessed as presenting the most serious threats, the percentage with an active diagnosis, some mental health history, or some contact with the mental health care system is far higher, approximately 90% (Coggins, Steadman, & Veysey, 1996; Fein & Vossekuil, 1999). As an example, Mr. S. had been hospitalized numerous times and monitored by MHPs between hospitalizations for symptoms related to schizoaffective disorder. Similarly, research on people who have been investigated by the U.S. Capitol Police for threats and other inappropriate interest in members of Congress or congressional staff has indicated that 60% showed evidence of serious mental illness or were actively symptomatic at the time of their contact with their congressional targets (Scalora et al., 2002).

It is likely that an MHP may be the first professional to make an assessment of his or her client's risk for targeted violence, even before the individual has come to the attention of law enforcement personnel. It has been argued that a threat to a public official represents a *Tarasoff*-type (*Tarasoff v. Regents of the University of California*, 1976) situation for a clinician in that the public official is an identifiable victim or potential victim (Borum & Reddy, 2001). In most jurisdictions, if a client threatens a public official and the clinician determines (or should determine) that the client poses a serious danger to the public official (or another target), a duty to warn, disclose, or protect exists (see chap. 2, this volume).

In circumstances in which a client threatens a public official, some have recommended that the standard of care for evaluation of the client's dangerousness to the public official is the performance of a threat assessment (Borum et al., 1999; Borum & Reddy, 2001; Gelles, Sasaki-Swindle, & Palarea, 2002; Scalora et al., 2002) as opposed to a clinical assessment of more general violence risk (Borum & Reddy, 2001). Threat assessment activities are distinguished from more traditional clinical assessments of violence risk in that they are designed to assess the risk of *targeted violence*—violence to an identified or identifiable target—rather than the more general risk of violent behavior per se (Borum et al., 1999; Borum & Reddy, 2001; Fein & Vosskuil, 1998). In a threat assessment, the appraisal of risk is primarily deductive and fact based, compared with the more inductive method of appraisal for general violence risk, which is guided primarily by base rates and historical risk factors (for a full discussion of threat assessments in *Tarasoff*-type situations, see Borum & Reddy, 2001). The emerging standard of care for evaluating threats against public officials suggests the use of a threat assessment approach that examines the threatener's attitudes that support or facilitate violence, his or her capacity to act on ideas or plans to harm, thresholds crossed with respect to breaking laws or rules, intent to do harm, others' reactions with respect to the threatener's ability to carry out an idea or plan to harm, and noncompliance with treatment or other risk reduction interventions (Borum & Reddy, 2001). The goal of a threat assessment is to determine whether the threatener is on a pathway toward attacking an identifiable, high-profile target; how fast he or she is moving toward an attack; and where intervention might be possible to stop the progression (Baumgartner et al., 2001; Borum et al., 1999; Fein & Vossekuil, 1998; Gelles et al., 2002; Scalora et al., 2002).

The argument for conducting a threat assessment is based on research conducted on assassinations of and attacks on public officials, which has shown that factors traditionally considered in clinical assessments of risk—including reliance on threats conveyed and on a previous history of violence—may lead MHPs to miss signs of a possible planned attack against an identified or identifiable public official (Borum & Reddy, 2001; Fein & Vossekuil, 1998). Moreover, demographic characteristics (e.g., gender) that are strongly correlated with risk of general violence are not correlated with risk of targeted violence to a public official, and as such are seen as less informative for gauging risk of such violence than is behavior suggesting an idea or plan to attack (Borum et al., 1999; Fein & Vossekuil, 1999). With respect to diversity issues specifically, this research has shown that there is no accurate or useful profile of a public official attacker or assassin (Fein & Vossekuil, 1998, 1999). Rather than focusing on demographics, researchers have emphasized the importance of relying on "attack-related behavior" for assessing risk to public official targets (Borum et al., 1999; Fein & Vossekuil, 1998).

Although a clinician is advised to conduct a threat assessment to evaluate the potential for targeted violence against a public official, such an assessment should be viewed as an addition to, rather than a substitute for, a more traditional clinical assessment of the client's overall risk of violence. This is because MHPs are responsible for assessing the level of violence risk their clients pose irrespective of the nature of the potential target. Thus, a thorough evaluation would involve both types of assessment. It is important for supervisors to be aware of the various issues involved with threat assessments for targeted violence and to ensure that their supervisees are familiar with these issues as well.

Information Collection for Assessment of Dangerousness

In working with cases in which a client poses a potential threat to public officials, clinicians should consider additional ways to collect needed information and encourage the client to allow others to be supportive in his or her care. As part of sound professional practice, clinicians work with new clients to understand their previous mental health treatment. They also have new clients sign consent forms so that clinicians can not only request prior treatment records but also speak with the MHPs who worked with those clients previously. Reviewing records of previous mental health treatment is particularly important in working with clients who may pose a threat to public officials because they may have complicated histories. Records provide independent corroborative information as the clinician assesses the client's current level of risk (Borum et al., 1999; Fein & Vossekuil, 1998).

For example, Mr. S. signed consent forms to allow the release of his previous treatment records. The records indicated that Mr. S. had been hospitalized at least 12 times from 1994 through 1999. The records also showed that he eloped on at least two occasions without permission from hospital personnel. He was hospitalized for posing a danger to self and others, for reasons including assaults against various family members, a young woman, police officers, and a security guard; threatening to blow up numerous federal buildings and important individuals; and driving at speeds in excess of 120 miles per hour. The records also noted that his treatment compliance had been poor.

Reviewing these records provided information to understand several areas of Mr. S.'s threat assessment for targeted violence. In particular, Mr. S. had a history of breaking laws or rules (e.g., eloping from psychiatric hospitals without permission, threatening public officials), a history of carrying through on his intent to do harm (e.g., history of assaults against family members and others), and a history of noncompliance with treatment. Information documented in the records also corroborated the history that Mr. S. had shared during his evaluation. Understanding the veracity of a client's personal account of his or her history, and the implications of this history for the client's threat assessment, is an additional reason why working with the client to obtain consent forms to review records of previous treatment is so important at the outset of treatment.

In addition, when assessing a client's potential for targeted violence, it may be helpful for the clinician to gain the client's consent for the clinician to speak with other persons familiar with the client's current functioning. This option is not one that clinicians generally pursue in traditional therapeutic contexts because of the need to maintain confidentiality and the integrity of the therapeutic relationship. However, neither of these important tenets need be compromised if the decisions for engaging others in the client's care are reasonable and the clinician is able to convey to the client the benefit of involving others in the client's care. The extent of this involvement and the content will vary depending on the desires of the client and the scope of the consent to release information, but at a minimum it is helpful for the clinician to be able to receive information from people in the client's life who may have knowledge about changes in the client's functioning that would influence the clinician's assessment of the client's level of dangerousness and other important professional decisions the clinician will make in managing the case. The clinician may also want to consider interviewing third parties with the client present, as this may serve to alleviate some of the client's concerns. Caution is advised, however, because third parties may not feel as free to discuss their concerns with the client present.

As an example, Mr. S. signed consent forms to allow the clinician to speak with his estranged wife. When reached by phone, she reported that Mr. S.'s condition had deteriorated over the past 2 years and that he had often not followed through with treatment recommendations. She also reported that he had fired a shotgun in their home, bound her and held a knife to her throat, and held a gun on her. As with the treatment records, the information gathered from Mr. S.'s estranged wife added substantively to the evaluation.

It is often beneficial to speak with several individuals because the people in the client's life may have various motives for describing the client's propensity for violence, organizational ability, and mental health in differing terms. Information from multiple sources can be used to develop a picture of the client's functioning that is corroborated by many people rather than a single source (Borum et al., 1999; Borum & Reddy, 2001; Fein & Vossekuil, 1998). Also, reviews of research on clinicians' decision making suggest that using multiple sources of information in clinical decision making helps to reduce a range of judgment errors, including errors resulting from overreliance on the memory of clients and other informants, relying on heuristics for decision making, the introduction of confirmatory and hindsight biases, and other cognitive deficiencies in decision making (Borum, 1996; Borum, Otto, & Golding, 1993; Garb, 2005). Multiple sources can include consultation with other clinicians, particularly those who have treated the client in the past (Garb, 2005).

To complete a thorough threat assessment, it is helpful when clinicians have access to previous treatment records, have signed consent to speak with others familiar with the client's past and current functioning, and attempt to corroborate as much of the information related to the threat assessment as they are able. Some of these activities are not part of traditional clinical assessments of dangerousness, which often rely on the client's statements to the clinician and description of his or her behavior, thoughts, and plans in evaluating the level of violence risk. These efforts highlight the importance of the therapeutic relationship, particularly during the early phases of assessment, when gaining the client's trust and conveying a desire to protect him or her from harm is essential to gaining the client's consent to gather more information in support of the client's care and the clinician's evaluation.

In those situations in which the client does not provide consent for the clinician to speak with third parties, the clinician's ability to release information is governed by the legal criteria that outline the confidentiality of mental health treatment and records, and the exceptions to confidentiality, in the jurisdiction in which the clinician practices. Such exceptions may include the disclosure of information in situations in which the client is deemed a threat to self or others.

REPORTING OF THREATS AGAINST PUBLIC OFFICIALS

Threats against and inappropriate interest in public officials that are reported to law enforcement agencies come from a variety of sources, including the threateners themselves and others who may know of the threat or otherwise have concerns about the threatener because of behavior he or she has exhibited that suggests some risk. Persons reporting such concerns include friends or family of the threatener, coworkers, neighbors, local law enforcement personnel, prison staff, health care workers, MHPs, and persons not known to the threatener.

Professional Considerations in Reporting Threats
Against Public Officials

At any point during the threat assessment process, a clinician may find him- or herself in a situation in which he or she must make a decision as to whether to report the potential threat the client may pose to a public official and, if so, to whom. Despite the prevalence of mental illness and contact with the mental health care system among those who threaten or show inappropriate interest in public officials, only a small percentage of threats reported to law enforcement agencies are typically reported by therapists (e.g., 12% of reports of threats against Secret Service protectees come from MHPs; Coggins et al., 1996).

The low percentage of reporting from these professionals may result from the multiple mechanisms that therapists often have with which to discharge a duty to protect in this type of situation, one of which is reporting to law enforcement (e.g., Borum & Reddy, 2001). It may also reflect some disagreement within the field regarding the appropriateness of reporting threats against public officials to law enforcement agencies. For example, some MHPs have argued that any and all threats against the president should be reported to the Secret Service (e.g., Coggins et al., 1996; Menninger, 1982). Others have suggested that the decision to report a threat to law enforcement should strike a balance with the client's civil rights and should be based on an assessment of the client's dangerousness, imminence of the threat, confinement status, right to privacy, and MHP–patient confidentiality and strength of the therapeutic alliance (Griffith, Zonana, Pinsince, & Adams, 1988, cited in Coggins et al., 1996).

Research has suggested that a myriad of factors may influence a clinician's decision to report such threats. In a survey of psychologists, psychiatrists, and social workers regarding their attitudes about reporting threats against the president, respondents indicated that factors that would affect their decision to report a threat included whether their client had a viable plan for the attack, had the opportunity to attack, and had a history of violence (Coggins et al., 1996). Results also indicated that the majority of respondents would report a threat only if they thought the threat was real. More than half of respondents indicated they would only report information they believed to be clinically relevant (Coggins et al., 1996).

What is unknown is the extent to which MHPs may be reluctant to report because of concerns regarding the outcome of threat cases reported for law enforcement investigation and the clinician's desire to retain involvement in the case. One major theme that has arisen in the threat assessment field in the past decade has been recognition within the law enforcement community of the importance of mental health consultation and input in threat cases, for case management and assessment (Coggins & Reddy Pynchon,

1998; Gelles et al., 2002). In large part, this interest has arisen because of the importance of the therapeutic alliance in managing those cases in which an individual is assessed as posing a threat to a public official. Partnership between MHPs and law enforcement agencies is now widely recognized as vital to the prevention of harm to public officials and the successful management of those threateners who have some history of mental illness.

In recent years, the agencies charged with protecting major public officials, including the Secret Service and the Capitol Police, have engaged in extensive liaison efforts to educate the mental health community regarding the nature of their threat investigations and the importance of consultation from MHPs in assessing and managing individuals who threaten public officials (Coggins & Reddy Pynchon, 1998; Coggins et al., 1998; Gelles et al., 2002). These agencies depend on reporting from a range of sources, including MHPs, to learn about threats to the public officials they protect. The earlier they learn about such threats, the greater their opportunity to assess the threat in advance of any potential harm and work with the treating MHPs, where necessary, to craft a case management strategy (Coggins et al., 1998; Gelles et al., 2002).

Legal and Ethical Considerations in Reporting Threats Against Public Officials

MHPs also have to consider legal and ethical requirements when determining whether to report a client who may pose a threat to a public official. Generally, these decisions are guided by traditional legal and ethical proscriptions. These include the *Tarasoff* duty that has been enacted through legislation in certain states or established via case law in others (see chap. 2, this volume) and confidentiality restrictions and exceptions as outlined in statutes and ethical codes that guide the practice of various MHPs (see, e.g., Section 4.05[b] of the American Psychological Association's [2002] "Ethical Principles of Psychologists and Code of Conduct," which states that "psychologists disclose confidential information . . . where permitted by law for a valid purpose such as to . . . protect the client/patient . . . or others from harm").

Threats posed by clients to public officials are subject to the same considerations as those posed by clients against other, less high-profile individuals (Borum & Reddy, 2001). Thus, depending on the law in the jurisdiction in which the clinician is practicing, he or she may be mandated and/or authorized to report the client's potential dangerousness. Certain states provide the option of notifying law enforcement as one of the mechanisms by which the clinician's duty to protect (perhaps by warning) the potential target may be discharged (e.g., Del. Stat. title 16, ch. 54, § 5401, stating that the clinician may notify a law enforcement agency or arrange for the client's hospitalization). Other states require the clinician to communicate the threat to law enforcement to discharge the clinician's duty to protect or warn the potential victim (e.g., Al. Stat. § 34-8A-24: "If there is a duty to warn and protect . . . the duty shall be discharged by . . . making reasonable efforts to communicate the threat to the victim . . . and to a law enforcement agency"). In either of these states, the clinician would likely be able to discharge his or her duty by contacting the law enforcement agency charged with protective responsibility for the public official to whom the client poses a threat. However, it is essential for clinicians to be familiar with the nuanced reporting requirements outlined in the relevant laws covering the jurisdiction in which they practice.

INTERVENTION OPTIONS WITH PERSONS WHO MAY POSE A THREAT TO PUBLIC OFFICIALS

One of the biggest misconceptions about how law enforcement agencies handle threat cases is that their focus is on prosecution of the threatener. The reality is that only a small minority of threats to public officials are prosecuted (e.g., on average fewer than 5% of all threats investigated each year; Coggins et al., 1998). The Secret Service, for example, has long recognized that prosecution of threat cases carries only short-term penalties and does little to solve the longer term personal problems that drive many people to threaten the president in the first place (Coggins et al., 1998; Fein & Vossekuil, 1998). In fact, the vast majority of cases investigated by the Secret Service, for example, are closed without arrest or other intervention. For the small percentage of cases each year in which the person is thought to pose a potential risk to a public official, agencies such as the Secret Service focus much more on successful assessment and management of the cases through involvement of the threatener's family, other social support systems, and MHPs than on prosecution (Borum & Reddy, 2001; Scalora et al., 2002). Typically, intervention in such cases involves the law enforcement agency developing and implementing an individualized case management plan to move the person away from thoughts and plans of violence, frequently focusing on connecting the person with resources and social support to solve whatever personal problems motivated the individual to consider threatening or attacking a public official in the first place (Coggins et al., 1996, 1998). In a similar way, MHPs establish individual treatment plans designed to improve a client's functioning and keep their clients and others safe from harm. At times, these treatment plans may benefit from, rather than be harmed by, the participation of law enforcement officials in the client's case management.

Case Study 2: A Public Official Stalker

Several years ago a woman, Ms. R., visited a state capitol repeatedly in an effort to see and meet the governor.[2] She was a student attending college in a different state and on occasion would travel the considerable distance in the hope of meeting him. She also sent numerous letters and gifts to him, expressing a persistent delusional belief that he was in love with her and wanted to meet her. Over time, she continued her efforts to gain access to events at which the governor was to appear, often traveling hundreds or even thousands of miles across the country to do so, and attempted to breach security at sites where he appeared. Her behavior prompted a law enforcement investigation to determine whether she posed a threat to the governor.

In the course of the investigation, it was determined that Ms. R. had been seeing a therapist for several years, including throughout the duration of her known interest in and pursuit of the governor. The law enforcement agency conducting the threat assessment investigation contacted her clinician to ask about her. However, because Ms. R. had refused to give consent for the clinician to release any information about her, the clinician could not answer any questions, including whether she was even a client.

The investigating law enforcement officials recognized that even though the clinician could not release any information to them, there was no prohibition against them providing information to the clinician. The law enforcement officials were able to document for the clinician Ms. R.'s delusional belief that the governor was in love with her and her love interest in him—something of which the clinician had been unaware, as Ms. R. had never mentioned the governor or her interest in him at any point in her several years of therapy. The law enforcement officials also documented the numerous times Ms. R. had traveled to try to see the governor, including trips across the country. The clinician had been unaware of the extent of his client's travel, knowing only that she had failed to appear for her sessions with him on the same dates that the law enforcement officials showed she was several hundred miles away trying to gain access to a secure site where the governor was scheduled to appear. Finally, the law enforcement officials were able to share with the clinician information they had gained from Ms. R.'s housemate that Ms. R. had talked of wanting to kill herself in front of the governor and had recently purchased a handgun. After her repeated efforts to pursue a romantic relationship with him had been thwarted, they were concerned that she might be considering harm to the governor and killing herself.

The case study of Ms. R. is presented to illustrate the benefit of a joint case management approach in which the MHP teams with law enforcement

---

[2]This case study reflects a compilation of fact patterns from multiple case studies. The facts were combined to protect confidentiality in the individual cases.

for the protection of the client and the protectee. The case study illustrates that a partnership between mental health and law enforcement professionals can be mutually beneficial in a threat case even when the treating clinician cannot release any information about his or her client. It also underscores how communication between a treating MHP and an investigating law enforcement agency in the case of a threat against a public official can enhance the clinician's assessment of dangerousness and provide a framework for a more effective intervention. Because of a successful partnership between the MHP and the investigating law enforcement official, the woman received treatment that was tailored to address her delusions. Moreover, the clinician was thereafter used by the law enforcement officials as a key resource in devising a case management plan to move the woman away from thoughts of harming herself or the governor. Without the information the clinician received from the law enforcement officials, he would have had a less comprehensive understanding of Ms. R.'s behavior outside of their sessions.

Indeed, a similar situation occurred in the case of John Hinckley Jr., who stalked President Carter before he eventually tried to assassinate President Reagan. Before he became interested in President Reagan, Hinckley was seeing a psychiatrist at the request of his parents, who were concerned that he was despondent and suicidal. Hinckley was being treated during the same time period that he was stalking President Carter and leaving letters for actress Jodie Foster in the hope of attracting her interest. Although he saw the psychiatrist for 4 months, Hinckley never revealed to him that he had appeared at President Carter's campaign sites, his thoughts of or plans for assassination, or his love interest in Foster (Phillips, 2006).

As MHPs become more familiar with the case management efforts of agencies charged with protecting public officials at the federal, state, and local levels, they may feel more at ease sharing in these efforts, within the bounds of legal and ethical restrictions, to best meet the needs of their clients. In this respect, MHPs share similar goals with those agencies charged with protective responsibilities—the safety of the client and the safety of those with whom the client comes in contact. Consideration of this mutual aim sets the basis for a collaborative framework in which clinicians play a vital role in managing their clients' safety while having access to the multiple resources that investigators assigned to protective intelligence cases may bring to bear. It may be that these resources include additional case management skills and opportunities, such as assistance with housing and employment, that serve the client's needs and create a more stable support network for the client than the clinician would be able to create on his or her own. Also, the clinician may have more access to information about the client's functioning outside of the therapeutic relationship, which may enhance the clinician's work with the client and ultimately the client's well-being.

CONCLUSION

Research on targeted violence directed toward public officials has pro-vided clinicians with additional guidance as to how to assess their clients' potential for causing harm. In conducting such assessments, it is critical to obtain corroborating information from multiple sources by obtaining the client's consent to review previous treatment records and to discuss the client's care with other persons familiar with the client's functioning. The threat assessment process will be in addition to the clinician's more general vio-lence risk assessment, as both are important in assessing the myriad issues and risks that a potential client may pose and they are focused on different types of risk.

Once a clinician has completed his or her assessment of the client's potential threat to a public official, the clinician must determine whether he or she is mandated and/or authorized to report the client's risk of violence. Threats to public officials are similar to more traditional dangerousness as-sessments, and the same issues related to the 1976 *Tarasoff* duty to protect or warn situations arise, as well as the confidentiality protections and exceptions that guide disclosures of information related to a client's risk of violence. Laws vary depending on the jurisdiction in which the clinician practices, so knowl-edge of those laws is essential in guiding possible disclosures. If a clinician does report his or her client's potential for targeted violence to a public official, it may be possible for the clinician to gain helpful information from the investi-gating agencies such that the clinician's care of the patient is enhanced.

Finally, partnership with law enforcement to manage a client who may pose a threat to a public official does not mean certain arrest or prosecution for the client. MHPs may serve vital roles in creating and implementing case management plans to move the client away from thoughts or plans of vio-lence. A strong therapeutic alliance makes MHPs a key resource in encour-aging compliance from clients and preventing them from doing something harmful.

REFERENCES

American Psychiatric Association. (1994). *Diagnostic and statistical manual of mental disorders* (4th ed.). Washington, DC: Author.

American Psychological Association. (2002). Ethical principles of psychologists and code of conduct. *American Psychologist, 57,* 1060–1073.

Baumgartner, J., Scalora, M., & Plank, G. (2001). Case characteristics of threats toward state government targets investigated by a Midwestern state. *Journal of Threat Assessment, 1,* 41–60.

Borum, R. (1996). Improving the clinical practice of violence risk assessment: Tech-nology, guidelines and training. *American Psychologist, 51,* 945–956.

Borum, R., Fein, R., Vossekuil, B., & Berglund, J. (1999). Threat assessment: Defining an approach for evaluating risk of targeted violence. *Behavioral Sciences & the Law, 17,* 323–337.

Borum, R., Otto, R., & Golding, S. (1993). Improving clinical judgment and decision making in forensic evaluation. *Journal of Psychiatry and Law, 21,* 35–76.

Borum, R., & Reddy, M. (2001). Assessing violence risk in *Tarasoff* situations: A fact-based model of inquiry. *Behavioral Sciences & the Law, 19,* 375–385.

Calhoun, F. (1998). *Hunters and howlers: Threats and violence against federal judicial officials in the United States, 1798-1993.* Washington, DC: U.S. Department of Justice, U.S. Marshals Service.

Coggins, M., & Reddy Pynchon, M. (1998). Mental health consultation to law enforcement: Secret Service development of a mental health liaison program. *Behavioral Sciences & the Law, 16,* 407–422.

Coggins, M., Pynchon, M., & Dvoskin, J. (1998). Integrating research and practice in federal law enforcement: Secret Service applications of behavioral science expertise to protect the president. *Behavioral Sciences & the Law, 16,* 51–70.

Coggins, M., Steadman, H., & Veysey, B. (1996). Mental health clinicians' attitudes about reporting threats against the president. *Psychiatric Services, 47,* 832–836.

Fein, R., & Vossekuil, B. (1998). *Protective intelligence and threat assessment investigations: A guide for state and local law enforcement officials.* Washington, DC: U.S. Department of Justice, Office of Justice Programs, National Institute of Justice.

Fein, R., & Vossekuil, B. (1999). Assassination in the United States: An operational study of recent assassins, attackers, and near-lethal approachers. *Journal of Forensic Sciences, 44,* 321–333.

Garb, H. N. (2005). Clinical judgment and decision making. *Annual Review of Clinical Psychology, 1,* 67–89.

Gelles, M., Sasaki-Swindle, K., & Palarea, R. (2002). Threat assessment: A partnership between law enforcement and mental health. *Journal of Threat Assessment, 2,* 55–66.

Menninger, W. (1982). Threatening the president. *Hospital and Community Psychiatry, 33,* 436–437.

Phillips, R. (2006). Assessing presidential stalkers and assassins. *Journal of the American Academy of Psychiatry and the Law, 34,* 154–164.

Scalora, M., Baumgartner, J., Zimmerman, W., Callaway, D., Hatch Mailette, M., Covell, C., et al. (2002). Risk factors for approach behavior toward the U.S. Congress. *Journal of Threat Assessment, 2,* 35–56.

Tarasoff v. Regents of the University of California, 131 Cal. Rptr. 14, 551 P.2d 334 (1976).

Vossekuil, B., Borum, R., Fein, R., & Reddy, M. (2001). Preventing targeted violence against judicial officials and courts. *Annals of the American Academy of Political and Social Science, 576,* 78–90.

9

DRIVING AND OPERATING OTHER EQUIPMENT: LEGAL AND ETHICAL ISSUES

SAMUEL KNAPP[1] AND LEON VANDECREEK

In the course of treatment, Dr. Rodriguez learns that the older client he is treating for bereavement has had two recent fender-bender traffic accidents. Later, he receives a note from the client's daughter indicating that her mother appeared to be more forgetful and disoriented than usual. Among other concerns, the psychologist wonders whether his client is a safe driver; whether he should assess her safety as a driver and if so, how he would do that; and how to broach the issue with her without damaging the therapeutic relationship. If the client is an impaired driver, Dr. Rodriguez wonders about his legal and ethical obligations.

Traffic accidents are the third leading cause of death in the United States and the leading cause of death of people under the age of 34. Approximately 40% of Americans will sustain some kind of injury in an automobile accident sometime in their lives. Many accidents are caused by drivers who are impaired through drug and alcohol abuse, dementia, or other mental health or medical problems (American Medical Association & National Highway

[1]These views do not necessarily represent those of the Pennsylvania Psychological Association.

Traffic Safety Administration, 2006). These impairments may occur at any age, although they are more likely to occur with older adults because the likelihood of physical or mental impairments increases with age. As the population of older adults (persons older than 65 years of age) continues to increase, mental health professionals (MHPs) will treat more adults who will face decisions about driving and operating other types of dangerous equipment (Knapp & VandeCreek, 2005).

This chapter reviews the legal, ethical, and professional issues that MHPs face when counseling clients who present safety concerns when they drive or operate other equipment. Because questions about how to respond to older clients with driving impairments are increasingly raised by MHPs and this topic has received the most attention in the legal and clinical literature, we focus primarily on this population. In some instances, we broaden our discussion to include clients who operate other types of equipment. As we discuss later, the traditional duty to protect is, on the one hand, not likely to arise in these circumstances because these clients do not express intent to harm others and potential victims are not usually identifiable. On the other hand, principles of general professional negligence are relevant to work with these clients.

IMPAIRMENT FROM ALCOHOL OR OTHER DRUGS

Clients who abuse alcohol and other drugs represent an important subset of individuals who are at high risk for causing traffic accidents. In 2006, there were more than 17,602 alcohol-related traffic fatalities in the United States (National Highway Traffic Safety Administration, 2008). Drivers impaired by alcohol and other drugs are predominately men between the ages of 21 and 34. Drivers between the ages of 35 and 64 have a rate about 50% to 55% that of the younger group, and those older than age 65 have about 1% as many fatalities resulting from alcohol impairment.

Drivers impaired by alcohol and other drugs represent a special subset of impaired drivers. For example, the laws governing privacy and reporting for such individuals may be governed by the strict confidentiality rules found in federal or state confidentiality statutes.

DRIVING IMPAIRMENTS

Many drivers, regardless of age, have impairments that affect their ability to drive. However, older adults have crash rates per mile that are three times higher than those of middle-aged drivers (Foley, Harley, Heimovitz, Guralnik, & Brock, 2002). Although older adults made up 12% of the population in 2006, they accounted for 14% of all vehicle occupant fatalities and 19% of all pedestrian fatalities (National Highway Traffic Safety Administration, 2008). The death rate from motor vehicle accidents is higher for people 75 or older than for any other age group except those younger than 25 (Centers for Disease Control & Prevention [CDC], 2001). These rates occur even though older adults almost always wear seat belts, are less likely to speed, and are less likely to drive while intoxicated. However, they are more likely to die of crashes because their bodies are less able to withstand the injuries than are those of younger people (CDC, 2001).

The number of older drivers is expected to continue to increase dramatically in the future (Straight & Jackson, 1999). Although 10% of current drivers are older than age 65, by 2030 20% to 25% of drivers will be older than age 65. The increase in older drivers in part reflects the general aging of the population. In addition, a higher percentage of adults drive now than in the past, primarily because of an increase in the percentage of female drivers. Finally, public transportation is less available, increasing the reliance on private driving. The driving abilities of most older adults will decrease as vision, working memory, hearing, reaction time, and body strength decline. Furthermore, they are more likely to take medication and thus be at risk for side effects such as drowsiness or disorientation. Also, older adults are more likely to have conditions that affect driving ability, such as diabetes or dementia (American Medical Association & National Highway Traffic Safety Administration, 2006).

Most older adults self-regulate their driving and restrict or give it up when they notice an increased risk in their driving. Many take compensatory measures such as avoiding driving in heavy traffic, in bad weather, to unfamiliar places, or over long distances (American Medical Association & National Highway Traffic Safety Administration, 2006). Giving up driving may be a difficult transition for older adults in part because it involves a loss of independence and reliance on others to meet their safety and social needs. Those who discontinue driving are more likely to become depressed (Marottoli et al., 1997), although factors beyond driving are likely to be implicated.

MHPs who treat older adults will eventually encounter clients who appear to have limitations in their ability to drive safely. In those situations, MHPs, such as Dr. Rodriguez, appropriately ask what steps they need to take to fulfill their legal and ethical responsibilities.

WHAT ARE THE LEGAL OBLIGATIONS?

When encountering clients who may have impairments that reduce their ability to drive or operate dangerous equipment, MHPs should consider their responsibilities toward their clients and toward the public in general. MHPs need to be knowledgeable about their state laws that provide direction for working with impaired clients and must adhere to reasonable minimal standards of professional conduct. Accordingly, courts have on the one hand held that physicians are liable for harm that comes to their clients when they should have, according to the standards of the profession, alerted drivers to the foreseeable impact of their disabilities or medication on their driving abilities (e.g., see *Schuster v. Altenberg*, 1988). Using the same standard of reasonable professional conduct, the courts could ask whether a reasonable MHP should have known that the client's mental condition was such that he or she could not drive safely or operate dangerous equipment and whether the client was so advised.

On the other hand, courts have generally not held MHPs liable for harm their clients caused to third parties. Typically, negligence can only occur in the context of a professional relationship, and the professional does not have a relationship with the client's victim. There are limited exceptions, however, such as when an MHP owes a duty to an identifiable third party threatened with imminent and substantial physical harm by an angry client (often called the "duty to protect"). In addition, a few state courts (e.g., California, Delaware, Michigan) have held that physicians have a special duty to the public when they have reason to believe that a medical disorder or a medication could make it dangerous for the client to drive (Booth, 2006). In these cases, courts have held that the physician should have warned the client against driving and that accident victims in these instances had the right to recover damages. Other state courts (e.g., Iowa, Florida, Kansas, Missouri, Texas) have drawn the opposite conclusion. This is an area of case law that is evolving, but it seems unlikely that the duty to protect will be widely applied to such cases.

Accordingly, physicians or prescribing MHPs could be liable if they failed to inform clients who drive or operate machinery of the possible relevant side effects of medication. Similarly, it could be assumed that MHPs could be liable if they failed to inform older adults with early onset dementia that they will experience a gradual decline in cognitive skills that will make driving or operating equipment dangerous or if they failed to raise the issue in the treatment of a person who is known to drink and drive or operate dangerous equipment. Of course, MHPs may not have the legal ability to control the actions of their clients and would not be liable only because clients failed to follow instructions. Nonetheless, the failure to inform clients of the likely course of the disorder could be grounds for negligence.

Another area in which the law affects practice is related to clients who are being treated in substance use treatment facilities. For example, federal laws governing the confidentiality of records in federally assisted drug and alcohol treatment facilities do not include an exception to confidentiality for impaired drivers without the client's consent or a court order (Comprehensive Alcohol Abuse and Alcoholism Prevention, Treatment, and Rehabilitation Act of 1970).

Insofar as supervisors are responsible for the behavior of their supervisees, they could be held negligent for any misconduct on the part of their supervisees. Consequently, it is important for supervisors to ensure that their supervisees are alert to the possibility of impairments and the proper ways to assess and intervene when such impairments are suspected.

To reduce the frequency of traffic accidents by impaired drivers, a few states mandate that physicians, or sometimes other health care professionals, report impaired drivers. Other states permit, but do not require, such reports (Kane, 2002). Information about state laws concerning driving can be found at the Insurance Information Institute Web site (http://www.iii.org/media/hottopics/insurance/olderdrivers/). We are not aware of a similar source that reviews state laws on reporting requirements for people who operate dangerous equipment.

WHAT ARE THE ETHICAL OBLIGATIONS?

Although courts have commonly held that MHPs have no common-law duty to the victims of accidents caused by impaired drivers, MHPs such as Dr. Rodriguez nonetheless feel a concern for their clients and the public. Generally speaking, ethics codes of MHPs are primarily founded on the moral principles of beneficence, general beneficence, and respect for client autonomy, among others, in dealing with clients. Each moral principle needs to be considered when determining how to respond to a potentially impaired driver. Beneficence is the moral aspect of working to help others, a quality assumed to be essential in professional relationships (Beauchamp & Childress, 2001). Beneficence is most commonly operationalized when MHPs select and conscientiously implement appropriate services for their clients. A good therapeutic relationship is generally necessary for MHPs to fulfill their beneficent goals.

General beneficence (Knapp & VandeCreek, 2004) requires MHPs to be aware of their obligations to members of the public in general. Laws about reporting contagious diseases or a duty to protect are based on the moral obligation of general beneficence.

Respect for autonomy means acknowledging the freedom of clients to think or choose as they please. "Personal autonomy is, at the minimum, self-rule that is free from both controlling interference by others and from limitations, such as inadequate understanding, that prevent meaningful choice" (Beauchamp & Childress, 2001, p. 58). MHPs should generally treat clients as autonomous and independent agents who can participate as full partners in determining treatment goals and methods. Even when treating adolescents who may not be able to give legal consent for treatment, professionals should make efforts to get their assent, or general agreement, with the goals and methods of treatment. The concepts of beneficence and respect for client autonomy are intertwined. For example, clients tend to feel more invested and do better in treatment when they have some control over the methods and focus of treatment.

However, moral principles such as beneficence, general beneficence, and respect for client autonomy are not absolute guides to human behavior and may be superseded if other superior obligations override them. Beauchamp and Childress (2001) noted that when a moral principle is overridden, "the form of the infringement selected is the least possible, commensurate with achieving the primary goal of the action" and "the agent seeks to limit the negative effects of the infringement" (p. 34).

For example, respect for client autonomy is not absolute and may sometimes be overridden by beneficence, or the need to act on behalf of the client's welfare (Knapp & VandeCreek, 2007). As it applies to elderly clients, MHPs will generally respect the client's autonomy to make decisions about driving and operating equipment and the content, goals, and direction of therapy in general. Nonetheless, when the welfare of the client or others is at risk, it may be necessary to allow beneficence to temporarily trump respect for client autonomy. That is, the MHP may redirect the focus of treatment to the ability to drive and operate equipment, even though that may not be the focus of therapy for the client. In such situations, it is desirable to minimize the violation to client autonomy as much as possible, such as by attempting to enlist the cooperation of the client in addressing the issue.

Similarly, the treatment of adolescents requires special skills and a delicate balance in that parents or guardians are also interested parties in the treatment setting. At times, they may also be directly involved in the treatment itself. Many MHPs only accept adolescent clients when parents or guardians permit them to reserve the option of informing parents or guardians, if necessary, of high-risk behaviors, such as repeated driving while intoxicated (or being a passenger in a car with a driver impaired by drugs or alcohol).

HOW TO ASSESS AND INTERVENE WITH IMPAIRED DRIVERS

The question facing MHPs is how to determine when the potential harm to the client or the public is high enough that beneficence or general beneficence trumps respect for client autonomy. We propose three steps to help in that decision: Screen clients with potential driving problems, gather more information about the client's driving ability, and intervene when necessary. The intervention stage may involve recommending compensatory strategies for driving and operating equipment, preparing the client for the eventual need to discontinue driving or operating equipment, or counseling the client to discontinue driving or operating equipment immediately. These stages are not necessarily sequential. For example, MHPs who are preparing elderly clients to stop driving in the future may acquire information that will cause them to alter their intervention plan. As we describe later, it may sometimes be necessary to report driving impairment to a state department of motor vehicles or to involve family members or employers in a decision to stop the client from driving or operating equipment. Unless the client expresses intent to harm another person and a potential victim is readily identifiable, such clients do not trigger a traditional duty to protect in which the professional would need to notify a potential victim or public officials. In the unlikely event that a client does express intent to harm an identifiable family member or fellow employee, then the professional should follow the guidelines provided by the state's duty-to-protect law or other relevant literature, if any are available.

Step 1: Screening for Potential Driving Problems

Clients will seldom enter treatment with the expressed intent to address their ability to drive or operate equipment, although that issue may sometimes emerge in treatment. Even if a client does not raise the issue of driving safety, for example, we recommend that MHPs initiate that discussion if (a) the client or a family member reports substantial difficulty in driving or operating equipment; (b) the client has a serious physical or mental illness (or is abusing alcohol or other drugs) that involves substantial functional limitations and the client is not receptive to adopting compensatory driving strategies or to stopping driving or operating equipment; or (c) the client has a dementia, especially if it is a progressive dementia that has been present and diagnosed for more than 2 years.

Reports from the client, members of the client's family, and others who know the client well are triggers if they represent a pattern of difficulties. Often a single incident, such as an accident, represents nothing more than a random occurrence. However, it is productive to discuss these incidents and assess their implications for the client's ability to drive and work.

A serious physical or mental illness is a trigger only if it involves a substantial functional impairment. Most persons with severe disorders compensate for their disability or know to refrain from driving or working, even if only temporarily. When treating individuals who abuse alcohol or other drugs, it is prudent to inquire into their driving and working habits. The interviewer should appreciate a tendency of people in the acute phases of alcoholism or drug abuse to underreport problems. The health care professional is more likely to obtain accurate information if a trusting relationship has developed.

Although individuals with advanced dementia of the Alzheimer's type or other advanced dementias should not drive (Dubinsky, Stein, & Luyon, 2000), it is difficult to make such decisions about individuals who have mild dementias. Carr, Duchek, and Morris (2000) found that individuals with mild dementia of the Alzheimer's type had crash rates similar to same-age controls. The issue is how to determine whether the client with dementia has reached a stage when driving is no longer advisable. These decision makers need to recognize that the rate of cognitive decline for individuals with dementia varies considerably. Some may become highly impaired only a few months after their initial diagnoses, whereas others may retain most of their cognitive capacities and ability to function for many years.

Because the factors cited above only trigger further investigation by the MHP into the client's driving and working habits, we recommend adopting a low threshold for these triggers. The greatest harm that could come to clients from activating one of these triggers is that there would be further inquiry or information gathering into the client's capacity to drive and work safely.

In the example given at the start of the chapter, Dr. Rodriguez became concerned by his client's two accidents and the note from the client's daughter. He had sufficient information to move to Step 2 and do a more in-depth assessment of the client's driving abilities. Similarly, psychologists may want to gather more information on functional capacity when they encounter younger clients with serious impairments who drive or operate dangerous machinery.

Step 2: Gathering More Information About Driving Skills

If a client is positive on the screening, then the clinician needs to gather more information to determine whether the client can drive or work safely. MHPs can gather more information from neuropsychological tests, a driver evaluation, a referral to other health care professionals, and more detailed inquiries into the person's driving and work history.

Neuropsychological Tests

Common sense suggests that neurological impairments of selective attention, speed of information processing, and visuospatial orientation would negatively affect the ability to drive and operate dangerous equipment. However, studies using neuropsychological tests to identify unsafe drivers have found a high number of false positives. Continued research is leading to greater usefulness for these tests. At this time, however, neuropsychological tests are often suggestive of driving and working impairment, but are seldom sufficient, in and of themselves, for deciding about safety.

Driver Evaluation Programs

Another option for gathering data about driving safety is to refer the client to a driver evaluation program. Many hospitals and rehabilitation centers have such programs, usually run by driver rehabilitation specialists (who are usually, but not necessarily, occupational therapists). The nature of these programs varies, but they generally include measurements of visual acuity and perception, night vision, eye–foot and hand–eye coordination, and other physical movements related to driving, memory, judgment, and understanding of traffic signs and rules. These evaluations last from 1 to 4 hours and cost between $200 and $800, depending on the needs of the client and the standards of the driving rehabilitation specialist. The Association for Driver Rehabilitation Specialists has an online directory of members (available at http://www.driver-ed.org or http://www.ADED.net).

The driver evaluation may include performance on driver simulation instruments, closed-course off-road driving tests, and in-traffic evaluations. Despite efforts at standardization, driving evaluators often use discretion and vary in how they score these tests. Nonetheless, the tests can identify the more seriously impaired drivers and can often lead to the identification and correction of driving errors.

Referrals to Other Health Care Professionals

Sometimes the decision about driving safety needs to be informed by evaluations by other health care professionals such as physicians, podiatrists, or optometrists. Some medical conditions, such as sleep apnea, narcolepsy, and epilepsy, are risk factors for driving and working accidents regardless of age. Fortunately, most cases of epilepsy can be adequately controlled with medications if the client takes them as prescribed and avoids abusing alcohol. The American Medical Association, in cooperation with the National Highway Traffic Safety Administration (2006), has developed a comprehensive guide for physicians that lists many medical conditions and medications that may impair driving ability. The assessment of driving safety depends more on the client's functional limitations and receptiveness to compensatory strategies than the presence or absence of any specific disease.

Sometimes providers can treat the underlying problem and thus allow the client to continue to drive or work. For example, a physician may be able to change or reduce a strongly sedating medication or at least change the times during the day when the medication is taken.

Driving History

Taking a driving history is important in helping MHPs to evaluate clients' driving skills. The general rule is to predict future behavior on the basis of past behavior. Events that should raise concern include accidents and reports that other drivers frequently honk their horn at the driver (presumably because the driver almost caused an accident). Other important self-reported client behaviors include getting lost, not seeing oncoming traffic, driving far slower than the flow of traffic (American Psychological Association, 1998), confusion, loss of direction, weaving in and out of traffic, failure to use turn signals, and tailgating. Family members are often (but not always) a good source of information about the client's driving ability.

A driving diary may sometimes be helpful as well. The diary might include special events or perceptions related to the ability to drive safely. The results could be used to help develop compensatory strategies or to counsel the client to stop driving entirely. The Hartford Insurance Company has developed a checklist that can assist family members in monitoring the older adult's driving ability (http://www.thehartford.com/talkwitholderdrivers/ or http://www.thehartford.com/alzheimers/).

Step 3: Monitoring, Prevention, and Intervention

Most clients will not need to discontinue driving or working immediately when safety questions are first raised. For those clients, the MHP can suggest monitoring by a family member and/or compensatory driving programs. In addition, MHPs can prepare the client for the time when he or she will need to discontinue driving and working. Client- or family-oriented brochures may be helpful.[2] As noted above, a traditional duty-to-protect obligation typically does not arise unless the client expresses intent to harm an identifiable victim, but the principles of general professional negligence are important to consider.

Compensatory Strategies

Sometimes the safety of drivers depends on their use of compensatory strategies. For example, some drivers may voluntarily restrict their driving to daytime hours, familiar locations, or times and locations when the volume of traffic is low. Computer-based training sessions can help some older adults improve their cognitive processing ability and keep driving safely (Clay, 2000). Also, the American Automobile Association and the American Association of Retired Persons offer refresher courses for older drivers in some locations.

Another compensatory strategy described in the literature is the use of copilots or codrivers, which refers to the use of individuals who assist the driver by performing navigational tasks such as alerting them to hazards or telling them where to drive. Although the use of copilots is common, it has limitations. Copilots are often unable to assist drivers who need to detect or to alert a driver quickly enough to avoid accidents, so we do not recommend their use.

Preparation for Driving Cessation

The general rule is that unless contraindicated, older adults should maintain their lifestyle and activities, including driving. The question be-

---

[2]Available brochures on older driver safety include *At the Crossroads: Family Conversations About Alzheimer's Disease, Dementia and Driving* (available from http://www.thehartford.com/alzheimers/brochure.html or from The Hartford, *At the Crossroads,* 200 Executive Boulevard, Southington, CT 06489; specify English or Spanish version), the National Highway Traffic Safety Administration's "Driving Safely While Aging Gracefully" (available from http://www.nhtsa.dot.gov/people/injury/olddrive/Driving%20Safely%20Aging%20Web/), and various publications from AARP's Driver Safety Program (available at http://www.aarp.org/families/driver_safety/).

comes, When does driving become contraindicated? When dealing with clients in the early stages of dementia or who have or are at risk of developing functional limitations affecting their driving or working, it may be desirable to talk with them about ceasing to drive well in advance of when the actual decision has to be made. Such initial discussions will encourage clients to critically evaluate driving skills and to consider alternative transportation arrangements. The topic of driving may be introduced in the context of how the client and the family are going to cope with the expected gradual decline in independent functioning and cognitive abilities.

Hartford Insurance Company has developed a "family agreement" in which the older adult signs an acknowledgment that a family member will tell him or her when driving constitutes a safety risk (available at http://www.thehartford.com/talkwitholderdrivers/ or http://www.thehartford.com/alzheimers/). Although this agreement is not legally binding, it serves as a therapeutic tool to get older drivers and their family members to think about driving cessation and commits the older driver to receive feedback from family members as to when he or she should discontinue driving. Like other documents of this nature, it is likely to be effective only if it reflects the wishes of the client. Pressured signatures are countertherapeutic.

From a clinical perspective, MHPs need to recognize that driving cessation can be a volatile and emotionally charged issue. A sudden prohibition on driving could precipitate or aggravate isolation or depression, increase the person's dependency on others, or shift family dynamics (Berger & Rosner, 2000). An older adult who once contributed greatly to the family and who was, at least until recently, self-sufficient may now be dependent on others. The lack of transportation may be the final straw that causes older adults to leave their family homes and move into an assisted living facility. Consequently, it is desirable to discuss the implications of discontinuation of driving and alternative transportation options.

The success of alternative transportation will increase if the planning considers the places to which the older adult goes and the social, personal, or business needs that driving fulfills. For some older adults, many of these tasks could be accomplished through the use of public transportation (buses or trains), taxis, or community- or church-supported van services.

For adults with advanced dementia, public transportation can be confusing. However, taxis can be used with persons with advanced dementia if the older adult has no behavioral problems, the taxi driver is given explicit directions, and someone is available to meet the person at the beginning and end of the trip. Some taxi companies set up accounts for older adults.

Counseling Clients to Discontinue Driving

Under rare circumstances, such as when a client presents an imminent danger of self-harm (or harm to others), MHPs may temporarily "trump" the principle of respecting client autonomy (Knapp & VandeCreek, 2007). The confrontation should be honest, but tactful, and may require gentle persistence (American Medical Association, 1999). Indirect methods, such as surreptitiously hiding car keys or disabling cars, are to be avoided because clients often find ways to circumvent them, such as having an extra set of keys or getting the car repaired. It is generally better to confront the issue directly and explain the concerns up front.

For clients who are currently in rehabilitation hospitals, discussions of driving are usually less of a problem because clients expect that the facility will be evaluating their functioning in many domains. Outpatients vary in their response to such inquiries. Some clients are already aware of the deterioration in their driving abilities and are open to discussion. Others react with indignation or anger. Lack of insight and poor self-control should raise the threshold of concern for the MHP. Persons with advanced dementias may be unable to appreciate the degree to which their driving is impaired. Rashness, impulsiveness, and a refusal to consider compensatory strategies make for a poor driving prognosis. If clients still resist voluntarily giving up or curtailing their driving, then it may be desirable to involve family members as much as is clinically appropriate. Family members sometimes feel relief that the MHP is addressing the issue openly and will support efforts to get the client to withdraw from driving.

In those states in which reporting is required or permitted, therapists should be hesitant or cautious about reporting drivers with a mild increase in driving risk (Berger & Rosner, 2000). Psychologists need to understand their state law regarding making reports, especially whether making a report is required or permitted and where the report is filed. It is desirable to involve the client in the decision making as much as possible. Many clients respond to the inquiries about their driving favorably and voluntarily give up driving. Even in those situations, it is desirable to minimize the infringement of autonomy and to involve the client as much as possible in selecting the intervention designed to reduce the likelihood of self-harm. For example, if the desired intervention requires notifying the client's spouse of the danger of driving, then the MHP can ask the client, "How should we go about informing your spouse? Do you want to be present when I share the information?"

When MHPs are treating clients conjointly with another health care professional, they need to decide between themselves who is to counsel the client to discontinue driving. In deciding which professional is going to confront the client, it is often desirable to consider who will have the most important long-term relationship with the client. Often, it is most important to protect the psychologist–client relationship. In other circumstances, such as when the psychologist has a brief relationship with the client for a neuropsychological evaluation, it may be more important to protect the physician–client relationship.

CONCLUSION

As the United States population ages, MHPs will inevitably treat clients who present with questions about impairment that may make driving and operating equipment increasingly dangerous. We have described some of the ethical and legal issues that arise in these cases. We have detailed a series of steps that professionals can take to screen, evaluate, monitor, and intervene with these clients. Several helpful resources are available for professionals.

REFERENCES

American Medical Association. (1999). *E2.24: Impaired drivers and their physicians*. Retrieved December 8, 2006, from http://www.ama-assn.org/apps/pf_new/pf_online?f_n=resultLink&doc=policyfiles/HnE/E-2.24.HTM&s_t=impaired+drivers&catg=AMA/HnE&catg=AMA/BnGnC&catg=AMA/DIR&&nth=1&&st_p=0&nth=1&

American Medical Association & National Highway Traffic Safety Administration. (2006). *Physician's guide to assessing and counseling older drivers*. Retrieved December 8, 2006, from http://www.ama-assn.org/ama/pub/category/10791.html

American Psychological Association. (1998). *Older adults' health and age-related changes: Reality versus myth*. Washington, DC: Author.

Beauchamp, T., & Childress, J. (2001). *Principles of biomedical ethics* (5th ed.). New York: Oxford University Press.

Berger, J., & Rosner, F. (2000). Ethical challenges posed by dementia and driving. *Journal of Clinical Ethics, 11*, 304–308.

Booth, B. (2006, December 6). Massachusetts judge allows liability claim by plaintiff who was not a patient. *American Medical News, 49*, 46.

Carr, D. B., Duchek, J., & Morris, J. C. (2000). Characteristics of motor vehicle crashes of drivers with dementia of the Alzheimer type. *Journal of the American Geriatrics Society, 48*, 18–22.

Centers for Disease Control & Prevention. (2001). *Older adult drivers: Fact sheet*. Atlanta, GA: Author. Retrieved December 8, 2006, from http://www.cdc.gov/ncipc/factsheets/older.htm

Clay, R. (2000, January). Staying in control. *APA Monitor*, pp. 32–34.

Comprehensive Alcohol Abuse and Alcoholism Prevention, Treatment, and Rehabilitation Act of 1970, Pub. L. No. 91-616 (1970).

Dubinsky, R., Stein, A. C., & Luyon, K. (2000). Practice parameter: Risk of driving and Alzheimer's disease (an evidence-based review): Report of the Quality Standards Subcommittee of the American Academy of Neurology. *Neurology, 54*, 2205–2211.

Foley, D., Harley, K., Heimovitz, H., Guralnik, J., & Brock, D. (2002). Driving life expectancy of persons aged 70 years and older in the United States. *American Journal of Public Health, 92*, 1284–1289.

Kane, K. (2002). Driving in the sunset: A proposal for mandated reporting to the DMV by physicians treating unsafe elderly drivers. *University of Hawai'i Law Review, 25*, 59–83.

Knapp, S., & VandeCreek, L. (2004). A principle-based analysis of the 2002 American Psychological Association's Ethics Code. *Psychotherapy: Theory, Research, Practice, Training, 41*, 247–254.

Knapp, S., & VandeCreek, L. (2005). Ethical and patient management issues with older, impaired drivers. *Professional Psychology: Research and Practice, 36*, 197–202.

Knapp, S., & VandeCreek, L. (2007). Balancing respect for autonomy with competing values using principle-based ethics. *Psychotherapy: Theory, Research, Practice, Training, 44*, 397–404.

Marottoli, R. A., Mendes de Leon, C. F., Glass, T. A., Williams, C. S., Cooney, L. M., Jr., Berkman, L. F., et al. (1997). Driving cessation and increased depressive symptoms: Prospective evidence from the New Haven EPESE. *Journal of the American Geriatrics Society, 45*, 202–206.

National Highway Traffic Safety Administration. (2008). *Traffic safety facts 2006 data.* Washington, DC: Author. Retrieved July 28, 2008, from http://www.nrd.nhtsa.dot.gov/Pubs/810809.pdf

Schuster v. Altenberg, 414 N.W.2d 159 (1988).

Straight, A., & Jackson, A. M. (1999). *Older drivers.* Washington, DC: AARP.

10

THE DUTY TO PROTECT: MENTAL HEALTH PRACTITIONERS AND COMMUNICABLE DISEASES

LESLIE KOOYMAN AND BOB BARRET

For many practicing mental health professionals (MHPs), clients who present with communicable diseases pose complex challenges. Most clients understand the risks of passing on a disease and can be expected to act accordingly, at least within their knowledge base. In those instances, the role of the MHP is focused on educating or finding resources for education about the particular disease and assisting in the development of coping strategies. However, a much more complex challenge occurs when the client truly does not show concern that her or his behavior might result in another person becoming infected.

The complexity of providing services to clients who have a communicable disease may bewilder some practitioners. The limits of confidentiality are set out in professional ethics codes, and their primacy in terms of protecting clients is well understood. The duty to protect likewise implies steps that the MHP must keep in mind in situations in which there is risk to others or to the client. Nonpsychiatric MHPs are clearly not physicians and should never dispense medical advice, yet in many instances they find themselves the primary person who knows their clients' efforts to understand and plan for a medical condition that may place others at risk. For example, the HIV crisis propelled many mental health workers into a domain that demanded they learn about this disease and its transmission to deliver effective mental health services. When a medical condition may place others at risk, there can be a perception that the practitioner must take immediate action that may protect others, even though this violates the principle of confidentiality. Thus, although comfort with ambiguity is a quality encouraged in the training of MHPs, a sense of urgency when dealing with noncompliant clients with infectious diseases may lead to initiating a plan of action prematurely.

Questions such as the following may arise: Who is responsible for an individual's health? The state or the individual? How do I know for sure that my client does, in fact, have a communicable disease? Does the *Tarasoff v. Regents of the University of California* (1976) case apply here? Am I obligated or mandated to help my client come to a decision that protects the health of others? Or must I report the client to public agencies and risk losing his or her trust, or must I take steps to protect others who may or may not be at risk? How much time do I have to work with the client while others are at risk? Where are the trusted professionals to whom I can turn for support and guidance? How do my own biases affect my decision making in these situations? Finding a balance between taking steps that protect others from undue risk while maintaining a successful therapeutic relationship can be quite daunting. To help answer these and other questions, we present in this chapter an ethical decision-making model, two cases involving infectious disease, a practitioner's response to the cases, and some of the issues inherent in situations such as these.

AN ETHICAL DECISION-MAKING MODEL

MHPs who work with clients with communicable diseases may find themselves in situations in which therapeutic decisions and actions regarding health and safety and individual responsibility are not always clear. To assist service providers, Bob Barret participated in the development of a decision-making model that can be useful as a tool for the MHP who faces clients with communicable diseases (Barret, Kitchener, & Burris, 2001; see Exhibit 10.1). This model involves nine steps that carefully describe a process that will assist in the development of a well-reasoned response that supports the standards of confidentiality and the duty to protect.

A quick review of this model reveals that the practitioner is led to reflect, review the facts, conceptualize a plan, and consult before taking action. These steps slow down the process and minimize the likelihood of acting too quickly. The fifth step highlights five foundational principles that have frequently been discussed in the decision-making literature (Kitchener, 1984) and form the foundation for the aspirational aspects of the American Psy-

EXHIBIT 10.1
A Model for Making Ethical Decisions: Application

1. Pause and identify your personal responses to the case.
2. Review the facts of the case.
3. Conceptualize an initial plan based on clinical issues.
4. Consult the ethics code and assess the ethical issues based on the five foundational principles:
   - autonomy
   - beneficence
   - do no harm
   - fidelity
   - justice.
5. Identify the legal issues.
6. Identify and assess the options.
7. Choose a course of action and share it with your client.
8. Implement the course of action: monitor and discuss outcomes.

Note. Consultation should take place whenever you have any doubts or questions about the legal or ethical issues or your own ability to be objective. Consultation with co-workers, colleagues, supervisors, professional ethics committees, and attorneys should be an integral part throughout the process. Each step of the decision-making process must be carefully documented. From "A Decision Model for Ethical Dilemmas in HIV-Related Psychotherapy and Its Application in the Case of Jerry" by B. Barret, K. Kitchener, and S. Burris (p. 134), in J. Anderson and B. Barret (Eds.), *Ethics in HIV-Related Psychotherapy: Clinical Decision-Making in Complex Cases,* 2001, Washington, DC: American Psychological Association. Copyright 2001 by the American Psychological Association.

chological Association's (APA's; 2002) and American Counseling Association's (ACA's; 2005) ethics codes. These foundational principles—autonomy, fidelity, minimize harm, beneficence, and justice—lead the practitioner to reflect on the ways a particular course of action may support or violate the client's rights. These principles can affect a specific clinical situation in apparently contradictory ways, which can create tension. For example, supporting the client's autonomy and demonstrating fidelity may clash with the need to minimize harm because it expands consideration to include not only not harming the client but also being aware of possible harm to others. It is not within the scope of this chapter to discuss the model or the foundational principles in detail, and the reader is encouraged to seek other sources such as Anderson and Barret (2001) for an in-depth presentation. Both the model and the foundational principles are used in the cases that follow. Although not applicable as a tool for all ethical dilemmas, we use this model here because it does assist in cases in which communicable diseases are a focus.

In cases involving a client's privacy and potential duty to protect, such as when a communicable disease may be the issue, any ethical decision-making model must be applied in combination with consultation and careful documentation. Consultation should take place whenever the clinician has any questions about the legal or ethical issues or the ability to be objective. Colleagues, ethics committees, medical personnel, and attorneys should be consulted throughout the process. In addition, the actions taken in each step of the decision-making model process must be carefully documented (Barret et al., 2001, p. 134).

TWO DIFFICULT CASES

Benitia

Benitia,[1] 34, has been your client for the past 4 months. She contacted the local mental health clinic shortly after moving to your city from a rural part of Louisiana. She came to this area to seek work because she is the sole support for her grandmother and her two children, who remain with her grandmother in Louisiana. Unfortunately, finding work has been difficult. She stays with a friend and takes care of her friend's two young children 3 days a week. The other days she spends diligently seeking work. You have been impressed with her determination to improve the lives of her children and grandmother, and the relationship between the two of you is solid and mutually respectful. She is on time for every appointment, neatly dressed, and focused on finding work. Unfortunately, she has few marketable skills.

After you noticed that she seemed to have a chronic cold (she coughed a lot), she went to the medical clinic where she said she was told that she has tuberculosis (TB). This crisis overwhelmed her, and she did not say anything to the friend with whom she lives or even explore the implications TB might have on her goals. She says, "This TB is not important. I have much more important things to worry about." She has not returned to the medical clinic for a follow-up visit. Instead, she continues to look for work and to provide child care, desperate to find a way to assist her family back in Louisiana.

The case of Benitia reflects the situation of many clients whose efforts to support themselves and their families override their concern about their own health. For these clients, the demands of finding work and income may be their only focus. Dealing with issues such as a communicable disease may overwhelm them and distract them from their goal of finding income. At times, the MHP may likewise be overcome and get confused. Assisting Benitia in stabilizing the financial resources for her dependents is critical for the family, and the health crisis may threaten to worsen the family's plight. There are several issues the professional may face, such as how to support Benitia, who is trying very hard to solve the family financial problem. At the same time, her illness threatens all those who come in contact with her, including her friend and the children for whom she is caring, and possibly even the practitioner. How can the practitioner balance these competing demands?

---

[1]For purposes of confidentiality, all names are fictitious, and clinical material is significantly disguised or loosely based on actual cases.

Jake

Jake, 27 and unemployed, has been your client for 3 weeks. He came in complaining of depression and has primarily talked about not being able to find work and living without any cash resources. You suspect he is either dealing drugs or involved with trading sex for money. His anger is evident, along with a lack of motivation or a sense of personal or family responsibility. He seems to live in the moment, doing just what he wants to do and little else. At the beginning of the fourth session, he reveals that he is HIV positive, something you have suspected in spite of his denial in the intake interview. He says he was tested at a public health clinic and was told to go for treatment at a hospital that serves citizens without resources. He has not initiated that contact, saying, "I have too much to do to spend the day over there waiting to see a doctor. Especially when there is not much they are going to do for me." When you ask about his success in having safer sex, he states, "I'm not going to do that. Why should I care about others? I have enough to do to take care of myself. Besides, real men don't use rubbers." He seems to know the information about safer sex but is just not interested in discussing that issue further.

Unlike Benitia, Jake knows he has a serious illness but seems to care little about infecting others. He is a relatively new client, so there has been little time to build a relationship, and acting too quickly may lead him to discontinue treatment altogether and resist further psychological help. Although seeming unconcerned about his own health, he has returned each week for his appointment. This may indicate that there is some trust being developed and that he wants emotional support, some form of medical or financial assistance, or both. At the same time, he is out in the community and may be infecting others. Clinicians working with clients like Jake must find a way to balance their perceived need for action with the time needed to build an effective therapeutic alliance.

A PRACTITIONER'S RESPONSE TO BENITIA AND JAKE

In this section, the ethical decision-making model described earlier (Barret et al., 2001) is applied to the two case scenarios to demonstrate the value of using a clear process regarding duty-to-protect issues with clients who present with a communicable disease. We present the complex, challenging, and sometimes controversial issues a clinician must face when acting in the best interests of the client. A comparison of the differing responses to each case also illustrates the significance of factual circumstances, personal bias, and cultural assumptions in developing a treatment plan with these clients.

Step 1: Pause and Identify Your Personal Response to the Case

As Benitia relays that she has been diagnosed with TB and states, "This TB is not important," the clinician's initial self-protective reaction may be anxiety about the possibility of contracting TB from physical closeness to Benitia. This is a normal and expected reaction given the contagiousness of active TB with coughing in an enclosed setting. The other typical reaction with either Benitia or Jake may be concern about the risk of liability if someone gets infected. However, a premature self-protective reaction by a practitioner to either client may create a legalistic relationship rather than a therapeutic one. Although these thoughts and feelings are expected, they need to be secondary to the more salient professional and ethical responsibilities regarding the client's welfare and the analysis of whether there is an immediate threat of harm to others. Recognizing one's personal reactions is essential to understanding and developing a sound professional response to the client. This self-awareness and the realization of the client's struggle in managing the diagnosis (e.g., TB, HIV) will, one hopes, enable the clinician to focus on the client's needs and proceed in developing an effective treatment plan.

In comparing these two scenarios, the reader may detect a bias toward working more earnestly with Benitia than with Jake; however, a clinician needs to consider the principle of justice here in treating all clients equally and fairly. Benitia has a longer history in therapy, and her drive to improve her living circumstances may create a greater feeling of admiration and likableness in the clinician. These reactions and perhaps sympathy for her situation may influence how the therapist proceeds through the ethical decision-making model. Allowing this personal bias to guide the therapy process with Benitia may result in not gathering all the information necessary to create an effective plan, or the clinician may favor the trusting relationship with Benitia over possibly protecting others. Thus, even though various approaches may be ethical, personal bias may negatively affect the degree to which a variety of alternatives are considered.

On the basis of Jake's attitude in therapy, the practitioner might be more defensive and more assertive in interactions. The assumption may be that Jake will be more resistant and less motivated to address the issue of potential harm to others, leading to a premature response that is viewed by Jake as invasive, shaming, and legalistic regarding his behavior. A more investigative response may be influenced by safety but may also be the result of bias regarding gender and sexual orientation. Palma and Iannelli (2002) found that clinicians experience greater reactivity to unsafe sexual disclosures by heterosexual men than to those by women or gay men. The fact that Jake presents as a heterosexual man may inadvertently raise the clinician's reactivity to his disclosure that "real men do not use rubbers."

One must be aware of these assumptions and biases and proceed with the same ethical decision-making process for each client. Consultation with a peer or supervisor will assist the clinician in assessing his or her own emotional responses guiding the process. In consultation, the clinician also needs to explore and understand his or her boundaries of competence as presented in ethics codes (APA, 2002, Standard 2.01b; ACA, 2005, C.2.a.). Perhaps the clinician needs to refer each client to another, more qualified MHP.

Step 2: Review the Facts of the Case

The practitioner will more than likely need consultation from medical personnel regarding each disease to assess the likelihood and lethality of contagion to others. Most practitioners are not knowledgeable about communicable disease, so getting the facts involves understanding these diseases. This information can be obtained from or through medical personnel at clinics, but the best resource for consultation may be the medical director of the local health department or the state health department. This information will assist the practitioner in assessing the degree of urgency associated with addressing the potential ethical dilemma of client privacy versus a duty to protect others. The local health department should be able to provide the MHP with appropriate physician referrals for each client. A clinician must not give medical advice, but he or she can refer the client to the appropriate medical personnel. This consultation must be carefully documented in the client's record.

In addition, the practitioner must review all the pertinent facts as presented by the client. This means discussing the client's potential risky behavior in detail and reviewing the client's understanding of the disease, its transmission, and legal responsibilities. In addition, a thorough assessment, including cultural norms and values, needs to be conducted to ascertain the client's ability to address the potential harm to others.

If the clinician is guided by a duty to protect others, then he or she cannot merely accept the client's report of a diagnosis. A release of information from the client needs to be obtained that allows the practitioner to contact the appropriate agency for a copy of the actual diagnosis in writing. For professional counselors, this confirmation of the diagnosis is part of the ACA (2005) *Code of Ethics* (Standard B.2.b.), but for any clinician this is simply part of gathering factual information and is probably the first step in addressing the issue of a duty to protect with a client who has a communicable disease.

Obtaining the actual written diagnosis may be essential with Benitia. The clinician needs to know whether she actually has TB because she has identified others (her friend, the children for whom she is caring, her own children, and her grandmother) who may be infected. Given her condition (coughing), there may be a sense of urgency because of the threat of contagion. In this case, the clinician needs to obtain consent from Benitia to get the actual diagnosis in writing from the clinic and assess the amount of close contact Benitia has had with her friend, her friend's children, her own children, and her grandmother. The clinician may also want to discuss the advisability of treatment with Benitia in an effort to get her to receive medication and thereby reduce her contagious state. These interventions would need to be done in coordination with a physician. We acknowledge that these actions are more directive and may challenge many clinicians' beliefs in the primacy of the therapeutic relationship.

Jake does not identify specific "others" in terms of contagion, and he has not discussed the behaviors in which he is engaging that may or may not be putting others at risk for infection. The clinician will need to gather more specific factual information from him to identify whether there is a duty to protect. The therapist will need to know and discuss certain sexual and drug-using behaviors that transmit HIV and then determine Jake's level of dangerousness to others. On the one hand, if Jake does not discuss specific partners, ethically there may not be a duty because there are no identifiable others (although this conclusion may vary depending on state law); however, a practitioner may still feel morally bound to report Jake's behavior to the public health authorities even without identified partners. On the other hand, the duty to protect may apply if Jake identifies a partner and reports unprotected intercourse. Clearly, in Jake's case, the clinician needs to gather facts by asking specific questions regarding sexual and drug activity to ascertain the potential for harm to others.

In both of these cases, gathering information may create tension in the counseling relationship. Rather than interrogate the client, a more therapeutic approach may be to explore the client's understanding of the particular disease and the possibility of transmission. This may lead to a better sense of the client's worldview regarding personal responsibility, cultural influences, and personal fears regarding the diagnosis. Then the clinician and client can begin to develop an effective treatment plan, which may include an educational component to help a client such as Benitia or Jake understand what is needed to protect others.

Although this seems to be a straightforward approach, in reality the gathering of information may be more complicated because of the professional's biases. A practitioner may view Benitia as less threatening because of her likeability and motivation for change, and he or she may overlook some of the information regarding her case. Or the clinician may be weighing the importance of Benitia's financial needs versus the health needs of others and delaying action to gather more information. In Jake's case, the practitioner may not feel comfortable with or knowledgeable in discussing sexual and drug-using behaviors, and this avoidance of fact finding may compromise meeting ethical and legal responsibilities. Regardless of whether the clinician thinks cases such as these may lead to a duty to protect, gathering of factual information is essential to making sound clinical and ethical decisions.

Step 3: Conceptualize an Initial Plan on the Basis of Clinical Issues

At this point, the therapist will begin formulating a plan on the basis of all the information gathered. The initial plan with Benitia will probably reflect an urgency related to the principle of minimizing harm because she may be actively contagious and has identified specific others who may have been exposed to TB. The initial plan with Jake, who has not identified specific partners, may involve more exploration of his depression and a better understanding of how he may be putting others at risk for HIV infection. In either case, the plan should be documented, and the clinician needs to consult with a knowledgeable colleague, physician, or both before creating the initial plan.

The initial plan for Benitia, given her motivation and strong relationship with the clinician, would probably involve exploring and understanding her reluctance to receive treatment and disclose her diagnosis. She is concerned about the welfare of her children and family. Clinically, this concern needs to be examined in the longer term context of maintaining her health so she can provide for her family. Given the relationship, this may be the first approach with Benitia. The goal of the initial plan is for her to maintain her health so she can provide for her family. This means the clinician will likely need to focus on her getting into treatment and disclosing her condition to others. One could begin by discussing her understanding of TB and encouraging her to explore her disclosure options. This initial plan could also include an honest and frank discussion of both her own and the professional's ethical, moral, and legal responsibilities. A discussion of the facts about TB, the need for immediate treatment, the need to potentially disclose information to the affected parties, and an exploration of Benitia's fears and resistance regarding these actions will be a part of the initial plan. Although this initial plan may seem too directive for some, clinically it follows Benitia's significant motivation of caring for her family. Her ultimate goal is to provide for her family, and helping her maintain her health would assist her in meeting this goal.

If Benitia remains resistant to treatment and disclosure, then the clinician needs to more clearly discuss the ethical and legal responsibilities with the client. However, the therapist must carefully weigh the potential harm to Benitia if she never returns for counseling against the potential harm to others. This initial plan needs to include a time frame (number of sessions) within which the clinician will work with Benitia in exploring her issues to get her to agree to treatment (reducing risk of transmission) before disclosing her condition to others. One positive aspect in this case is the trusting, ongoing, positive relationship with this client. The challenge to clinicians is having the courage to risk losing that trusting relationship when others may be harmed by the client's actions.

The initial plan with Jake may be less clear. It appears as if Jake has not integrated his HIV diagnosis into his identity, and these issues may take time to explore. Clinically, the focus could be on his depression and anger. There may be some sessions devoted to gathering information about his sexual behavior and addressing his possible resistance. Because there are no identified persons at risk and he has not specifically described his unsafe sexual behavior, a clinician may initially want to explore Jake's apparent anger and depression. This exploration will allow the clinician to better understand Jake's defensiveness and build a more trusting relationship. However, if he does identify partners and discuss unprotected intercourse, then a more directive plan similar to the one described with Benitia may be appropriate. This involves moving the process toward Jake's self-disclosure or the clinician's notifying a third party. Given the case as presented, the initial plan with Jake could focus on the clinical issues of exploring his anger, depression, and sense of identity as it relates to HIV. The challenge in this initial plan may be the clinician's limited knowledge of HIV and possible inability to discuss intimate sexual and drug-using behavior with a less likable client.

Step 4: Consult Ethics Code and Assess Ethical Issues

After gathering the factual information and developing an initial plan, the practitioner needs to consult the ethics code of his or her profession (e.g., ACA, 2005; APA, 2002). A clinician working with clients infected with a communicable disease must review these guidelines periodically and be knowledgeable of his or her organization's policies in working with these populations. Furthermore, as noted above, a therapist must also be aware of the role of personal values and cultural beliefs in reviewing these guidelines and policies. In the cases of Benitia and Jake, a psychologist faces the dilemma of protecting the client's confidentiality according to the APA "Ethical Principles of Psychologists and Code of Conduct" (APA, 2002, Standard 4.01) versus permission to disclose confidential information without the client's consent for the purposes of protecting the client, the clinician, or others from harm (Standard 4.05). These two standards make up the practitioner's ethical dilemma. Does client confidentiality outweigh the duty to protect others? In the APA Ethics Code, the general principles also provide a template for analysis. But nowhere in this code does one find any mention of communicable disease.

However, as discussed in chapter 3 of this book, the ACA's *Code of Ethics* (ACA, 2005, p. 7) does include this issue.

B.2.b. Contagious, Life-Threatening Diseases
When clients disclose that they have a disease commonly known to be both communicable and life threatening, counselors may be justified in disclosing information to identifiable third parties, if they are known to be at demonstrable and high risk of contracting the disease. Prior to making a disclosure, counselors confirm that there is such a diagnosis and assess the intent of clients to inform the third parties about their

disease or to engage in any behaviors that may be harmful to an identifiable third party.

The ACA (2005) *Code of Ethics* also identifies the respect for privacy (B.1.b.), the respect for confidentiality (B.1.c.), and the limitations of confidentiality when harm to self or others is serious and foreseeable (B.2.a.). Referring to the codes of two professional organizations may assist the practitioner who is beginning to be overwhelmed. It is not that one code is better than another, for all are guidelines for ethical and professional behavior. In this instance, using both codes does assist in decision making. The ACA *Code of Ethics* points out that verifying the diagnosis of a communicable disease is a necessary first step. Both the ACA *Code of Ethics* and APA's (2002) Ethics Code support a client's right to privacy and the ability to disclose without consent when harm to self or others is present.

Although codes provide direction for what to do and what not to do, they do not give specific guidance for how to do something. However, when faced with a difficult ethical situation, therapists can often find some guidance in the literature. Unfortunately, there are few articles on how to balance duties to the client and others when dealing with communicable diseases, and most of those that are available focus on clients with HIV disease. This may be because of the crisis HIV posed in its early days when infection led quickly to death (Barret, 1989), or it may reflect the general lack of specificity in codes of ethics. Today, HIV disease has become more of a chronic condition, so the decision to not break confidentiality appears to have less dire consequences; therefore, practitioners may not feel such an intense need to act, and a variety of actions may be considered ethical (see, e.g., Huprich, Fuller, & Schneider, 2003).

Step 5: Analyze the Plan in Terms of the Five Foundational Principles

As noted earlier, the five foundational principles (Kitchener, 1984) guiding MHPs include autonomy (client's right to self-rule), beneficence (promoting the client's welfare), nonmaleficence (minimize harm), fidelity (being faithful), and justice (being fair). Nonmaleficence is the primary principle in medical ethics and seems to override other principles, but all must be considered in ethical decision making. The goal in this step of the model is to consider each principle to yield a decision that balances and maximizes all the ethical principles.

At first glance, the guiding principles appear to clearly address the issue of client protection. Helping Benitia gain control over her life (autonomy), approaching her nonjudgmentally, protecting the constructive quality of the relationship (fidelity), being faithful to her (integrity), and making sure she is treated fairly and justly (justice) characterize the essence of an effective professional relationship in the mental health field. Yet, however sympathetic one may be to Benitia's desire to provide financial support to her family, the need to protect others may be the overriding concern (nonmaleficence). MHPs faced with an "irresponsible" client with a communicable disease are likely to stumble over this dilemma. The initial plan with Benitia as described above seems to maximize the principles. The clinician will attempt to maintain the strong therapeutic relationship (autonomy, fidelity, and beneficence) by exploring Benitia's needs and focusing on her desire to care for her family while also suggesting nonmaleficence in getting her to treatment and disclosing her diagnosis. Balancing these ethical principles with the ethics codes may create tension for the clinician because of the need to decide which principle is primarily guiding his or her actions. In the end, does the duty to protect others outweigh the integrity of the relationship?

If the therapist solely considers client welfare, it would appear that the client's well-being is the paramount concern. For example, in the case of Benitia, the conflicting concerns about her own health and her need to generate income for her family create tension. When applying the five foundational principles, several courses of action emerge, and determining which is in the best interests of the client's welfare is difficult. It seems clear that her entire situation will worsen if her disease progresses. But helping her to see illness as a priority at this time may not be easy. If action is too quickly initiated, Benitia may leave therapy and not return for either emotional or physical treatment. Yet, every day that action is delayed increases the risk to those she may infect. Finding a balance between these two concerns is challenging.

In Jake's case, the clinician may not experience the same sense of connection and need to be faithful as with Benitia. The clinician has only seen Jake for four sessions. He or she may not have a feeling of closeness to him, and this may influence the clinician's sense of fidelity to the relationship. In addition, Jake presents as a more resistant client, and the clinician's emotional response to his attitude may deter the clinician from adhering to the principles of beneficence, fidelity, and justice. However, in reviewing the initial plan with Jake it appears that these principles and autonomy are guiding the therapeutic process. The clinician will spend more time with Jake exploring the clinical issues of anger, depression, and identity, and therefore the initial plan seems to follow the primary principles of autonomy and beneficence. If Jake were to become more resistant to therapy and more forthcoming in reporting his disregard for his unsafe sex behavior, then the clinician may tend to shift his or her initial plan, placing primary importance on the principle of nonmaleficence rather than autonomy or beneficence. The clinician's personal values may influence which ethical principle primarily guides this step in the process. Self-awareness of one's own values and bias is a critical component of sound ethical decision making. This may be found in consultation with a colleague, as suggested earlier. Again, balancing these principles while maintaining the client's best interest will reflect best practice.

Step 6: Identify the Legal Issues

The legal ramifications of ethical decision making also need to be considered. There is little consistency between various state and even local laws (see chap. 2, this volume). In both of these cases, a legal consultation (perhaps with a public health attorney at the state health department) will provide the most valuable and reliable interpretation of state communicable disease law. This consultation will be crucial in determining whether there is a legal justification for breaching confidentiality. This legal consultation must be carefully documented in the record.

In regard to HIV, the literature deals with issues related to the *Tarasoff* (1976) ruling in the California Supreme Court. The *Tarasoff* ruling and subsequent cases suggest that the duty to protect third parties and breach client confidentiality may be warranted when there is active, imminent danger to specific persons. Although it might appear that *Tarasoff* demands breaching confidentiality with clients who have HIV and have not informed sexual or needle-sharing partners, Burris (2001) and others have presented comprehensive legal reviews indicating that there is no legal or ethical imperative to break confidentiality to warn others who may be at risk. Each case must be considered on its own merits, and it is possible for two highly competent professionals to follow different courses of action and both be acting within sound ethical practice. The clinician serving Benitia or Jake will likely struggle with this dilemma within the context of minimizing harm because there is no perfect ethical solution given the myriad variables affecting each case.

Most states have a mechanism for partner notification with communicable diseases. Notifying others of potential risk is usually left to local health departments, who report to state department of public health personnel, who then conduct contact tracing. Learning that state or local agencies are mandated to provide contact tracing (partner notification) in situations in which someone with a communicable disease is potentially exposing others may reduce the sense of isolation for the practitioner. Through legal consultation, the counselor working with Benitia may find that TB is a reportable communicable disease, and the physician is responsible for reporting to the health department. If the practitioner feels the need to breach confidentiality, the first step might be to seek Benitia's permission to discuss her situation with her physician. This may be a less threatening approach for her and may preserve the therapeutic relationship. If Benitia refuses to cooperate in notifying anyone, then a state program may begin the process of notifying the affected persons. This may also appear to eliminate the demand to take some action with Benitia regarding talking with others about her condition. However, although this may resolve the issue of disclosure responsibility, a thorough exploration of the client's awareness of the contagiousness of her disease is necessary. Having Benitia review her understanding of TB and its danger to the health of those around her as well as her knowledge of treatment options will assist the therapist in determining the appropriate course of action in this case.

With Jake, the situation might seem very different. Unlike TB, HIV is not highly contagious, yet Jake's attitude suggests that he is unconcerned about infecting others. Jake's sexual or drug-using partners are not identifiable. Again, knowledge of state communicable disease law may, in some states, warrant breaching confidentiality with Jake (e.g., reporting him to the public health department) even though he has not identified specific sexual or drug-using partners.

In summary, a clinician considering either of these two cases needs to be familiar with communicable disease laws as well as any specific state statutes on HIV or TB confidentiality requirements (see chap. 2, this volume). Chenneville (2000) provided a fairly clear, general description of state guidelines, along with a resource listing of statutes on confidentiality by state. For most practitioners, this is a challenging area to understand (Simone & Fulero, 2001), thus consulting with the medical director of the local health department or an attorney with the state health department is highly recommended. This legal consultation should be considered before developing the final plan of action.

Step 7: Refine the Initial Plan and Assess the Options

Having considered personal values and beliefs, the factual information presented by the client, ethics codes, foundational principles, and legal ramifications, the clinician is now prepared to assess options for a final treatment plan in which the initial plan will be more fully developed. At this step in the process, the clinician needs to refine the initial plan so that it (a) is congruent with his or her personal values, (b) advances the clinical interests of the client, (c) permits the clinician to operate within the ethics codes and agency policies, (d) minimizes harm to the client and relevant others, (e) maximizes the ethical principles to the extent possible, and (f) allows the clinician to work within the law.

The clinician needs to review the consultation notes and consider the consequences of the various options. One real challenge at this step is to assess whether breaching confidentiality with Benitia or Jake will result in their termination of therapy. The practitioner needs to consider the benefit of maintaining the client in the therapeutic process in the hope that the client will initiate personal responsibility for her or his behavior. At the same time, delaying a plan of action allows for possible continued harm to the client and others. The clinician thus needs to weigh the consequences of any plan carefully.

Given a review of these steps in the process, the clinician may want to revise the initial plan with Benitia and focus more on the strength of the relationship. The therapeutic relationship and the foundational principles of autonomy and fidelity may guide Benitia to take more personal responsibility for her actions. The counseling process will still involve allowing Benitia to discuss her understanding of TB and how she wants to proceed with this responsibly. The clinician will be empowering Benitia to see medical treatment and disclosure of her diagnosis as a way of doing what is best for her family. The specific plan for Benitia may still involve the following: (a) reviewing the ethical and legal consequences of her actions, (b) identifying how she or someone can notify her friend and family about her diagnosis, (c) pursuing treatment for TB immediately so she can get back to her job search, and (d) assisting her with the emotional and financial challenge of not working while she is in treatment. The approach, however, may be refined to allow the relationship rather than the clinician's sense of urgency to guide the process. This process will probably occur over a few sessions, but in the revised plan Benitia's sense of personal responsibility may guide the process to resolution. Timing of when to focus on the duty to protect others in this relationship will still be the challenge, and each clinician will vary on this time frame. If Benitia continues to deny her personal responsibility, then the clinician, on the basis of ethical and legal consultations, may need to breach confidentiality and proceed as described above without Benitia's consent.

The initial plan for Jake involved addressing his resistance and anger. Jake is complaining of depression, and that needs to be taken into consideration in identifying options. Jake seems to be more emotionally volatile compared with Benitia. Clinically, this warrants taking more time with Jake to establish a more trusting relationship. Given a review of the steps of this model, Jake's initial plan will remain essentially the same, with a focus on clinical issues rather than the ethical dilemma. Certainly, the issue of sexual and drug-using behavior needs to be addressed. If Jake continues to be vague about his risky behavior and does not identify specific partners, then the clinician may adopt a more psychoeducational approach in assisting Jake to take more personal responsibility for his behavior. The goal here would be to get him to commit to safer sex and safer drug use only, possibly including the use of a formalized agreement. If Jake does identify partners, then a more directed approach similar to Benitia's plan needs to be considered.

Step 8: Choose a Course of Action and Share It With the Client

Once the course of action is determined, the clinician carefully explains the suggested treatment plan to the client. Naturally, this is an interactive process that will, one hopes, lead to a collaborative treatment plan. The practitioner needs to be prepared for a volatile reaction if the client strongly disagrees with the course of action. The clinician must watch the client carefully during this process. The person may verbally agree to the treatment plan, but body language, eye contact, or tone of voice may indicate otherwise. The clinician will probably want to focus on the therapeutic relationship and promote empowerment of the client during this step in the model. The options for a course of action are discussed and decided on with the client. The clinician may decide that there is a duty to protect, and the client may choose not to notify third parties as suggested. One hopes that in this case, communication between the client and practitioner has been open and honest, and the client will at least be informed as to the rationale for why the clinician will need to take action.

A treatment plan would likely be developed and discussed with Benitia within one to four sessions, given her contagious condition and her identification of other people who are at risk of infection. Benitia is clearly devoted to her children and family, and her sense of obligation to them may need to be the focal point of discussion in creating her treatment plan. If Benitia agrees to seek treatment and then notifies her friend and family, and the clinician confirms the disclosures occurred, then the clinician continues to assist her in managing these challenges and may be present for the actual disclosures. Benitia may opt for state health personnel to notify family and friends.

What if Benitia refuses treatment and refuses to disclose her condition to others? The clinician must then decide whether he or she will breach confidentiality. On the basis of the guiding principle of nonmaleficence, the APA Ethics Code (APA, 2002, Standard 4.05) and the ACA *Code of Ethics* (ACA, 2005, Standards B.2.a. and B.2.b.), and the legal case (*Tarasoff*, 1976), the clinician certainly has the support to breach confidentiality. If the clinician is a licensed professional counselor, he or she will need to get proof of Benitia's diagnosis (this is not necessary for other MHPs, although it is advised). The clinician must discuss the need to breach confidentiality with Benitia. The clinician can notify her physician or perhaps notify the local health department. The clinician will need to review his or her actions carefully with Benitia and make sure she is informed of each step that is to be taken. The clinician must focus on Benitia's best interests here and help her to understand how these actions are empowering rather than disempowering her. The clinician needs to be confident that this decision is not based on his or her own sense of urgency or fear of legal liability. Benitia may actively agree with this action plan (given the trusting relationship); she may passively agree with the actions, but resent this new direction in the relationship; or she may simply get angry and not return for therapy. The practitioner needs to be prepared for any and all reactions.

Clearly, this process will need to be done in consultation with a respected colleague session by session. Documentation of the process and the client's noncompliance is essential. Breaching confidentiality will generate many conflicting emotions for the clinician. Personal counseling may be advised on the basis of the particular client's circumstances.

Jake's plan may involve more sessions before the duty to protect is discussed, given his resistance and anger issues. To approach him prematurely could result in his not returning for therapy. Furthermore, with Jake the course of action may need to be communicated in a less directive manner. Because Jake has not identified any specific sexual or drug-using partners and has not divulged the behaviors in which he is engaging, the clinician is probably wise to maintain confidentiality. After reviewing the legal issues (e.g., *Tarasoff*, 1976), reviewing the APA Ethics Code (APA, 2002, Standard 4.01) and the ACA *Code of Ethics* (ACA, 2005, Standard B.1.c.), and being guided by the principles of beneficence, fidelity, and autonomy, a clinician could justify maintaining Jake's confidentiality with regard to his behavior. If Jake does identify specific partners whom he may be putting at risk for HIV infection and he is unwilling to disclose his HIV status to these partners, then the clinician may need to follow a similar course of action as discussed regarding Benitia's refusal to seek treatment and disclose to others. Again, the local health department is the best source for consultation and guidance in these matters of public health law and notification. Even after reviewing legal, ethical, and guiding principles, each practitioner may vary in the length of time he or she will work with the client to balance the need of maintaining confidentiality and notifying others.

Step 9: Implement the Course of Action: Monitor and Discuss Outcomes

Monitoring both these clients as the treatment plan is implemented will allow the practitioner to adjust and revise the plan. The clinician can evaluate the plan by assessing the client's self-report on progress with the plan. The client may be more engaged in the therapeutic relationship as a result of managing a crisis honestly with the clinician. Client engagement with the clinician needs to be carefully monitored and documented during this process. If the client appears to be withdrawing from the clinician, a new treatment plan will have to be developed. The client may report better coping and conflict resolution skills as a result of this process. The clinician can also discuss the experience of addressing the duty-to-protect issue through the ethical decision-making model as an educational process on which the client can reflect for personal growth. A discussion of progress and outcomes in regard to the plan need to be discussed in each subsequent session and documented in case notes.

CONSULTATION AND DOCUMENTATION

Clearly, in cases such as these, it is important to remember that the best resource for the clinician is consultation. Consultation will be needed with other MHPs on the ethical dilemma(s) presented in each case, and medical consultation will be needed regarding communicable diseases. Most MHPs are not trained in communicable diseases and must not engage in medical advice giving with the client. Thus, best practice would encourage the practitioner to receive consultation from medical personnel or the medical director of the local health department to gain a better understanding of disease transmission, contagion, treatment, and partner notification. This consultation will allow the practitioner to discuss the issues of contagion with clients and enable appropriate referrals to medical personnel. Consultation is also needed with regard to legal issues. This may be best done through public health attorneys in the state health department. Consultation enables the practitioner to think through her or his own ethical decision making regarding client privacy and the duty to protect others. Consultation will also lengthen the amount of time for making a decision, which can allow for a more thoughtful and ethically sound decision. Finally, documentation of consultation needs to be included in the client's record, including any material provided by the various consultants.

CONCLUSION

These possible responses to the scenarios of Benitia and Jake illustrate how a model of ethical decision making can be applied to varying client situations. Clearly, in any duty-to-protect situation there may be divergent treatment options that are ethically sound. The circumstances affecting Benitia and Jake were dissimilar and the treatment plan for each varied; however, the ethical decision-making process for addressing the duty-to-protect issues remained the same. When the client does not respond positively in changing behaviors that place others at risk, the clinician will have to develop a plan that may include breaking confidentiality. This is best done with the assistance of a clinical supervisor or a consultant and would require thorough documentation.

As illustrated through these cases, clients with communicable diseases that place others at risk can pose significant difficulties for the clinician. A basic rule to follow is to have a decision-making model (Barret et al., 2001) and to carefully cover each step. Consultation and supervision are additional resources. Although possibly difficult and challenging, clients with communicable diseases offer opportunities for clinicians to grow in their understanding of the use and importance of ethical standards.

REFERENCES

American Counseling Association. (2005). ACA *code of ethics*. Alexandria, VA: Author.

American Psychological Association. (2002). Ethical principles of psychologists and code of conduct. *American Psychologist, 57,* 1060–1073.

Anderson, J., & Barret, B. (2001). *Ethics in HIV-related psychotherapy: Clinical decision-making in complex cases.* Washington, DC: American Psychological Association.

Barret, B., Kitchener, K., & Burris, S. (2001). A decision model for ethical dilemmas in HIV-related psychotherapy and its application in the case of Jerry. In J. Anderson & B. Barret (Eds.), *Ethics in HIV-related psychotherapy: Clinical decision-making in complex cases* (pp. 133–154). Washington, DC: American Psychological Association.

Barret, R. L. (1989). Counseling gay men with AIDS: Human dimensions. *Journal of Counseling & Development, 67,* 573–575.

Burris, S. (2001). Clinical decision-making in the shadow of the law. In J. Anderson & B. Barret (Eds.), *Ethics in HIV-related psychotherapy: Clinical decision-making in complex cases* (pp. 99–129). Washington, DC: American Psychological Association.

Chenneville, T. (2000). HIV, confidentiality, and duty to protect: A decision-making model. *Professional Psychology: Research and Practice, 31,* 661–670.

Huprich, S. K., Fuller, K. M., & Schneider, R. B. (2003). Divergent ethical perspectives on the duty-to-warn principle with HIV patients. *Ethics & Behavior, 13,* 263–278.

Kitchener, K. S. (1984). Intuition, critical evaluation, and ethical principles: The foundation for ethical decisions in counseling psychology. *Counseling Psychologist, 12*(3), 43–55.

Palma, T. V., & Iannelli, R. J. (2002). Therapeutic reactivity to confidentiality with HIV positive clients: Bias or epidemiology? *Ethics & Behavior, 12,* 353–370.

Simone, S. J., & Fulero, S. M. (2001). Psychologists' perceptions of their duty to protect uninformed sex partners of HIV-positive clients. *Behavioral Sciences & the Law, 19,* 423–436.

Tarasoff v. Board of Regents of the University of California, 551 P.2d 334 (1976).

III

HARM TO SELF

11

THE DUTY TO PROTECT SUICIDAL CLIENTS: ETHICAL, LEGAL, AND PROFESSIONAL CONSIDERATIONS

DAVID A. JOBES AND STEPHEN S. O'CONNOR

Sylvia[1] was a straight-A National Merit Scholar in high school. Outstanding in both academics and extracurricular activities, Sylvia looked like a most promising college student. She was admitted to all the top schools and ultimately opted to attend a prestigious Ivy League university at which she would major in electrical engineering. Her parents packed her off to school with great expectations; she was their only child, and they had poured everything into her education and success. Her 1st year began with the typical adjustment issues that come with being away from home for the first time—the freedom, the lack of a parentally imposed schedule, the dorm room parties, the sexual acting out, the drinking, and the drug use were all a bit overwhelming to Sylvia. In spite of these issues, her academic gifts enabled her to excel in her coursework. Her first-semester midterm grades were excellent, and she was feeling confident about her academic prospects as many of her other peers toiled away.

---

[1]For purposes of confidentiality, all names are fictitious, and clinical material is significantly disguised or loosely based on actual cases.

However, things began to shift after midterm break. Perhaps feeling overly confident, Sylvia began to party with some of the girls in her hall, discovering alcohol, marijuana, and designer drugs. Having had little exposure to these in her private coed high school, Sylvia quickly immersed herself in heavy drinking and drug use. By the end of the first semester, she salvaged a 3.00 GPA, but more than one professor pulled her aside to express concern about the sudden drop in her performance.

The semester break was difficult for Sylvia. Cut off from her new college friends, she was sullen and avoided interacting with her parents. Relieved to be back at school after the break, Sylvia promptly picked up where she had left off. Classes were more often skipped than attended, and she began to drink heavily, even more than her friends. She lapsed into feelings of depression, sleeping long hours, and noticeably losing weight. By mid-semester, her friends were sufficiently concerned to talk to the resident assistant about Sylvia's depression and overall decline. The resident assistant referred Sylvia to the university counseling center, where she was seen for a total of two sessions.

Her counselor was a doctoral-level psychologist who did not conduct an evaluation of her psychosocial history or her symptoms; no formal *Diagnostic and Statistical Manual of Mental Disorders* (American Psychiatric Association, 1994) diagnosis was given, and he only reluctantly referred her for a medication consultation. It was not his habit to assess suicidal risk, but he considered her sufficiently troubled to inquire about suicide. Sylvia acknowledged passive suicidal fantasies but said she was "too chicken" to do anything about it. She played down her substance abuse. Sylvia verbally committed to her safety and agreed to return for once-per-week "supportive counseling." She saw a nurse practitioner in the health center who diagnosed her as depressed and prescribed Zoloft.

At her next outpatient counseling appointment, Sylvia and the counselor discussed her family. She did not attend her third session; her counselor sent a routine follow-up form letter encouraging her to reschedule, but she did not reply. A week later, Sylvia was found dead in her dorm room bed, lying in a pool of her own blood. Her wounds had been self-inflicted. There were two deep slits in her wrists and one on the side of her throat that was lethal, severing her carotid artery. A suicide note was discovered on her laptop, apologizing to her parents but insisting they would be better off without her. She said that no one knew the depths of her pain and no one ever could. She felt there was no other way out of the hell she was in.

Although a fictitious rendering of a suicide death, the case of Sylvia is realistic in terms of content and tragic aftermath. The dramatic descent of such an apparently outstanding and successful young person into the abyss of misery and suicidal despair is stunning. However, what is most troublesome about this particular case is the underresponse of the system and the mental health clinician to a seriously disturbed young woman who was actually receptive and willing to seek professional help. Although mental health practitioners (MHPs) are not soothsayers, all states in the United States have explicit expectations of a *duty to protect* that requires clinical recognition of the severity of clients' emotional and behavioral problems when these struggles pose an imminent danger to self. As is discussed throughout this chapter, the potential life-and-death seriousness of suicidality demands a responsible and competent clinical reaction. Yet, all too often responses to suicidal individuals are uninformed and inadequate and may even directly or indirectly contribute to a tragic fatal outcome (Berman, Jobes, & Silverman, 2006).

OVERVIEW

Generally speaking, the essential purpose of professional mental health care is the provision of sound clinical assessment and treatment to patients seeking care. Diagnosing and treating cases involving suicidal risk can be particularly complex. This is especially true because suicidal states are inherently difficult to assess in valid and reliable ways (Jobes, 2006), and the field's knowledge base about effective treatments remains remarkably limited (Linehan, 2005).

Given the pervasiveness of suicidality in general mental health practice, it is likely that most MHPs will have numerous encounters with suicidal clients (whether they want to or not). Yet, survey research has shown that MHPs across professional disciplines rarely receive training in clinical suicidology in their curricula (Bongar, 2002). Even though the highest level of clinical acumen does not guarantee that a client will not take his or her own life, MHPs can learn to make a meaningful difference in the life of a suicidal client. Beyond clinical considerations, however, the various actions an MHP chooses to take (or not take) while performing assessment and treatment with any suicidal person may have important implications for ethics complaints or professional liability (i.e., malpractice) if a mental health client ends her or his life by suicide. Thus, our aim in this chapter is to provide useful guidance that applies to various MHPs practicing in a range of settings and that will lead to better assessment and treatment of suicidal patients (Berman et al., 2006; Jobes, 2006; Jobes & Berman, 1993). To accomplish this, we guide the reader through the following: (a) the duty to protect, (b) the therapeutic relationship, (c) diversity issues, (d) malpractice and effective clinical care, and (e) supervisory issues.

THE DUTY TO PROTECT

As described elsewhere, there exists a fundamental duty for MHPs to protect suicidal patients from themselves (Berman et al., 2006; Bongar, 2002). As described by Millon (2004), this moral and subsequent legal duty to protect dates back to the philosophical notions of the Europeans who championed the development of asylums for individuals with mental illness as a means to protect the vulnerable "lunatic" from the potentially harmful influences of larger society. Since the advent of psychoanalysis in the late 19th century, the notion that MHPs must do everything in their power to avert any prospective suicide has been widely embraced. As discussed by Jobes (2006), for most contemporary providers there is a pervasive assumption that suicidal patients properly belong in protected inpatient environments. However, this way of thinking has been increasingly challenged over the past decade by the exponentially increasing costs of inpatient care, which have compelled managed care insurance providers to raise the bar for obtaining a precertification for inpatient insurance coverage. Admissions are tougher to effect; lengths of stay have dwindled into a matter of a few days. Yet the duty to protect remains.

It is our sense that this long-standing duty is becoming an evolving expectation in relation to certain reality-based constraints. As ever, the operative professional judgment still hinges on one's clinical assessment of "clear and imminent danger to self" (which is essentially a 0/1 binary decision). Increasingly, however, even in cases in which an MHP clinically determines the presence of imminent suicidal risk, thereby triggering efforts to pursue a voluntary or involuntary inpatient hospital stay, the prospect of actually being able to admit such a patient and keep her or him in the hospital has become quite daunting. Indeed, acute and imminent suicidal ideation alone may be insufficient to precertify a hospitalization in the absence of suicide attempt behavior. Given this changing clinical reality, we guide the reader through considerations that are relevant to the evolving expectations of contemporary care that will satisfy the duty to protect.

THE THERAPEUTIC RELATIONSHIP

Reducing suicidal risk is largely dependent on the strength of the therapeutic relationship between clinician and client (Jobes, 2006). The foundation of a potentially effective clinical relationship begins during the initial interview assessment, in which new clients invariably "test the waters" of a clinician's personality and reactivity to certain issues that the client presents. As with any clinical presentation, the clinician should adopt an open, supportive, nonjudgmental, and understanding approach when getting to know the client. When suicide is a consideration for the client, it is particularly important to be balanced, relatively neutral, and noncoercive; there should be no hint of moralizing, intimidating, or patronizing behavior on the clinician's part. A matter-of-fact and forthright approach to talking about suicide puts the client at ease and thereby less inclined to engage in a clinical power struggle with the provider (Jobes, 2006). Carl Rogers's (1957) ground-breaking work emphasized the importance of empathic listening, and such an approach is particularly germane when sitting with someone entertaining thoughts of suicide. Indeed, Orbach (2001) wrote eloquently about the value of having empathy for the suicidal wish as a critical element to successfully forming an alliance with the suicidal client.

Jobes and Maltsberger (1995) noted several methods for clinical interviewing to help improve the therapeutic relationship, which will in turn assist in proper treatment planning for suicidal individuals. A crucial interview goal must center on the development of an understanding as to how suicide "works" or functions within the client's cognitive, emotional, and behavioral world. As Shneidman (1996) pointed out, suicidal thinking fundamentally involves a certain kind of problem-solving cognitive process, which tends to eliminate all possible options but suicide. In this sense, the clinician can usually come to appreciate the process whereby suicide becomes viable—even compelling—to the client. One must carefully cultivate a working knowledge of the sequence of events and the emotions and thoughts that land the client in a suicidal state. Although risk factors for suicide are of course important, the life-versus-death struggle must be thoughtfully assessed and examined: Why does the client see suicide as an option? Why has the client not already taken his or her life? In this regard, research examining wishes to live versus die, or similar consideration of reasons for living versus reasons for dying, helps MHPs appreciate the ambivalence that many suicidal people experience (Brown et al., 2005; Jobes & Mann, 1999; Kovacs & Beck, 1977; Linehan, Goodstein, Nielsen, & Chiles, 1983).

Unfortunately, many suicidal individuals report that although they presented in a suicidal state, their symptoms were treated in a reductionistic manner by the attending clinician (Jobes, 2003). Finding themselves subjected to a barrage of probing questions targeting the diagnostic variables of major psychiatric disorders, such clients often feel that the heart of their suicidal struggle is not recognized (Jobes, 2000). To this end, recent empirical work by Jobes et al. (2004) has shown that treatment-seeking suicidal clients are much more preoccupied with issues of relationships, work, and self than they are with symptoms of mental disorders. Both high recidivism rates in emergency rooms for individuals with a history of either suicide ideation or behaviors and the characteristically poor follow-through for recommended outpatient treatment strongly suggest that current standard practices may not be meeting the needs of suicidal clients (Jobes, 2003). As is discussed elsewhere, pervasive use of ineffective "no-suicide" or "no-harm" contracts and overreliance on increasingly short hospital stays, as well as an overemphasis on psychotropic medications, may not be adequately addressing contemporary challenges posed by suicidal clients (Jobes, 2003, 2006; Rudd, 2006).

DIVERSITY ISSUES

Current epidemiologic research implies that older European American men represent the largest portion of deaths by suicide in the United States annually (Garlow, Purselle, & Heninger, 2005). However, the field of applied mental health has become increasingly sensitive to ethnic and cultural differences among mental health consumers, many of whom experience specific risk factors related to suicide-related behaviors. For example, Garlow et al. (2005) conducted a study using two separate data sets to compare the life cycles of men and women of differing ethnicities in terms of suicide deaths. Their data demonstrated a significant difference in mean age of suicide deaths for adults who were European American (46 years of age) and those who were African American (36 years) or of "other" race (36 years). Additionally, their study showed that African American women have the lowest rate of suicide of all demographic groups in the United States.

As the United States continues to become increasingly diverse, MHPs should be mindful of cultural considerations when conducting risk assessments. The American Psychological Association (APA, 2003) has listed multiple guidelines to follow when providing services for ethnic minorities. Cultural sensitivity is not simply part of the treatment plan; rather, it is reflected throughout the formulation and provision of treatment. MHPs should consider cultural differences in worldview and interpersonal style when discussing suicidal behaviors to ensure the greatest likelihood of ascertaining the client's level of risk. Trends in suicide among different groups have been well documented in the professional literature (McKenzie, Serfaty, & Crawford, 2003; Rudmin, Ferrada-Noli, & Skolbekken, 2003) and underscore the need to be mindful of acculturation when assessing suicidal risk. For example, Hjern (2002) showed that in comparison with their country of origin, recent immigrants have increased rates of suicide, and the risk generally increases for their offspring. In addition to both racial and cultural issues, a client's sexual orientation also provides meaningful information regarding risk of suicide-related behaviors.

The current literature reflects increased rates of suicidal ideation among adult gay men and lesbians (Bagley & Tremblay, 1997; Herrell et al., 1999), with approximately 12% of individuals reporting a history of at least one suicide attempt (Paul et al., 2002). The genetic influence of sexual orientation on suicide-related behavior was earlier studied using the Vietnam Era Twin Registry (Herrell et al., 1999), which after controlling for substance abuse and nonrelated symptoms of depression found a significantly higher rate of suicide-related symptoms for twins who reported lifetime homosexual relations than for twins reporting no same-sex relations. Furthermore, age has been shown to moderate the risk of suicidal behaviors in gay and bisexual men, with young men being at an increased risk for exhibiting both self-harm behaviors and symptoms of depression (Paul et al., 2002).

Given these data, we recommend sensitively discussing any psychosocial stressors that may be associated with gender, ethnic, cultural, and sexual orientation issues in the course of conducting a suicide risk assessment. As noted, suicidal clients may experience an increased level of stress related to family and peer relationships, as well as environmental, cultural, and health-related issues not normally experienced by the majority of the population. Mental illness is often stigmatized in society, and the additional stigma related to same-sex relationships or practicing different beliefs has the potential to raise the risk of lethality in minority mental health consumers. MHPs have a responsibility to expand their own worldview in an attempt to better serve individuals within specific minority groups, which will most likely improve clinical rapport and openness throughout the therapeutic process.

MALPRACTICE AND EFFECTIVE CLINICAL CARE

The literature suggests that one out of six annual suicides in the United States involves persons receiving psychotherapy at the time of their death, and one half of all suicides involve individuals who had received prior psychotherapeutic treatment (Berman, 1986); more recent research has shown that many suicidal patients routinely see health providers in the weeks or months before their death (Luoma, Martin, & Pearson, 2003). These statistics have become increasingly pertinent to MHPs as litigation involving suicide-related malpractice claims results in the highest percentage of monetary awards involving psychologists and psychiatrists (Robertson, 1988). Additionally, Jobes and Berman (1993) reported that these are the second most costly kind of lawsuit filed against psychologists in the United States.

If a client does die by suicide, the risk of an ethics complaint or a negligence action being filed can be substantially reduced if a reasonable assessment and treatment process occurred. The following methods will increase the likelihood that proper techniques and judgments are used and therefore considerably reduce the risk of a successful complaint: (a) thorough and contemporaneous documentation, (b) appropriate methods of clinical assessment and triangulation of data, (c) reasonable treatments and interventions, (d) professional consultation, and (e) clinical referrals (Jobes, 2006; Simpson & Stacey, 2004).

Thorough and Contemporaneous Documentation

When determining whether to pursue malpractice litigation, plaintiff attorneys spend many hours carefully reviewing clinical case notes and discharge summaries checking for proper (and contemporaneous) information regarding the clinical care that was rendered to the deceased client (Simpson & Stacey, 2004). Simpson and Stacey (2004) contended that either missing data or information entered well after the actual assessment are viewed very unfavorably by a jury and leave the door open for questions regarding the efforts put forth by the clinician. Wise, Jobes, Simpson, and Berman (2005) further asserted that MHPs should never rely on undocumented proof of competent clinical care, such as recollections of conversations with the dead client. As any plaintiff attorney will glibly tell you, "If it wasn't written down, it didn't happen." Particularly in the aftermath of the Health Insurance Portability and Accountability Act of 1996, there is an expectation that certain key elements must be noted in the medical record (e.g., description and history of the problem, mental status exam results, social and family history, prior treatment history, significant medical and psychosocial problems, brief formulation, *Diagnostic and Statistical Manual of Mental Disorders* diagnosis, treatment plan).

Methods of Clinical Assessment and Triangulation of Data

Risk Assessment

It is our opinion that all MHPs conducting mental health assessments, especially those focused on risk of lethality, have a duty to protect the client. Fundamentally, no clinician is pleased to see another person suffer, much less endorse thoughts of suicide. However, MHPs choosing to skirt the issue of suicide, as in the case of Sylvia, are directly failing their clients. Although each person's suicidal ideation is individualized and unique to his or her own issues, the literature on suicide clearly provides resources for proper assessment, with which all MHPs should familiarize themselves before being thrust into a position in which they have a duty to protect. Furthermore, informing the client about protocol for handling instances of suicide-related behaviors before conducting an assessment results in a more transparent dialogue regarding what is believed to be in the client's best interest and also serves to normalize thoughts of suicide as something discussed with all clients. Thus, we strongly suggest thinking proactively and mentioning your own protocol for handling suicide-related behaviors during the initial informed consent process, including when confidentiality can be broken and hospitalization is most likely to occur. The informed consent process aspects of suicide risk should be written and, depending on the case, verbal as well.

Joiner, Walker, Rudd, and Jobes (1999) established a hierarchy for assessing suicidal risk based on current scientific literature. These authors presented an ordinal scale of threshold for suicidal risk, placing individuals who have a history of multiple attempts (at least two attempts that could have led to death) at the ceiling, followed by individuals with a history of one attempt, with nonattempters at the bottom of the scale. The presence of one or more risk factors elevates the risk of suicide attempt for all three groups. Diagnoses, psychosocial stressors, and personality traits are also examined and rated in relation to their potential influence on suicidal ideation, behaviors, or both.

Beyond the significance of the client's attempt history, any client who presents with resolved plans and preparation for an attempt needs to be taken very seriously. For example, evidence of mustering courage and the gathering of suicidal resources (e.g., a stash of pills or the presence of a loaded firearm in the home) is cause for serious concern. As Joiner, Rudd, and Rajab (1997) showed, suicide attempts are more highly correlated with evidence of resolved plans and preparation than with suicidal ideation (which is often considered the benchmark for suicide risk assessment; see Joiner et al., 1999). Additional factors a clinician should consider when assessing potential for suicide include current psychosocial stressors, such as interpersonal problems or financial difficulties (see review by Maris, Berman, & Silverman, 2000).

In this vein, de Moore and Robertson (1999) found that psychosocial stressors were related to the attempter's resolve and to the severity of attempt. Their findings showed that attempters who survived a firearm-related suicide attempt reported increased domestic disputes, alcohol abuse, despair, and tension for a short time period (several days to a few weeks) before the attempt. Individuals with a severe Axis I diagnosis but without an increase in psychosocial stressors were more likely to abort an attempt if faced with relatively trivial barriers, such as short guardrails on a rooftop. These findings suggest that MHPs must investigate recent psychosocial stressors while conducting suicide assessments, regardless of current psychopathology.

Although we highlight the importance of psychosocial variables, we still note that any complete assessment must include a thorough investigation of Axis I or II symptomatology (e.g., mood disorder, substance dependence or abuse, anxiety disorder, personality disorder). Despite the inability to predict suicide risk solely on the basis of diagnostic considerations, the relationship between psychopathology and suicide is still important to appreciate. Kessler, Berglund, Borges, Nock, and Wang (2005) reported that data from the National Comorbidity Survey (1990–1992) and the National Comorbidity Survey Replication (2001–2003) showed that major depressive disorder was the most frequent single disorder in individuals reporting suicidal behaviors within the previous 12 months. The study also suggested that the anxiety disorder spectrum was the highest class of disorders reported by individuals with suicidal behaviors within the previous 12 months. Both findings are largely based on odds ratio statistics and suggest that major depressive disorder is the mental health disorder most commonly associated with suicidal behaviors, whereas anxiety disorders are most highly correlated with suicidal behaviors when measuring each entire spectrum of disorders (i.e., mood disorder or substance use disorder). Moreover, Cornelius et al. (1995) noted the significance of diagnostic comorbidity, suggesting that individuals with unipolar depression are at increased risk for self-harm while concurrently abusing alcohol.

Sometimes, clinical assessments of suicidal risk may be overly focused on current events at the expense of appreciating more historical influences and events. Joiner et al. (1999) referred to a chaotic family history and a history of sexual or physical abuse as two important factors to investigate while conducting a thorough assessment of risk to harm. Indeed, as Linehan (1993) noted, an unstable childhood marked by an invalidating environment is a crucial factor in the development of borderline personality disorder, a diagnosis that often involves suicidal and self-harming behaviors.

Impulsivity is another critical risk factor noted by Joiner et al. (1999). Bryan and Rudd (2006) observed that multiple attempters are often marked by notably increased levels of impulsivity. Historic suicide attempts are often seen to occur in response to obvious environmental triggers. Therefore, the clinical assessment should investigate both current psychosocial stressors, as mentioned above, and an individual's historic response to certain triggering stressors. In this regard, Oquendo et al. (2004) indicated that the presence of aggressive and impulsive behaviors predicted suicidal behaviors in an outpatient population of adults with bipolar disorder and major depressive disorder.

Finally, Joiner et al. (1999) concluded their considerations of suicidal risk assessment by mentioning several protective factors that tend to limit the risk of suicidality. The presence of a strong support system and/or the potential presence of problem solving or self-control can help reduce the risk of suicidal behaviors. Relying on a strong therapeutic alliance and the development of personal goals targeting interpersonal, vocational, and coping skills can increase personal self-efficacy to cope with tremendous pain and thereby decrease self-harm behaviors.

Triangulation of the Data

An adequate clinical assessment of suicidal risk depends on use of multiple sources of data, known as "triangulation of data" (refer to Shea, 1999). The importance of including family information in the overall risk assessment cannot be overstressed for two reasons. First, additional collateral information always provides a larger database from which the clinician is able to draw conclusions regarding client lethality. Second, engaging the family as part of the assessment and treatment builds rapport and decreases the likelihood of clinician scapegoating should the client die by suicide. Skip Simpson, a well-known malpractice plaintiff attorney, argued that MHPs should try to obtain a release of information early in the treatment of any high-risk person so that the therapist can discuss her or his concerns with the client's family so they know the seriousness of the situation (Simpson & Stacey, 2004).

Reasonable Treatments and Interventions

Generally speaking, the treatment plan serves as the critical roadmap for clinical care, reflecting both short- and long-term goals for treatment and evolving considerations that emerge over the course of care. Documentation of goals aimed specifically at reducing suicidal behavior should always be included in the treatment plan. Obviously, the treatment plans for suicidal individuals stand a higher likelihood of intense legal scrutiny should a suicide occur. In this regard, the treatment and "dose" (the number and amount of clinical contacts) should be commensurate with the assessed level of risk. Amend the treatment plan as necessary on the basis of the most current level of suicidal risk. A well-conceived and appropriately executed treatment plan will likely increase the chances for improvement within a relatively limited time frame for most cases and should include the full range of clinical resources.

When working with suicidal clients, the use of a treatment team is invariably better than flying solo, particularly if the suicidal risk is more chronic in nature. By *team*, we mean the use of a consulting psychiatrist along with additional adjunctive professionals (e.g., group treatment or a dietician if there are eating problems) and perhaps nonprofessionals (e.g., the additional support of a 12-step group). In this regard, it is important to obtain relevant releases to coordinate appropriate communications with members of the team, and efforts must be made to keep colleagues up to date on the client's suicide risk so they are prepared for any crises they may observe. A team approach is crucial for averting the burnout that often accompanies these challenging cases. Linehan (1993) asserted that MHPs working with difficult chronic cases should be required to attend weekly consultation meetings to improve clinical vitality and their ability to effectively treat high-risk clients. The potential for burnout becomes more pronounced in work settings in which providers carry heavy caseloads with several suicidal or self-harming clients, most notably community mental health centers.

Jobes (2006) recommended the use of suicide-specific treatment plans that consider both psychological and biological underpinning of suicidal states. Although the literature related to suicidal ideation is focused heavily on major psychiatric illnesses and psychopathology (for a summary, see Maris et al., 2000), more recent research has considered potentially crucial interactions between the central nervous system and the endocrine system. For example, some attention has been given to the hypothalamic–pituitary–adrenal axis, a key interactive system involved in stress management, including the flight-or-fight response (Bostwick, 2005; Pfennig et al., 2005).

However, what has been more traditional in this area of research is a focus on mood spectrum disorders, particularly those linked to seratonergic and norandregenic systems of the brain, which have been shown to respond to certain psychotropic medications. Yet, consistent with the larger treatment literature, combining psychosocial treatments and medication can prove to be therapeutically synergistic. For example, a recent study by the Treatment of Adolescent Depression Team (2004), consisting of specialists at several locations on the East Coast, showed that a combination of fluoxetine and cognitive–behavioral therapy was significantly more effective at reducing depressive symptoms than was either treatment alone. The study's authors described the sample as moderately severe, with 27% of participants reporting suicidal ideation at pretreatment.

In contrast to historic approaches to suicidal clients, there is an increasing emphasis on working with suicidal patients in outpatient settings. As discussed by Jobes (2003, 2006) and noted earlier, this trend reflects pressures imposed by managed mental health care given exponential increases in inpatient costs. However, there is also accumulating evidence that outpatient treatment of suicidal behavior can lead to more rapid decreases in suicidal ideation than inpatient treatment (Rudd, Joiner, Jobes, & King, 1999). It follows that involuntary hospitalization should only be used in the most dire of cases in which intensive outpatient treatment is not sufficient to ensure immediate safety and stability. Should any hospitalization occur, the therapist should immediately establish contact with the hospital staff to plan for discharge that usually occurs in a few short days.

However, when considering various approaches, it is important to know that there are remarkably few clinical trial studies of what actually works in the treatment of suicidal states (Linehan, 2005). To date, relatively structured cognitive–behavioral/skill-building approaches have had the most empirical support (e.g., Brown et al., 2005; Chiles & Strohsal, 1995; Linehan, 2005; Rudd, Joiner, & Rajab, 2001). Alternatively, there are various humanistic and psychodynamic approaches with intuitive clinical appeal (e.g., Jobes, 1995; Jobes & Karmel, 1996; Leenaars, 2004; Maltsberger, 1986), but such approaches need further empirical investigation.

Straddling some of these various perspectives is the Collaborative Assessment and Management of Suicidality, a relatively new clinical framework developed by Jobes (2006). Built on 15 years of empirical clinical research, the Collaborative Assessment and Management of Suicidality approach emphasizes the use of a multipurpose clinical tool called the Suicide Status Form, which serves to guide the clinical dyad through a collaborative assessment of the client's suicidal risk, leading to the development of a suicide-specific treatment plan that is coauthored with the client (Jobes & Drozd, 2004). Collaborative Assessment and Management of Suicidality is designed to enhance the clinical alliance while increasing client motivation; the approach guides the clinical interchange without dictating the nature of treatment or usurping the clinician's judgment. Critically, use of the Suicide Status Form provides a comprehensive medical record tracing the course of care from assessment to treatment to clinical outcomes.

After reviewing the treatment options mentioned previously, an MHP may still find that he or she faces an impossible case. Many clinicians have experienced trying everything they can think of to assist a complex client, all for naught. For example, if the fictitious clinician in the case of Sylvia had properly addressed suicide-related behaviors in his treatment plan and had used all realistic resources, he might still feel discouraged about Sylvia's prognosis. The bottom line is this: There is always a duty to protect, but relevant legal language invariably invokes an expectation of reasonableness. Frankly, one can do what one can do. Although clinicians' ability to guarantee safety has been increasingly challenged by contemporary limitations on hospitalizations, there is an evolving expectation that clinicians nevertheless must do their very best to thoughtfully assess, consult, document, and treat a suicidal client within the realities of the situation. At the end of the day, only the suicidal client can determine the final life-or-death outcome. What we can do is support, guide, teach, and optimize the therapeutic conditions for life-saving changes that may in the best scenarios help lead to a life worth living.

Professional Consultation

The importance of professional consultation cannot be overemphasized. This is true in a general sense and especially germane in cases of suicidal risk (Jobes & Berman, 1993). The pursuit and documentation of consultation naturally reflects a level of thoughtfulness and concern on the part of the practicing clinician. It indicates that the therapist was not working in isolation but rather was seeking the input of a trusted colleague who would naturally have more objectivity on the case (being one step removed). Thus, clinicians should always and regularly seek professional consultation in high-risk cases—it is a part of our ethical traditions and emblematic of competent clinical care.

The use of contemporaneous consultation with a qualified consultant in high-risk cases helps establish that a thorough assessment and a reasonable course of action were pursued. The information received should be clearly documented and can even be sent back to the consultant to establish that agreement about how to proceed occurred (Simpson & Stacey, 2004). Selection of an appropriate consultant may depend on the case; typically, a good consultant will be an established MHP of similar training who is clearly experienced with the kind of case in question. In a particularly complex situation, it may make sense to seek consultation from an MHP and an attorney who is familiar with mental health law.

Clinical Referrals

The health and mental health fields are made up of professionals from many disciplines; each type of health provider has unique skills and areas of expertise. Thus, the appropriate use of clinical referrals is critical to competent care, particularly in high-risk cases of suicidality. For example, a primary care physician, psychiatrist, neurologist, or dietician can provide additional insights into client behaviors and potential biological stressors to nonmedical providers. The MHP should routinely refer the client to a psychiatrist, psychiatric nurse practitioner, or medical psychologist for a psychopharmacological evaluation if apparent symptoms could have a potential biological basis. For example, classic vegetative symptoms associated with major depression, symptoms of bipolar disorder, any evidence of psychosis, or serious anxiety should automatically trigger a referral to an appropriate health professional for evaluation and possible pharmacological care. In cases of eating disorders (e.g., anorexia or bulimia nervosa), referral to an appropriate physician is always critical to monitoring and maintaining the patient's ongoing medical stability. Alternatively, social workers, counselors, or medical practitioners may need to refer patients to a psychologist for diagnostic assessment and psychological testing. Knowing the limits and strengths of each discipline is critical to making appropriate and informed clinical referrals.

SUPERVISORY ISSUES

A widely overlooked area of clinical responsibility and the duty to protect involves supervision issues with unlicensed clinicians or clinicians-in-training. Supervisory responsibilities of licensed providers in cases of suicide are considerable and cannot be overstated. Invariably, licensed professionals are ultimately responsible for the clinical practices of their supervisees. In cases of suicidal risk, the supervisor must be closely involved in care and should consider countersigning all documentation. For trainees, the burden of losing a client during the start of one's career can be extremely traumatic. It is essential that students in graduate programs receive proper training to deal with suicidal clients, as well as support after the unfortunate circumstance in which a client takes his or her own life.

In this vein, Ellis and Dickey (1998) examined psychology and psychiatry internship programs across the United States to capture the degree to which graduate students and medical residents receive formalized training on issues related to client suicide. Their study showed that although the majority of both psychiatry and psychology programs conducted some form of suicide training, fewer than 50% of all training programs offer workshops specific to treating suicidal clients or training in coping with the suicide of a client. Although it is not widely known, supervisory discussion after a suicide may need to be limited in content because of potential concerns about malpractice-related issues (i.e., a supervisor's being compelled to divulge postsuicide debriefing regarding supervisee mistakes). It is important for MHPs-in-training to receive adequate training before working with suicidal clients (refer to Ellis & Dickey, 1998).

CONCLUSION

This chapter began with the tragic case of Sylvia, a promising college student who tumbled into the depths of a severe depression, substance abuse, and suicidal thoughts. Sylvia was clearly someone who could have been helped by proper clinical assessment and treatment. Hindsight is almost always 20/20. However, the clinician in this case clearly failed in his duty to protect his client by thoroughly assessing and appropriately treating Sylvia's life-threatening distress. It is plain that there should have been a much more comprehensive assessment of her depression and substance abuse; her suicidal ideation should also have been much more thoroughly assessed. A thoughtfully developed treatment plan that included a psychiatric referral plus structured support, problem solving, and plans for coping with her distress and suicidal impulses could have made a life-saving difference. An emphasis on intensive suicide-focused outpatient treatment, coupled with more intensive measures (e.g., inpatient hospitalization) might have averted this tragedy, but the clinician in this case neglected his duty to protect this otherwise promising young woman from her suicidal despair.

As described throughout this book, MHPs have certain and distinct professional duties toward their clients. Few issues in mental health prompt the level of clinical responsibility that a suicidal client demands. Indeed, one's professional duty to respond to any suicidal risk in a reasonable and competent manner can potentially make a profound difference with clear implications for malpractice liability should the clinician fail in carrying out this duty. Given the potential repercussions, we believe that all suicidal clients deserve competent clinical assessments and treatments that may well prove to be part of a life-saving endeavor.

REFERENCES

American Psychiatric Association. (1994). *Diagnostic and statistical manual of mental disorders* (4th ed.). Washington, DC: Author.

American Psychological Association. (2003). Guidelines on multicultural education, training, research, practice, and organizational change for psychologists. *American Psychologist, 58,* 377–402.

Bagley, C., & Tremblay, P. (1997). Suicidal behaviors in homosexual and bisexual males. *Crisis, 18,* 24–34.

Berman, A. L. (1986). Notes on turning 18 (and 75): A critical look at our adolescence. *Suicide and Life-Threatening Behavior, 12,* 1–12.

Berman, A. L., Jobes, D. A., & Silverman, M. M. (2006). *Adolescent suicide: Assessment and intervention* (2nd ed.). Washington, DC: American Psychological Association.

Bongar, B. (2002). *The suicidal patient: Clinical and legal standards of care* (2nd ed.). Washington, DC: American Psychological Association.

Bostwick, J. M. (2005). The stress axis gone awry: A possible neuroendocrine explanation for increased risk of completed suicide. *Primary Psychiatry, 12*, 49–52.

Brown, G. K., Ten Have, T., Henriques, G. R., Xie, S., Hollander, J. E., & Beck, A. T. (2005, August 3). Cognitive therapy for the prevention of suicide attempts. *JAMA, 294*, 563–570.

Bryan, C. J., & Rudd, M. D. (2006). Advances in the assessment of suicide risk. *Journal of Clinical Psychology: In Session, 62*, 185–200.

Chiles, J. A., & Strosahl, K. D. (1995). *The suicidal patient: Principles of assessment, treatment, and case management.* Washington, DC: American Psychiatric Association.

Cornelius, J. R., Salloum, I. M., Mezzich, J., Cornelius, M. D., Fabrega, H., Jr., Ehler, J. G., et al. (1995). Disproportionate suicidality in patients with comorbid major depression and alcoholism. *American Journal of Psychiatry, 152*, 358–364.

de Moore, G. M., & Robertson, A. R. (1999). Suicide attempts by firearms and by leaping from heights: A comparative study of survivors. *American Journal of Psychiatry, 156*, 1425–1431.

Ellis, T. E., & Dickey, T. O. (1998). Procedures surrounding the suicide of a trainee's patient: A national survey of psychology internships and psychiatry residency programs. *Professional Psychology: Research and Practice, 29*, 492–497.

Garlow, S. J., Purselle, D., & Heninger, M. (2005). Ethnic differences in patterns of suicide across the life cycle. *American Journal of Psychiatry, 162*, 319–323.

Health Insurance Accountability & Portability Act of 1996, Public Law 104-191, 110 Stat. 1936 (1996).

Herrell, R., Goldberg, J., True, W. R., Ramakrishnan, V., Lyons, M., Eisen, S., et al. (1999). Sexual orientation and suicidality: A co-twin study in adult men. *Archives of General Psychiatry, 56*, 867–874.

Hjern, A. (2002). Suicide in first and second generation immigrants in Sweden: A comparative study. *Social Psychiatry and Psychiatric Epidemiology, 37*, 423–429.

Jobes, D. A. (1995). The challenge and promise of clinical suicidology. *Suicide and Life-Threatening Behavior, 25*, 437–449.

Jobes, D. A. (2000). Collaborating to prevent suicide: A clinical-research perspective. *Suicide and Life-Threatening Behavior, 30*, 8–17.

Jobes, D. A. (2003). Understanding suicide in the 21st century. *Preventing Suicide: The National Journal, 2*, 2–4.

Jobes, D. A. (2006). *Managing suicidal risk: A collaborative approach.* New York: Guilford Press.

Jobes, D. A., & Berman, A. L. (1993). Suicide and malpractice liability: Assessing and revising policies, procedures, and practice in outpatient settings. *Professional Psychology: Research and Practice, 24*, 91–99.

Jobes, D. A., & Drozd, J. F. (2004). The CAMS approach to working with suicidal patients. *Journal of Contemporary Psychotherapy, 34*, 73–85.

Jobes, D. A., & Karmel, M. P. (1996). Case consultation with a suicidal adolescent. In A. Leenaars & D. Lester (Eds.), *Suicide and the unconscious* (pp. 175–193). Northvale, NJ: Jason Aronson.

Jobes, D. A., & Maltsberger, J. T. (1995). The hazards of treating suicidal patients. In B. M. Sussman (Ed.), *A perilous calling: The hazards of psychotherapy practice* (pp. 200–214). New York: Wiley.

Jobes, D. A., & Mann, R. E. (1999). Reasons for living versus reasons for dying: Examining the internal debate of suicide. *Suicide and Life-Threatening Behavior, 29,* 97–104.

Jobes, D. A., Nelson, K. N., Peterson, E. M., Pentiuc, D., Downing, V., Francini, K., et al. (2004). Describing suicidality: An investigation of qualitative SSF responses. *Suicide and Life-Threatening Behavior, 34,* 99–112.

Joiner, T. E., Rudd, M. D., & Rajab, M. H. (1997). The Modified Scale for Suicidal Ideation: Factors of suicidality and their relation to clinical and diagnostic variables. *Journal of Abnormal Psychology, 106,* 260–265.

Joiner, T. E., Walker, R. L., Rudd, M. D., & Jobes, D. A. (1999). Scientizing and routinizing the assessment of suicidality in outpatient practice. *Professional Psychology: Research and Practice, 30,* 447–453.

Kessler, R. C., Berglund, P., Borges, G., Nock, M., & Wang, P. S. (2005, May 25). Trends in suicide ideation, plans, gestures, and attempts in the United States, 1990–1992 to 2001–2003. *JAMA, 293,* 2487–2495.

Kovacs, M., & Beck, A. T. (1977). The wish to die and the wish to live in attempted suicides. *Journal of Clinical Psychology, 33,* 361–365.

Leenaars, A. A. (2004). *Psychotherapy with suicidal people: A person-centered approach.* New York: Wiley.

Linehan, M. M. (1993). *Cognitive–behavioral treatment of borderline personality disorder.* New York: Guilford Press.

Linehan, M. M. (2005, August). *Latest research on suicide and DBT.* Paper presented at the 113th Annual Convention of the American Psychological Association, Washington, DC.

Linehan, M. M., Goodstein, J. L., Nielsen, S. L., & Chiles, J. A. (1983). Reasons for staying alive when you are thinking of killing yourself: The Reasons for Living Inventory. *Journal of Consulting and Clinical Psychology, 51,* 276–286.

Luoma, J. B., Martin, C. E., & Pearson, J. L. (2003). Contact with mental health and primary care providers before suicide: A review of the evidence. *American Journal of Psychiatry, 159,* 909–916.

Maltsberger, J. T. (1986). *Suicide risk: The formulation of clinical judgment.* New York: New York University Press.

Maris, R. W., Berman, A. L., & Silverman, M. M. (2000). *Comprehensive textbook of suicidology.* New York: Guilford Press.

McKenzie, K., Serfaty, M., & Crawford, M. (2003). Suicide in ethnic minority groups. *British Journal of Psychiatry, 183,* 100–101.

Millon, T. (2004). *Masters of the mind: Exploring the story of mental illness from ancient times to the new millennium.* Hoboken, NJ: Wiley.

Oquendo, M. A., Galfalvy, H., Russo, S., Ellis, S. P., Grunebaum, M. F., Burke, A., et al. (2004). Prospective study of clinical predictors of suicidal acts after a major depressive episode in patients with major depressive disorder or bipolar disorder. *American Journal of Psychiatry, 161,* 1433–1441.

Orbach, I. (2001). Therapeutic empathy with the suicidal wish. *American Journal of Psychotherapy, 55,* 166–184.

Paul, J. P., Catania, J., Pollack, L., Moskowitz, J., Canchola, J., Mills, T., et al. (2002). Suicide attempts among gay and bisexual men: Lifetime prevalence and antecedents. *American Journal of Public Health, 92,* 1338–1345.

Pfennig, A., Kunzel, H. E., Kern, N., Ising, M., Majer, M., Fuchs, B., et al. (2005). Hypothalamus–pituitary–adrenal system regulation and suicidal behavior in depression. *Biological Psychiatry, 57,* 336–342.

Robertson, J. D. (1988). *Psychiatric malpractice: Liability of mental health professionals.* New York: Wiley.

Rogers, C. R. (1957). The necessary and sufficient conditions of therapeutic personality change. *Journal of Consulting Psychology, 21,* 95–103.

Rudd, M. D. (2006). Suicidality in clinical practice: Anxieties and answers. *Journal of Clinical Psychology, 62,* 157–159.

Rudd, M. D., Joiner, T. E., Jobes, D. A., & King, C. A. (1999). The outpatient treatment of suicidality: An integration of science and recognition of its limitations. *Professional Psychology: Research and Practice, 30,* 437–446.

Rudd, M. D., Joiner, T., & Rajab, M. H. (2001). *Treating suicidal behavior: An effective time limited approach.* New York: Guilford Press.

Rudmin, F. L., Ferrada-Noli, M., & Skolbekken, J. (2003). Questions of culture, age and gender in the epidemiology of suicide. *Scandinavian Journal of Psychology, 44,* 373–381.

Shea, S. C. (1999). *The practical art of suicide assessment: A guide for mental health professionals and substance abuse counselors.* New York: Wiley.

Shneidman, E. S. (1996). *The suicidal mind.* New York: Oxford University Press.

Simpson, S., & Stacey, M. (2004). Avoiding the malpractice snare: Documenting suicide risk assessment. *Journal of Psychiatric Practice, 10,* 185–189.

Treatment of Adolescent Depression Team. (2004, August 18). Fluoxetine, cognitive–behavioral therapy, and their combination for adolescents with depression: Treatment for Adolescents With Depression Study (TADS) randomized controlled trial. *JAMA, 292,* 807–820.

Wise, T. L., Jobes, D. A., Simpson, S., & Berman, A. L. (2005, April). *Suicidal client and clinician: Approach or avoidance.* Panel presentation at the annual conference of the American Association of Suicidology, Denver, CO.

12

STRATEGIES FOR RESPONDING TO SELF-INJURY: WHEN DOES THE DUTY TO PROTECT APPLY?

BARENT WALSH

Self-injury has been defined as when people deliberately harm their bodies, usually without suicidal intent, to reduce psychological distress (Walsh, 2006). Common forms of self-injury include wrist, arm, and body cutting; self-hitting; burning and branding; self-biting and excoriation of wounds; and picking, scratching, abrading, and hair pulling (Simeon & Hollander, 2001). Self-injury should be differentiated from diverse forms of body modification such as professionally obtained tattoos, body piercings, and brandings because these are imposed by others and are usually not used to manage psychological distress. Self-injury often poses complex challenges for professional caregivers. Consider the following two anecdotes, which have been modified considerably to protect confidentiality:

> Cheryl is a 16-year-old adolescent whose parents have brought her to the emergency room. She is a talented young woman who does well in school and sports and has many friends. The previous evening, Cheryl's parents discovered that she had inflicted six superficial cuts on her left wrist and forearm. They became quite worried that she might be suicidal. Cheryl tells the emergency room personnel that she did not want to die

181

but wanted to "get all the anxiety out." Her wounds do not require medical attention. The clinical questions regarding this incident are whether this behavior should be considered suicidal and what is an appropriate plan of action.

Abe is a 23-year-old who is living in a supported housing program for mentally ill adults. He was physically and sexually abused as a child and endured multiple foster home placements during his early years. He has a long history of self-injury dating back to age 14. In the past, Abe has usually cut or burned his arms or legs. His wounds have almost always not required medical intervention. On this occasion, however, Abe has done considerable damage. He lacerated his arm, requiring 11 stitches to close the wounds. The clinical questions in this case are whether, given his level of physical damage, Abe should be considered for psychiatric hospitalization or whether, because he has a long history of low-lethality self-injury, he should be returned directly to his supported housing program.

WHO SELF-INJURES?

Self-injury at present appears to be bimodally distributed in the United States. On one end of this distribution, it has for years been known that individuals who self-injure may come from backgrounds of loss, neglect, trauma, and abuse (Alderman, 1997; Favazza, 1996, 1998; Favazza & Conterio, 1988; Walsh & Rosen, 1988). Until the mid-1990s, the individuals who were identified as having self-injured tended to be individuals with serious psychological disturbance. Most frequently, self-injurers were

- outpatients with serious emotional disturbance or mental illness;
- persons recurrently presenting at psychiatric emergency rooms;
- seriously and persistently mentally ill persons in day treatment or partial hospitalization programs or those living in community-based residential or supported housing programs;
- patients in short- and long-term psychiatric and forensic units;
- youths in special education schools, residential treatment, or juvenile detention facilities; and
- inmates in correctional institutions.

It is not surprising that individuals served in such locations have tended to have serious psychiatric diagnoses such as borderline personality disorder, posttraumatic stress disorder, dissociative disorders, anorexia nervosa, bulimia, depression, anxiety, obsessive–compulsive disorder, antisocial personality disorder, and even a variety of psychoses (see Walsh, 2006, for a review of this literature).

Therefore, from the 1960s through the early 1990s, the assumption (correct or not) was that if someone self-injured, he or she was probably seriously disturbed and suffering from considerable functional impairment. Persons who self-injured were generally thought to have compromised social functioning and a diminished ability to deal with the demands of school or work. However, a new emerging phenomenon (and the other end of the bimodal distribution) is the self-injury of relatively healthy middle school, high school, and university students (S. Ross & Heath, 2002; Walsh, 2006; Whitlock, Eckenrode, & Silverman, 2006). For example, Whitlock et al. (2006) reported that in a sample of almost 3,000 students at Cornell and Princeton Universities, 17% indicated having self-injured. Even higher percentages have been reported in other college samples by Gratz, Conrad, and Roemer (2002) and Kokaliari (2005). The Cornell Research Program on Self-Injurious Behavior (n.d.) stated that

> the few studies which have been conducted in U.S. community samples of young adults and adolescents are limited by small convenience-based samples and vary in estimates of self-injury prevalence from 4% to 38% (Briere & Gil, 1998; Favazza, 1996; Gratz, Conrad, & Roemer, 2002; Kokaliari, 2005; Muehlenkamp & Gutierrez, 2004).

This emerging group of "healthier" self-injurers is intriguing because these individuals are able to function in school and society, including at highly competitive universities. Such capabilities suggest that old stereotypes about self-injurers being "borderlines with poor prognoses" have to be abandoned. Another stereotype that self-injurers are by and large female has also proved to be untrue. Most recent research samples have relatively high percentages of male self-injurers—ranging from 32% to 42% (e.g., Briere & Gil, 1998; Rodham, Hawton, & Evans, 2004)—with one (Gratz et al., 2002) actually having more male (56%) than female self-injurers.

RESPONDING TO SELF-INJURY

Regardless of whether one is dealing with seriously disturbed self-injurers or higher functioning individuals, it is important to learn how to respond strategically and effectively to the behavior. As noted later, in the majority of cases self-injurious behavior may not require a duty to protect. Nonetheless, in certain unusual instances, duty to protect regarding atypical self-injury may apply. The following sections detail making this key distinction.

Generally, responding strategically and effectively to self-injury requires a three-step process: (a) adequately understanding self-injury in relation to suicide, (b) skillfully assessing the behavior in all its details, and (c) developing a plan to manage and treat the behavior thereafter. In this chapter, I review these three steps in the order presented. I also return to the case examples presented at the outset.

Understanding Self-Injury

A key point in understanding self-injury is that the behavior is generally separate and distinct from suicide. As mentioned earlier, the most common forms of self-injury (e.g., cutting, scratching, carving; Alderman, 1997; Conterio & Lader, 1998; Favazza, 1996; Simeon & Hollander, 2001; Walsh, 2006) rarely result in death. More specifically, recent statistics compiled by the American Association of Suicidology (2006) demonstrated that cutting or piercing is a method of suicide for a very small percentage of people who die by suicide (1.8% vs. 53.7% who died by firearms and 21.1% who died by suffocation or hanging). However, cutting is the most common form of self-injury. Moreover, for those who do die, the cutting generally involves cutting the neck and severing the carotid artery or jugular vein. Most self-injurers cut the extremities or abdomen, not the neck. In addition, the other forms of self-injury listed above do not appear on the list of lethal methods. This characteristic argues for self-injury being considered a different form of self-harm than suicidal behavior, so the issues of when or whether the duty to protect applies deserve different consideration.

If self-injury is not about suicide, then what is it about? There is considerable evidence that most people self-injure to regulate emotional distress such as intense feelings of anxiety, anger, sadness, depression, guilt, shame, or even deadness. Emotion regulation is the most commonly cited reason for self-injuring (Alderman, 1997; Brown, Comtois, & Linehan, 2002; Conterio & Lader, 1998; Favazza, 1996; Walsh & Rosen, 1988).

However, self-injury can also be contagious, especially among teens (Favazza, 1996; Ross & McKay, 1979; Taiminen, Kallio-Soukainen, Nokso-Koivisto, Kaljonen, & Helenius, 1998; Walsh, 2006; Walsh & Rosen, 1985). In such cases, youths may trigger the behavior in each other by using it for diverse interpersonal reasons, including as a form of communication, controlling others via threat, competing with each other as to level of damage, resolving conflicts via self-harm, or generating intimacy by sharing the common problem of self-injury (Walsh, 2006). In other words, interpersonal factors can lead to the spread of self-injury in a peer group. In addition, Whitlock, Powers, and Eckenrode (2006) recently provided evidence that self-injury can be triggered via communication on the Internet. They reported that college students who self-injure spent substantially more time in Web sites, chatrooms, and message boards devoted to self-injury than did students who did not self-injure. Communications on the Internet can lead to competition, disinhibition, or triggering among self-injuring individuals. Therefore, understanding self-injury requires that one consider both intrapersonal functions (e.g., emotion regulation) and interpersonal functions (e.g., contagion influences; Nock & Prinstein, 2004; Walsh, 2006).

Assessing Self-Injury

Assessing self-injury generally involves an emphasis on the therapeutic alliance by initially responding to self-injury with a "low-key dispassionate demeanor" (Walsh, 2006, p. 76). Clients who self-injure are emotionally distressed and will not collaborate with the clinician if they are judged or criticized for their behavior. In addition, well-intended, effusive expressions of support may seem quite gratifying to such clients. However, these may lead to inadvertent reinforcement of the behavior. As a result, the most helpful strategy is to proceed in an understated, compassionate way that is neither reinforcing nor punitive.

Clients also generally find it helpful if professionals respond with "respectful curiosity" about the self-injury (Kettlewell, 1999). Asking clients, "What does self-injury do for you?" can open the door for useful information about the functions of the behavior. In contrast, quickly attempting to "contract for safety" may be contraindicated. Asking individuals to give up self-injury when it is their most efficacious emotion regulation technique can be unrealistic in the short term. Clients may also view efforts to contract for safety as an implicit form of condemnation, which would negatively affect the therapeutic alliance. Once the professional has set a nonjudgmental, respectfully curious tone, he or she can next launch into a more formal assessment. Key elements in conducting a thorough assessment include identifying the following:

1. *Environmental, biological, and psychological antecedents to the behavior.* These triggers are important in that they (a) can be used to predict future self-injury and (b) can become opportunities to practice replacement skills. For example, if self-injury typically follows a disagreement with a parent or peer, these incidents can be identified as high-risk periods. These incidents can then be targeted as opportunities to practice replacement skills as opposed to proceeding to the usual self-injurious outcomes.

2. *Number of wounds and extent of physical damage.* These details point to the level of distress and whether there is a need for protective intervention (see below). In general, the greater the number of wounds, the greater the level of distress. In addition, considerable research has indicated that most incidents of self-injury involve only modest tissue damage that does not require medical intervention (Favazza, 1996; Simeon & Hollander, 2001; Walsh, 2006). When individuals hurt

themselves in ways that require suturing or other medical response, this is atypical and points to the need for immediate psychiatric evaluation and protective interventions such as psychiatric hospitalization.

3. *Time*. This refers to both time of day and duration of episode. Many self-injurers harm themselves at bedtime to get to sleep; however, for others, time of day is far more random. Identifying high-risk times can be used to practice replacement skills and alter routines. Duration of episodes points to the amount of time it takes to achieve relief. Longer episodes suggest greater levels of distress and are thereby more alarming.

4. *Body area*. Most self-injurers harm the extremities or abdomen (Favazza & Conterio, 1988; Simeon & Hollander, 2001). Body areas that are alarming from an assessment point of view are face, eyes, and breasts in female clients and genitals in either sex (Walsh, 2006). Generally, people who injure these body areas are experiencing psychotic decompensation or some type of primitive trauma reenactment (Walsh, 2006). Such individuals should receive an emergency psychiatric assessment. Psychiatric hospitalizations are often indicated for these relatively rare types of self-injury.

5. *Pattern to wounds*. Some clients inflict words or symbols on their bodies. Common examples are words like *hate*, *pain*, a partner's name, or an inverted crucifix. It is useful to explore why the self-injurer has chosen to impose this specific content on his or her body.

6. *Use of a tool*. Generally, using a tool such as razor blade, lighter, brand, or knife indicates more control and sophistication than does using more primitive methods such as punching, scratching, or gouging oneself. There are notable exceptions, however, such as when someone randomly cuts all over his or her body.

7. *Physical location*. Determining where the acts of self-injury tend to occur is important to identifying situational triggers.

8. *Social context*. Does the self-injury occur alone or with others? Most people self-injure alone, but some teens and adults cut or burn together. Other individuals may be triggered to self-injure after participating in a self-injury chat room or message board (Whitlock, Powers, & Eckenrode, 2006). Some adolescents may self-injure in defiance of their parents. Therefore, identifying these social reinforcers is an important part of assessment.

9. *Aftermath*. It is important to determine the short- and long-term consequences of the self-injury. What does the behavior

accomplish for the individual? If it reduces anger or anxiety, then the client needs new skills in managing anger or anxiety. If it reengages a neglectful boyfriend or spouse, then the client needs more effective interpersonal skills. Individuals cannot be expected to give up self-injury unless the positive outcomes they receive from self-injury are obtainable by other means.

Duty to Protect in Response to Self-Injury

Central to the theme of this book is the topic of duty to protect. On the basis of the guidelines for assessment provided above, a number of recommendations can be made:

1. Self-injury should be clearly distinguished from suicidal behavior. More specifically, if clients disclose plans to or actually use potentially lethal methods, the duty to protect applies. These suicidal methods include use of a gun, pill or drug overdose, hanging, jumping from a height, self-poisoning such as carbon monoxide ingestion, self-drowning, and cutting the neck. Such individuals should be provided protective interventions immediately to ensure their safety.

2. In contrast, if the self-harm is common, low-lethality self-injury, emergency procedures including the duty to protect are generally not necessary. For example, if a high school student reports to a guidance counselor that he or she has been cutting, the response should generally not be to call an ambulance for transportation to a local emergency room. The self-injury can be handled on an outpatient basis without undue concern. In a school setting, the staff should notify the parents or guardians that their child is self-injuring. An explanation can be provided that indicates that the behavior is generally not about suicide but does point to emotional distress. The parents or guardians should be asked to follow up quickly with outpatient counseling. Specific names and phone numbers should be provided. A more detailed presentation of a school protocol is provided in Walsh (2006).

3. There are exceptions regarding self-injury that do require a duty to protect. These apply when the damage to the body requires medical attention such as suturing or other medical procedures. Research has shown that such damage is rare. Moreover, the physical damage in such situations is considerable and therefore should be assessed immediately. Protective intervention may be necessary to prevent additional bodily harm.

4. Another time the duty to protect may apply is when persons hurt atypical areas of the body, including the face, eyes, breasts, and genitals. These forms of self-harm are rare and are associated with psychotic decompensation or primitive trauma reenactment. In either case, there is a duty to protect these individuals until they are psychologically restabilized and behaviorally safe. Some might argue that using the term *duty to protect* exceeds proper legal usage here. I would argue otherwise because these types of self-injury can entail a severe level of bodily harm and, thereby, potential risk to life. Examples would be self-enucleation (self-inflicted eyeball removal) or autocastration that can certainly be life threatening. Therefore, I believe that a duty to protect does apply for these atypical and sometimes extreme forms of self-injurious behavior.

5. There can, however, be exceptions to the guideline about self-injury to certain body areas. For example, some adolescents may pierce their eyebrows or nostrils or lips—which technically involves the face and, thereby, an atypical and alarming part of the body. Such body modification may be more peer group experimentation than a truly atypical or extreme self-injury and, if so, will not require a duty to protect.

6. The range of protective interventions includes psychiatric hospitalizations, placement in short-term respite or stabilization settings, intense wraparound supervision, and residential placements. For atypical or extreme self-injury, psychopharmacological assessment and intervention are often an important aspect of treatment. After more intensive interventions, follow-up treatment on an outpatient basis is required, which is reviewed in the next section.

Treating Self-Injury

A few empirically supported treatments have emerged for working with clients who self-injure. The treatments that have shown the most promise to date are dialectical behavior therapy, developed by Linehan (1993a, 1993b, 2000; Linehan et al., 2006), and problem-solving therapy, developed by D'Zurilla (D'Zurilla & Goldfried, 1971; D'Zurilla & Nezu, 2001). See Muehlenkamp (2006) for a thorough review of the evidence in support of the efficacy of these treatments. Another therapy that has shown encouraging results in the treatment of self-injury is the acceptance-based emotion regulation group intervention developed by Gratz and Gunderson (2006). Although a thorough review of the details of these treatments is beyond the scope of this chapter, it is possible to indicate their common characteristics.

As noted by Muehlenkamp (2006, pp. 175–176), the common features of dialectical behavior therapy and problem-solving therapy are (a) an emphasis on an empathic, collaborative therapeutic relationship; (b) time-limited structured treatment (using a prescribed manual); (c) completion of a detailed functional behavioral analysis; (d) behavioral interventions, including attention to and modification of contingencies; (e) the teaching of new, more adaptive skills to regulate emotions and interact with others; and (f) modification of cognitive distortions and negative core beliefs.

Both dialectical behavior therapy and problem-solving therapy involve manualized treatments with specific protocols and intervention steps. Even for clinicians who do not implement such highly structured, prescribed treatments, there are basic steps that are highly recommended, which are summarized as follows:

1. Triggers are identified and, when they recur, are used to practice replacement skills in an effort to fend off self-injury.

2. Replacement skills that self-injurers typically find useful are those that help them regulate their emotions more effectively. Examples include mindful breathing and visualization techniques (Walsh, 2006); self-soothing skills for all five senses (Linehan, 1993b); writing and journaling (Conterio & Lader, 1998); and exercising (noncompetitively), creating artwork, playing or listening to music, communicating with others, and distracting oneself (Linehan, 1993b; Walsh, 2006). Clients need to practice these replacement skills when they are calm if the skills are to be effective when they become agitated and distressed.

3. Therapists should practice skills with clients during sessions and structure the practice for clients between sessions. Reinforcing clients for practicing skills is very important.

4. Many clients also require assistance with dysfunctional thoughts and beliefs that support their self-injury (Beck, 1995; Walsh, 2006; Walsh & Rosen, 1988). For example, some individuals are convinced that self-injury is the only thing that works or that they deserve this physical harm. These types of thoughts need to be compassionately challenged. The therapist can indicate that although self-injury does work in terms of regulating emotional distress, the client has learned other skills that work as well. In a similar vein, the therapist can compassionately dispute that anyone deserves self-injury. Rather, people deserve physical protection and nurturance, not self-damage. Such cognitive restructuring strategies often require that clients work on dysfunctional beliefs regarding their basic "unlovability" or "incompetence." Keeping logs of

one's dysfunctional thoughts and correcting them for more positive self-statements can be a useful ongoing exercise (Beck, 1995; Walsh, 2006).

5. For those self-injurers who have been mistreated and abused, an additional therapeutic step may be necessary. This is generally referred to as *exposure therapy*, a treatment for which there is considerable empirical evidence as to its efficacy (e.g., Foa, Keane, & Friedman, 2000; Follette, Ruzek, & Abueg, 1998). Exposure therapy involves systematically exposing clients to traumatic memories so that they can master emotional distress and related self-injury. In exposure treatment, clients first learn to understand the nature of their reactions to traumatic events. Next, they learn self-soothing techniques such as breathing retraining (Foa et al., 2000; Walsh, 2006). Then, they create a hierarchy or list of traumatic memories, ranking them from least to most upsetting. Next, clients retrieve these memories in session and practice breathing or other self-soothing strategies until the level of distress becomes tolerable (Foa at al., 2000). This practice is repeated over time until the traumatic content loses its power to dysregulate and disorganize. Finally, clients learn to generalize the practice to the real world so that they can deal with trauma-related experiences wherever and whenever these situations arise. Many of the more disturbed self-injurers may require this additional therapeutic strategy to overcome their traumatic past and give up self-injury (Favazza, 1998; Walsh, 2006).

CONCLUSION

In this chapter, I have described how self-injury is different from suicide, provided some detailed information about how to assess self-injury, and reviewed some basics in managing and treating the behavior. I have also discussed when a duty to protect applies and when it does not. Recalling the case examples presented earlier, I now offer some guidelines as to how to respond.

Cheryl is a high-functioning 16-year-old who is representative of the new generation of self-injuring persons. She is talented, competent in school and athletics, and socially connected. Her self-injury consisted of six superficial cuts on her wrist and forearm that required no medical attention. In addition, Cheryl has denied suicidal intent, saying she just wanted to "get all the anxiety out." For this incident, the evidence points to the behavior being an example of common low-lethality self-injury. Psychiatric hospitalization is not indicated. After a thorough assessment of her self-injury is completed, Cheryl should be referred to outpatient counseling that places an emphasis on her need to learn some replacement skills so that she can manage her anxiety and other intense emotions more effectively. She may also need some cognitive treatment to help her modify dysfunctional thoughts and beliefs that support her self-harm behavior. The only duty to protect (or inform) that would have been necessary is informing her parents of the self-injury so that they could obtain treatment for her; however, because they brought her in to the hospital, they are already aware of the behavior.

Abe poses far more complex treatment challenges than Cheryl. First, his level of functioning is much more compromised. He has a long history of abandonment, abuse, and placement. He also has been self-injuring for years and is a member of the adult mental health system. His most recent self-injury is concerning as well. The level of physical damage is atypical in that it required 11 stitches to repair the wounds. For Abe, a form of the duty to protect applies. The amount of physical damage he has inflicted argues for a short-term psychiatric hospitalization, which will provide protection and allow for a more detailed assessment of his mental status. A key unresolved assessment question is why Abe's level of physical damage has markedly increased at this time. This question should be addressed during the hospitalization. Psychopharmacological intervention or adjustment may be indicated.

Treatment for Abe is likely to be long term. He will need extensive skills training to combat his long history of self-injury. He will need cognitive restructuring to help him with core beliefs about unlovability and incompetence. He may also need exposure treatment to deal with his long history of abandonment and abuse. It is fortunate that he resides in a supported housing program because he is likely to require ongoing risk assessment and daily support as he goes through this complex treatment process.

REFERENCES

Alderman, T. (1997). *The scarred soul: Understanding and ending self-inflicted violence.* Oakland, CA: New Harbinger.

American Association of Suicidology. (2006). *U.S.A. suicide: 2003 official final data.* Washington, DC: Author. Retrieved November 27, 2006, from http://www.suicidology.org/associations/1045/files/2003data.pdf

Beck, J. S. (1995). *Cognitive therapy: Basics and beyond.* New York: Guilford Press.

Briere, J., & Gil, E. (1998). Self-mutilation in clinical and general population samples: Prevalence, correlates, and functions. *American Journal of Orthopsychiatry, 68,* 609–620.

Brown, M., Comtois, K. A., & Linehan, M. M. (2002). Reasons for suicide attempts and nonsuicidal self-injury in women with borderline personality disorder. *Journal of Abnormal Psychology, 111,* 198–202.

Conterio, K., & Lader, W. (1998). *Bodily harm.* New York: Hyperion.

Cornell Research Program on Self-Injurious Behavior. (n.d.). *What do we know about self-injury?* Retrieved November 27, 2006, from http://www.crpsib.com/whatissi.asp

D'Zurilla, T. J., & Goldfried, M. R. (1971). Problem solving and behavior modification. *Journal of Abnormal Psychology, 78,* 107–126.

D'Zurilla, T. J., & Nezu, A. M. (2001). Problem solving therapies. In K. Dobson (Ed.), *Handbook of cognitive-behavioral therapies* (2nd ed., pp. 211–245). New York: Guilford Press.

Favazza, A. (1996). *Bodies under siege* (2nd ed.). Baltimore: John Hopkins University Press.

Favazza, A. (1998). The coming of age of self-mutilation. *Journal of Nervous and Mental Disease, 186,* 259–268.

Favazza, A., & Conterio, K. (1988). The plight of chronic self-mutilators. *Community Mental Health Journal, 24,* 22–30.

Foa, E. B., Keane, T. M., & Friedman, M. J. (Eds.). (2000). *Effective treatments for PTSD.* New York: Guilford Press.

Follette, V. M., Ruzek, J. I., & Abueg, F. R. (Eds.). (1998). *Cognitive–behavioral therapies for trauma.* New York: Guilford Press.

Gratz, K. L., Conrad, S. D., & Roemer, L. (2002). Risk factors for deliberate self-harm among college students. *American Journal of Orthopsychiatry, 72,* 128–140.

Gratz, K. L., & Gunderson, J. G. (2006). Preliminary data on an acceptance-based emotion regulation group intervention for deliberate self-harm among women with borderline personality disorder. *Behavior Therapy, 37,* 25–35.

Kettlewell, C. (1999). *Skin game: A cutter's memoir.* New York: St. Martin's.

Kokaliari, E. D. (2005). *Deliberate self-injury: An investigation of the prevalence and psychosocial meanings in a non-clinical female college population.* Unpublished doctoral dissertation, Smith College School for Social Work.

Linehan, M. M. (1993a). *Cognitive–behavioral treatment of borderline personality disorder.* New York: Guilford Press.

Linehan, M. M. (1993b). *Skills training manual for treating borderline personality disorder.* New York: Guilford Press.

Linehan, M. M. (2000). The empirical basis of dialectical behavior therapy: Development of new treatments versus evaluation of existing treatments. *Clinical Psychology: Science and Practice, 7,* 114–119.

Linehan, M. M., Comtois, K. A., Murray, A. M., Brown, M. Z., Gallop, R. J., & Heard, H. L. (2006). Two-year randomized controlled trial and follow-up of dialectical behavior therapy vs. therapy by experts for suicidal behaviors and borderline personality disorder. *Archives of General Psychiatry, 63,* 757–766.

Muehlenkamp, J. J. (2006). Empirically supported treatments and general therapy guidelines for non-suicidal self-injury. *Journal of Mental Health Counseling, 28,* 166–185.

Muehlenkamp, J. J., & Gutierrez, P. M. (2004). An investigation of differences between self-injurious behavior and suicide attempts in a sample of adolescents. *Suicide and Life-Threatening Behavior, 34*, 12–23.

Nock, M. K., & Prinstein, M. J. (2004). A functional approach to the assessment of self-mutilative behavior. *Journal of Consulting and Clinical Psychology, 72*, 885–890.

Rodham, K., Hawton, K., & Evans, E. (2004). Reasons for deliberate self-harm: Comparison of self-poisoners and self-cutters in a community sample of adolescents. *Journal of the American Academy of Child & Adolescent Psychiatry, 43*, 80–87.

Ross, R. R., & McKay, H. R. (1979). *Self-mutilation*. Lexington, MA: Lexington Books.

Ross, S., & Heath, N. (2002). A study of the frequency of self-mutilation in a community sample of adolescents. *Journal of Youth and Adolescence, 1*, 67–77.

Simeon, D., & Hollander, E. (Eds.). (2001). *Self-injurious behaviors, assessment and treatment*. Washington, DC: American Psychiatric Press.

Taiminen, T. J., Kallio-Soukainen, K., Nokso-Koivisto, H., Kaljonen, A., & Helenius, H. (1998). Contagion of deliberate self-harm among adolescent inpatients. *Journal of the American Academy of Child & Adolescent Psychiatry, 37*, 211–217.

Walsh, B. (2006). *Treating self-injury: A practical guide*. New York: Guilford Press.

Walsh, B., & Rosen, P. (1985). Self-mutilation and contagion: An empirical test. *American Journal of Psychiatry, 142*, 119–120.

Walsh, B., & Rosen, P. (1988). *Self-mutilation: Theory, research and treatment*. New York: Guilford Press.

Whitlock, J., Eckenrode, J., & Silverman, D. (2006). Self-injurious behaviors in a college population. *Pediatrics, 117*, 1939–1948.

Whitlock, J. L., Powers, J. L., & Eckenrode, J. (2006). The virtual cutting edge: The Internet and adolescent self-injury. *Developmental Psychology, 42*, 1–11.

13

END-OF-LIFE DECISIONS AND THE DUTY TO PROTECT

JAMES L. WERTH JR. AND JESSICA M. RICHMOND

John,[1] a 41-year-old European American man, is on time for his first session, dressed casually in jeans, a short-sleeved t-shirt with a few stains, and tennis shoes. He does not wear any jewelry other than an earring in each ear and perhaps a necklace tucked under his shirt. His hair is covered by a baseball hat that he does not remove, but it appears to be short. He may have a tattoo on his left upper arm, but it is difficult to tell with the t-shirt. He appears to be rather thin, with sunken cheeks covered by stubble, and walks with a cane and a limp. He completes the paperwork without apparent problem. He uses the correct date and states that his presenting concern was "sent here by my AIDS doc"; however, he does not sign the informed consent form.

The standard verbal review of informed consent is conducted, but when the part about "harm to self or others" is discussed, John says, "Stop." John says that he believes it is his right to "end it all" if the quality of life because of his AIDS is so low that dying would be better than living. He continues by saying that he has advanced AIDS and has seen dozens of his friends die terrible, prolonged deaths. He has no intention of hanging

---

[1]This case is based on a combination of several of James L. Werth, Jr.'s, actual clients; specifics have been changed to protect the identities of these individuals.

195

on in misery, or being forced to stay alive by family and physicians, like they did. He then says that the only reason he came is to "get my doc off my back about being depressed" and states that he wants a referral to someone else if his views are a problem.

Psychologists and other mental health professionals (MHPs) who have worked with people with HIV disease and other chronic or terminal conditions probably have had a client present similarly to John. James L. Werth Jr., who had been doing HIV-specific work for more than 15 years, has a small pro bono practice with the local HIV services organization and a specialty HIV medical clinic. Of his 10 most recent clients, 4 made statements similar to John's, even though they were taking medications that may have lengthened their lives. In fact, one client, Pat, noted that he had done a Web search on Werth. He decided to follow up on the referral from both his physician and his case manager after reviewing a publication by Werth that took a contextual view of suicide intervention (i.e., Werth, 1992). The client stated that suicide was always an option for him. He was willing to come in and be honest about his nearly constant suicidality only because he believed no immediate attempt to hospitalize him would occur. He asserted that such an action would only make things worse for a variety of reasons (e.g., people would find out about the hospitalization, he would be charged for the treatment, he believed his family would overreact), and he said he was smart enough to know what to say and what not to say to prevent being admitted or at least being kept for very long. He said that his suicidal ideation was the result of a comorbid potentially terminal health condition and advanced HIV disease. Before these health problems, he had never considered suicide an option.

Ethical and legal obligations for a suicidal client must be considered in light of whether that client has developed impaired judgment as a result of a mental illness. Although we highlight suicide above, an entire chapter in this book focuses on the traditional conceptualization of suicide and the provider's options in such situations (see chap. 11, this volume). Often, clients with a terminal illness or condition who are considering hastening their deaths have means available beyond the typical suicidal person (e.g., they often have many very potent medications that could be fatal in excess or in combination, they may be receiving treatments that are keeping them alive that could be stopped), and therefore they do not need to (and may be physically unable to) resort to violent means such as firearms or hanging.

In this chapter, we provide information about a variety of ways in which the duty to protect may become a part of counseling in a case involving suicidal ideation as a result of a comorbid potentially terminal health condition. Ethical and legal requirements, and treatment options in such situations, are discussed. In addition, because cultural considerations are ubiquitous in therapy, diversity issues are identified in the next section.

END-OF-LIFE DECISIONS

The possibility of "rational suicide" for people who are dying has been discussed in the mental health and medical literature (see Werth, 1999a, for an overview from a variety of perspectives). Some have argued that "rational" suicide cannot exist and that people should not receive assistance in suicide. Others have stated that in some situations a person may be able to make a well-reasoned decision that ending her or his own life (with or without the assistance of others) is the best option available. Werth and Rogers (2005) extended this discussion by stating that the term used to describe the action that may end the person's life (i.e., calling an action "suicide" or "rational suicide") is not the crucial aspect; rather, the fact that the action may hasten death is the key. Thus, although the literature has tended to focus on mental health issues associated with suicide, rational suicide, and assisted suicide, Werth and Rogers stated that any decision a person may make that could foreseeably lead to death in a reasonably short period of time should be responded to by the therapist in the same way. These authors discussed suicide, rational suicide, withholding or withdrawing life-sustaining treatment, and voluntarily stopping eating and drinking as examples of end-of-life decisions that may hasten death through deliberate action or inaction by the person. An individual need not be terminally ill or have a condition that may lead to death to engage in any of these actions or inactions.

In this chapter, we restrict our discussion to situations in which the person is expected to die within 6 months regardless of the treatment provided or in which treatment is merely staving off the progression or effects of the underlying condition, and without intervention the condition will cause death. We emphasize that what sets these clients apart from the typical client who wants to harm or kill him- or herself is the fact that these clients know death is quickly approaching and their desire to hasten death is a reaction to this and the associated health conditions leading to their death (see chaps. 11 and 12, this volume). The focus of this chapter is the ethical and legal issues associated with the duty to protect for these clients; for treatment considerations, see Werth and Blevins (2006).

For example, a person with advanced pancreatic cancer will probably die quickly, regardless of what treatments are tried. An individual with advanced AIDS may be terminal if no medications slow or stop the devastation of that person's immune system, or she or he may decide to stop taking medication, resulting in progression of the disease. A person who has kidney failure may be kept alive for many years through dialysis, but if she or he discontinues dialysis, then death will be expected within a relatively short period of time. Similarly, a person with advanced amyotrophic lateral sclerosis (i.e., Lou Gehrig's disease) may live on a ventilator for a fairly long period of time, but if she or he is removed from the machine, death will occur quickly. Someone with any of these conditions may choose to stop eating and drinking to speed up the dying process, even if she or he continues with other treatments, such as the person with amyotrophic lateral sclerosis who does not want to go off a ventilator but makes a decision to stop artificial nutrition and hydration.

It is worth noting that members of several ethnic minority groups in the United States tend to not support or use actions that may appear to or actually do hasten death. Research has demonstrated that European Americans are more likely to develop attitudes that permit the use of advance directives (i.e., living wills and durable powers of attorney for health care), withholding and withdrawing life-sustaining treatment, "assisted suicide," and voluntary euthanasia; they are also more likely to use advance directives, to use assisted death where it is legal in Oregon,[2] and to enroll in hospice care (Werth, Blevins, Toussaint, & Durham, 2002). The potential reasons for the differences in attitudes and behaviors appear related to the following factors: the history of discrimination in this country, the lack of trust in the health care system, religious beliefs, and a focus on interpersonal relationships as opposed to independent decision making.

There are other end-of-life decisions that we do not discuss because these involve the actions of one or more individuals other than the dying person (see Kleespies, 2004; Werth & Blevins, 2009). For example, if a person is unable to make health care decisions for her- or himself, other people (either by designation such as through a durable power of attorney for health care or by default such as through a state's succession law) will make treatment decisions that may lead to prolonging life or hastening death. Alternatively, if the ill person or loved ones have requested treatment that the health care team considers futile, then the providers can decide to stop treatment, which will result in the earlier death of the ill person. Clearly, in these situations the MHP's roles are different than when working with the dying person who is making his or her own decisions regarding continuing or discontinuing treatment. Consequently, duty-to-protect considerations become more of a moral issue than an ethical or legal one, a topic that is beyond the purview of this chapter.

ETHICAL AND LEGAL CONSIDERATIONS

We begin with the assumption that the therapist is aware that the dying person is considering hastening death.[3] This knowledge can come from a

---

[2]Although not the focus of this chapter, it may be worth noting that the Oregon Death With Dignity Act has a provision for the involvement of a psychologist to conduct an evaluation if either the attending or the consulting physician of the patient requesting medicine to hasten death is concerned that the patient may have impaired judgment. Few evaluations by MHPs have been conducted, according to the official reports by the Oregon Department of Human Services (2008). Research examining the Death With Dignity Act has not revealed any significant problems with its use (Oregon Department of Human Services, 2008; Werth & Wineberg, 2005). For a more general discussion of assisted death, see Rosenfeld (2004).

[3]The material in this chapter should not be considered legal or ethical advice. Each case is unique, and changes in facts, in context, or in locality could change the outcome. As with any potentially

disclosure by the client (as in the case of John), by someone else such as a personal or professional caregiver, or as a result of inquiries by the therapist. On the one hand, broaching the topic of dying and end-of-life decision making is fairly easy when working with a person who has a terminal illness or condition because it is part of the person's daily experience. On the other hand, some dying individuals may be concerned about the therapist's potential reaction and may withhold information until they feel safe in revealing thoughts of hastening death.

A variety of ways of assessing a person's desire for death and consideration for hastening death exist, including a single direct question (Chochinov et al., 1995), a brief interview (Wilson et al., 2000), and a standardized instrument (Rosenfeld et al., 1999). One could also use instruments that are designed to assess depression and hopelessness, under the hypothesis that if a dying person is depressed or hopeless then she or he may be considering hastening death (see Rosenfeld, Abbey, & Pessin, 2006, for a review). Readers are urged to use more than one of these approaches and to consider the client's situation, cultural belief system, values, experiences, and extent of social support. Multiple-measure corroboration will lead to a more comprehensive understanding about what may be influencing the client's end-of-life decision making and whether hastening death is a reasonable option to consider (Werth, Benjamin, & Farrenkopf, 2000). Without a strong therapeutic alliance, it will in many cases be difficult for the therapist to elicit the degree to which the client is considering hastening death and the conditions associated with the possible decision to die sooner than would be expected. Part of creating this alliance is demonstrating to the client that one has not only a technical understanding and relevant experience related to the client's condition but also a willingness to appreciate the client's life circumstances that may make death appear to be a better option than continuing to live. Regardless of whether the therapist believes that hastening death is ever an appropriate or acceptable option for a particular client, the therapist will be best able to help the client by remaining focused on the client's experiences and struggles as opposed to an exclusive focus on the professional's ethical and legal obligations in this situation.

For more in-depth discussions of these issues, see books by Kleespies (2004), Rosenfeld (2004), and Werth and Blevins (2009). We primarily base the suggestions about how to work with such clients on previous publications by James L. Werth Jr., for there is little else in the literature on this topic (but

---

controversial situation that has legal ramifications, therapists are urged to consult with a knowledgeable attorney about applicable laws in the therapist's jurisdiction. The attorney could discuss any statutes that could be construed broadly (e.g., assisted suicide laws) or any case law that has developed since this chapter was written or could be extrapolated from other situations (e.g., nonprevention of suicide) or other professions (e.g., against physicians). Similarly, ethics consultation is recommended when these types of situations arise. These consultations would be especially important if anyone with standing to sue or bring ethics charges disagreed with the dying person's consideration of hastening death in some form.

see Barret, Kitchener, & Burris, 2001, for a case study that is consistent with the analysis we provide). Another limitation we want to note is that we focus on nonmedical practitioners because the issues are different for professionals who may actually play a role in implementing a person's decision to hasten death as opposed to those whose job is to provide counseling, assessment, and intervention but not provision of means. The issues for psychologists, professional counselors, and social workers are highlighted later in this chapter. Finally, although professional codes of ethics may be similar across countries, relevant court cases and laws likely differ significantly, so our emphasis is on practice in the United States.

Ethics Codes and Other Organizational Statements

All three of the national associations for MHPs have addressed end-of-life issues in ways that affect interpretation of ethical responsibilities when working with a dying client who is considering hastening death. The American Psychological Association's (APA's) Working Group on Assisted Suicide and End-of-Life Decisions issued a comprehensive report on end-of-life decisions in 2000. The authors of this report offered two resolutions, one on end-of-life care and one on assisted suicide. Both were slightly adapted and then accepted by the association's Council of Representatives in early 2001 (see http://www.apa.org/pi/eol). These resolutions indicated that psychologists have important roles to play when clients are making end-of-life decisions, including hastening death, a position consistent with a 1997 statement issued by the organization (see Farberman, 1997) that noted that psychologists could provide counseling and assessment but were not required to prevent people from following through with a decision to hasten death. APA revised its Ethics Code in 2002; notably, this was after the resolutions just mentioned. The Ethics Code does not specifically address end-of-life issues, and the section on breaking confidentiality that deals with harm to self was not changed in ways that affect the analysis related to the 1992 code (Werth, 1999b, 2002), which allowed for intervention but did not mandate it when clients were considering hastening death (see also Barret et al., 2001; Werth & Kleespies, 2006).

The National Association of Social Workers (NASW) was the first national mental health organization to address the role of its members in hastened death situations. Specifically, in 1994 NASW passed a statement on "Client Self-Determination in End-of-Life Situations" that stated that social workers could assist clients making end-of-life decisions, including hastening death (NASW, 1994/2003). However, Werth (1999b) noted that the NASW (1996/1999) *Code of Ethics* was ambiguous regarding whether breaking confidentiality was required or optional when clients were potentially engaging in harm to self. Given NASW's involvement in a recent court case associated with hastened death (see below), one now could reasonably assume that breaking confidentiality is not required. NASW (2004; Rosen & O'Neill, 1998) has also issued some statements providing direction to members working with clients who are dying. However, none of these explicitly addresses hastening death.

The American Counseling Association (ACA, 2005) recently revised its *Code of Ethics*, and it now includes a section (A.9.) specifically on working with terminally ill clients that offers guidance when a client is considering hastening death (see Werth & Crow, in press). Notably, in addition to stating that counselors can continue to work with clients making such decisions, the new code's section on breaching confidentiality notes that there are different considerations in end-of-life situations. It appears that this code of ethics permits professional counselors to work with dying clients considering hastening death and does not require preventing clients from following through with such decisions.

Court Cases

As noted earlier, some national mental health associations have been involved in end-of-life court cases. Specifically, both ACA and NASW's 1994/2003 statement, along with some state psychological associations, have signed on different *amicus curiae* (i.e., friend of the court) briefs for the U.S. Supreme Court when it has considered cases related to assisted suicide. In 1996, the ACA signed on a brief that took no position on assisted suicide but rather stated that MHPs have important roles when clients are considering hastening death (Werth & Gordon, 2002). This position is consistent with the current ACA (2005) *Code of Ethics*.

In 2005, NASW signed on a brief that again was neutral regarding assisted suicide but stated that MHPs can help individuals who are making end-of-life decisions, including possibly hastening death (Miller & Werth, 2006). This position is consistent with NASW's 1994 statement and may clarify the ambiguity in its *Code of Ethics* regarding whether a social worker is required to break confidentiality of a client who is perceived to be a potential harm to self. Given that NASW signed on this brief, it appears as if its *Code of Ethics* could be interpreted as allowing breaking of confidentiality but not mandating it.

There are other end-of-life cases that have had an impact on MHPs who are working with dying clients. Specifically, in another U.S. Supreme Court case, *Cruzan v. Director, Missouri Department of Health* (1990), the majority decision was that people and their surrogates have a constitutional right to withhold or withdraw life-sustaining treatment, including artificial food and fluids. Thus, clients (whether dying or not) are legally allowed to not start or to stop medical treatment that is designed to keep the person alive. A decision to refuse or to discontinue such treatment is not considered suicide. Thus, these types of decisions may appear to be outside the realm of intervention under duty-to-protect considerations. We return to this point later.

As noted elsewhere in this volume, the famous *Tarasoff v. Regents of the University of California* (1976) case does not apply to situations involving potential harm to self, but another California case, *Bellah v. Greenson* (1978), is often cited as an example that the same types of standard of care considerations and interventions that are present in homicide cases are important in suicide cases. Werth and Rogers (2005) argued that assessment of a person's decision making to determine whether the person's judgment is impaired is sufficient intervention to meet the standard of care in such situations, a point we examine in the next major section on treatment. Chapter 2 of this book and the review of state laws below suggest that MHPs are unlikely to have a legal obligation to intervene to prevent a dying person from making a decision that may hasten death.

State and Federal Laws

We are not aware of any federal laws that have implications for MHPs providing treatment to dying clients who are considering hastening death. Werth (2001) examined all state laws related to involuntary hospitalization in the specific situation of potential harm to self. He found that in virtually every state, the professional was not mandated to attempt to hospitalize a person who was considered to be at risk of harming her- or himself. Furthermore, he reported that the criteria for hospitalization nearly always specified that the self-harm thoughts or behavior must be the result of mental illness. Combining these results with the more recent review in chapter 2, it appears as if MHPs may have the option of trying to hospitalize a client who is considering hastening death, but only if the desire for death is the result of a diagnosable disorder.

Summary

Our review indicates that the expectations for MHPs working with dying clients who are considering end-of-life options that may include hastening death are different from the expectations related to working with clients who are suicidal. Specifically, on the basis of ethics codes, associated organizational statements, *amicus* briefs, and state laws, we believe that therapists are fairly free to explore a variety of end-of-life decisions with clients who are dying, without needing to assume that there is a duty to protect in the traditional sense (e.g., hospitalizing, breaking confidentiality). Yet, we think that clinicians do have some responsibilities in these situations, and it is to this topic that we turn next.

THERAPEUTIC RESPONSES

Rushing to the option of hospitalization and breaching confidentiality with a dying client who wants to discuss hastening death as a potential option should not be the clinician's first choice, even if he or she has moral concerns about suicide because at this point the client is merely bringing up the idea as hypothetical possibility. Furthermore, on the basis of the review in the previous section, such intervention would be based on moral beliefs, not ethical or legal obligations. Immediately planning to implement coercive and restrictive interventions will interfere with developing an alliance with the client. Rather, the counselor can focus on being present with the client, furthering the therapeutic relationship, and attempting to understand the client's situation—dying individuals may not have anyone else to whom they can talk; therefore, the therapist's empathy can be of great assistance to the client (Werth & Blevins, 2006). However, more is demanded of the therapist than merely listening for 50 minutes and sending the client on her or his way to act or not act as she or he so pleases. Werth and Rogers (2005) suggested that when working with a client who is near the end of life and is considering hastening death, the counselor should conduct a thorough assessment of the person's judgment to make such a decision. Sufficient evidence exists in the literature to recognize that some dying people's judgment may be impaired (e.g., by the disease or condition itself, by medications used to manage symptoms such as pain, by psychological conditions such as clinical depression), and their quality of life may be negatively affected by any number of psychological, interpersonal, and social issues; to fail to explore whether some changes can be made to help such a person would be professionally irresponsible (for reviews, see Gibson, Breitbart, Tomarken, Kosinski, & Nelson, 2006; Rosenfeld et al., 2006; Werth et al., 2000; Werth, Gordon, & Johnson, 2002).

The type of evaluation we support is too detailed to discuss, but we believe the set of issues identified by the APA Working Group on Assisted Suicide and End-of-Life Decisions (2000) and by Werth et al. (2000) provide comprehensive outlines of the areas we would want to include in an assessment. Many of the topics covered (e.g., delirium, mood disorders, anxiety disorders, hopelessness) can be addressed by empirically supported treatments (e.g., medication, cognitive–behavioral therapy, interpersonal therapy), and others (e.g., fear of loss of control, concern about being a burden) are amenable to intervention. Even if the person continues to consider hastening death as an option, her or his quality of life may be improved as a result of conducting the assessment and implementing associated interventions.

In addition, clinicians would be remiss if they did not consult with colleagues who have experience working with dying clients, especially with colleagues who have worked with clients who have considered hastening death. However, we believe it is important that the therapist choose a consultant who is not closed to certain options as a result of personal beliefs. A consultant is supposed to help identify options and help the counselor identify ways in which she or he may be missing important information, including ethical and legal responsibilities, not restricting treatment options on the basis of her or his own moral perspective. For example, we would not call a suicide prevention hotline for a consultation about what to do with a client such as John or Pat who is considering hastening death. Most hotline workers are volunteers with insufficient training or experience with hastening death. Nevertheless, a recommendation to hospitalize John or Pat immediately would create the impression that the therapist acted negligently or unethically if hospitalization did not occur. A contemporaneous peer consultation will demonstrate that the factors regarding a careful evaluation and a reasonable plan of action were considered in an independent manner.

However, if the provider is under the supervision of a professional, as would be the case for Jessica Richmond, then the supervisor's recommendations need to be implemented to the extent that they are directives and not merely options. In other words, if Richmond was providing counseling services under Werth's supervision, then if Werth tells Richmond to break confidentiality and call John's sister, Richmond must do so under the laws regulating supervisory relationships. A variety of ways of making such a call and involving John could be developed. For example, Richmond could remind John of the obligations discussed during informed consent and indicate that on the basis of consultation with her supervisor, she needs to make sure his sister knows that he is thinking of hastening his death. A call could be made by John, in Richmond's presence, asking his sister to come in for a joint session right then; John could tell his sister during a phone call about his desire for death (in Richmond's presence), and then Richmond could see whether his sister had any questions; or Richmond could call John's sister and talk with her in John's presence (Stadler, 1989). These options protect the therapeutic alliance while providing more data to (and possibly from) a member of John's family.

Finally, the clinician needs to write thorough case notes explaining decisions made and not made, interventions considered and implemented or considered and not used, and the peer consultant's views about these issues. If the counselor does not document that she or he thought about hospitalization but decided against it, then if an ethical or legal complaint is brought, the counselor will have little defense against the claim that she or he failed to meet the standard of care about considering hospitalization of a client who was talking about taking an action that would lead to death. Descriptions of these types of notes can be found in most risk management articles or texts (e.g., American Psychological Association, 2007).

CONCLUSION

The Case of John Revisited

The clinician responds to John's statements by proposing that they enter into a therapeutic contract stating that one of the purposes of their time together is to explore John's end-of-life options, including the possibility of ending medical treatment thus hastening death, and the issues that may be a part of his decision-making process (Werth, 1999b). Perhaps John would need to agree not to take any action that would affect the manner and timing of his death, and the counselor would agree to not break confidentiality or hospitalize John unless she believes that John's judgment is so impaired that he cannot make well-reasoned decisions and she is concerned about his taking an action that may lead to death. She could state that if, after exploring the issues, John believes that ending medical treatment in that way is his best option and she does not believe his judgment is impaired, she will not intervene to prevent him from hastening his death in that way.

After agreeing to this plan (or another plan that is documented), and after John signs the informed consent form, the therapist and John begin to explore the reasons for his desire for death. They decide to use the list developed by the APA Working Group on Assisted Suicide and End-of-Life Decisions (2000), and the counselor begins by making sure John has the mental capacity to make health care decisions for himself, proceeding to an exploration of his physical symptoms and the treatments he has received for his suffering. Although not a physician, she is knowledgeable enough to know to refer him for more discussion of treatment for his pain and nausea. In subsequent sessions, they explore whether any diagnosable psychological conditions exist that may be impairing his judgment as well as other mental health concerns such as hopelessness or fear of loss of autonomy. They also discuss his relationships with other people and the extent of their involvement in his life and, when possible, involve them in the counseling. Finally, they review larger systemic issues such as possible pressure to hasten his death.

As a result of this process of engaging the client in a thorough review of issues and options while evaluating his capacity to make decisions, we believe the therapist has met her obligation to protect the client (see Werth & Rogers, 2005). At this point, she would have no grounds for trying to hospitalize John (because there is no mental illness causing his desire for death), and because his family knows John is considering death as an option, there is no need to break confidentiality. As long as she has thoroughly documented (what she did or did not do and why or why not) and consulted (and documented her consultations), she will be able to defend her decisions. Furthermore, by involving the family, those people most likely to be upset and file legal or ethical charges are probably not going to do so. However, if she does believe she needs to intervene, the process described above gives her the leeway to consider options. Thus, in either case, the counselor and the client can focus on trying to help the client achieve as high a quality of life as possible, for as long as possible, while maximizing the counselor's respect for John's autonomy and self-determination.

REFERENCES

American Counseling Association. (2005). *ACA code of ethics*. Alexandria, VA: Author. Retrieved July 1, 2006, from http://www.counseling.org/Resources/CodeOfEthics/TP/Home/CT2.aspx

American Psychological Association. (2002). Ethical principles of psychologists and code of conduct. *American Psychologist, 57*, 1060–1073.

American Psychological Association. (2007). Record keeping guidelines. *American Psychologist, 62*, 993–1004.

Barret, B., Kitchener, K. S., & Burris, S. (2001). Suicide and confidentiality with the client with advanced AIDS: The case of Phil. In J. R. Anderson & B. Barret (Eds.), *Ethics in HIV-related psychotherapy* (pp. 299–314). Washington, DC: American Psychological Association.

Bellah v. Greenson, 146 Cal. Rptr. 535, 81 Cal.App.3d 614 (1978).

Chochinov, H. M., Wilson, K. G., Enns, M., Mowchun, N., Lander, S., Levitt, M., et al. (1995). Desire for death in the terminally ill. *American Journal of Psychiatry, 152*, 1185–1191.

Cruzan v. Director, Missouri Department of Health, 497 U.S. 261 (1990).

Farberman, R. K. (1997). Terminal illness and hastened death requests: The important role of the mental health professional. *Professional Psychology: Research and Practice, 28*, 544–547.

Gibson, C. A., Breitbart, W., Tomarken, A., Kosinski, A., & Nelson, C. J. (2006). Mental health issues near the end of life. In J. L. Werth, Jr., & D. Blevins (Eds.), *Psychosocial issues near the end of life: A resource for professional care providers* (pp. 137–162). Washington, DC: American Psychological Association.

Kleespies, P. M. (2004). *Life and death decisions: Psychological and ethical considerations in end-of-life care*. Washington, DC: American Psychological Association.

Miller, P. J., & Werth, J. L., Jr. (2006). *Amicus curiae* brief for the United States Supreme Court on mental health, terminal illness, and assisted death. *Journal of Social Work in End-of-Life and Palliative Care, 1*, 7–33.

National Association of Social Workers. (1994/2003). Client self-determination in end-of-life decisions. In *Social work speaks* (6th ed., pp. 46–49). Washington, DC: NASW Press.

National Association of Social Workers. (1996/1999). *NASW code of ethics* [approved in 1996, revised in 1999]. Washington, DC: Author

National Association of Social Workers. (2004). *NASW standards for social work practice in palliative and end of life care.* Washington, DC: Author. Retrieved November 1, 2005, from http://www.socialworkers.org/practice/bereavement/standards/default.asp

Oregon Department of Human Services. (2008). *Table 1: Characteristics and end-of-life care of 341 DWDA patients who died after ingesting a lethal dose of medication, Oregon, 1998-2007.* Portland, OR: Author. Retrieved April 29, 2008, from http://www.oregon.gov/DHS/ph/pas/docs/yr10-tbl-1.pdf

Rosen, A., & O'Neill, J. (1998). *Social work roles and opportunities in advanced directives and health care decision making.* Washington, DC: NASW Press.

Rosenfeld, B. (2004). *Assisted suicide and the right to die: The interface of social science, public policy, and medical ethics.* Washington, DC: American Psychological Association.

Rosenfeld, B., Abbey, J., & Pessin, H. (2006). Depression and hopelessness near the end of life: Assessment and treatment. In J. L. Werth, Jr., & D. Blevins (Eds.), *Psychosocial issues near the end of life: A resource for professional care providers* (pp. 163–182). Washington, DC: American Psychological Association.

Rosenfeld, B., Breitbart, W., Stein, K., Funesti-Esch, J., Kaim, M., Krivo, S., et al. (1999). Measuring desire for death among patients with HIV/AIDS: The Schedule of Attitudes Toward Hastened Death. *American Journal of Psychiatry, 156,* 94–100.

Stadler, H. (1989). Balancing ethical responsibilities: Reporting child abuse and neglect. *The Counseling Psychologist, 17,* 102–110.

Tarasoff v. Regents of the University of California, 13 Cal.3d 117, 529 P.2d 553 (1974), vacated 17 Cal.3d 425, 551 P.2d 334 (1976).

Werth, J. L., Jr. (1992). Rational suicide and AIDS: Considerations for the psychotherapist. *The Counseling Psychologist, 20,* 645–659.

Werth, J. L., Jr. (Ed.). (1999a). *Contemporary perspectives on rational suicide.* Philadelphia: Taylor & Francis.

Werth, J. L., Jr. (1999b). Mental health professionals and assisted death: Perceived ethical obligations and proposed guidelines for practice. *Ethics & Behavior, 9,* 159–183.

Werth, J. L., Jr. (2001). U.S. involuntary mental health commitment statutes: Requirements for persons perceived to be a potential harm to self. *Suicide and Life-Threatening Behavior, 31,* 348–357.

Werth, J. L., Jr. (2002). Legal and ethical considerations for mental health professionals related to end-of-life care and decision making. *American Behavioral Scientist, 46,* 373–388.

Werth, J. L., Jr., Benjamin, G. A. H., & Farrenkopf, T. (2000). Requests for physician-assisted death: Guidelines for assessing mental capacity and impaired judgment. *Psychology, Public Policy, and Law, 6,* 348–372.

Werth, J. L., Jr., & Blevins, D. (Eds.) (2006). *Psychosocial issues near the end of life: A resource for professional care providers.* Washington, DC: American Psychological Association.

Werth, J. L., Jr., & Blevins, D. (Eds.). (2009). *Decision-making near the end of life: Recent developments and future directions.* Philadelphia: Routledge.

Werth, J. L., Jr., Blevins, D., Toussaint, K. L., & Durham, M. R. (2002). The influence of cultural diversity on end-of-life care and decisions. *American Behavioral Scientist, 46,* 204–219.

Werth, J. L., Jr., & Crow, L. (in press). End-of-life care: An overview for professional counselors. *Journal of Counseling & Development.*

Werth, J. L., Jr., & Gordon, J. R. (2002). *Amicus curiae* brief for the United States Supreme Court on mental health issues associated with "physician-assisted suicide." *Journal of Counseling & Development, 80,* 160–172.

Werth, J. L., Jr., Gordon, J. R., & Johnson, R. R., Jr., (2002). Psychosocial issues near the end of life. *Aging and Mental Health, 6,* 402–412.

Werth, J. L., Jr., & Kleespies, P. M. (2006). Ethical considerations in providing psychological services in end-of-life care. In J. L. Werth, Jr., & D. Blevins (Eds.), *Psychosocial issues near the end of life: A resource for professional care providers* (pp. 57–87). Washington, DC: American Psychological Association.

Werth, J. L., Jr., & Rogers, J. R. (2005). Assessing for impaired judgment as a means of meeting the "duty to protect" when a client is a potential harm-to-self: Implications for clients making end-of-life decisions. *Mortality, 10,* 7–21.

Werth, J. L., Jr., & Wineberg, H. (2005). A critical analysis of criticisms of the Oregon Death With Dignity Act. *Death Studies, 29,* 1–27.

Wilson, K. G., Scott, J. F., Graham, I. D., Kozak, J. F., Chater, S., Viola, R. A., et al. (2000). Attitudes of terminally ill patients toward euthanasia and physician-assisted suicide. *Archives of Internal Medicine, 160,* 2454–2460.

Working Group on Assisted Suicide & End-of-Life Decisions. (2000). *Report to the board of directors.* Washington, DC: American Psychological Association. Retrieved November 1, 2005, from http://www.apa.org/pi/aseolf.html

IV

ADDITIONAL CONSIDERATIONS

14

SELF-CARE IN THE CONTEXT OF THREATS OF VIOLENCE OR SELF-HARM FROM CLIENTS

CHRISTIANE BREMS AND MARK E. JOHNSON

Consider the following three cases:

> Dr. Rollins, a psychologist at a university health service, has been seeing a 23-year-old physical therapy student named Jonathan, who has a dual diagnosis of bipolar disorder and alcohol dependency. For 9 months, the student has been sober and compliant with treatment. Last week, Jonathan learned that he failed two of his courses and is being dismissed from the program. He was furious and expressed his rage in the session with Dr. Rollins immediately after he learned of the dismissal. The psychologist immediately implemented a crisis treatment plan and using a standard risk assessment inventory, assessed Jonathan's risk of using alcohol, of harming himself, or of taking violent action against the faculty members who failed him. After an extended therapy session, Jonathan calmed down, agreed to all recommended portions of the new treatment plan, and dis-avowed any violent intent against himself or anyone else. Dr. Rollins also consulted with a colleague about the client before Jonathan left the office to ensure that he was acting responsibly. The client agreed to see Dr. Rollins the next morning and had contact information if the rage

reemerged during the night. At 8:00 a.m. the next morning, Dr. Rollins learned that Jonathan had driven his car into a tree in the wee hours of the morning, killing himself and seriously injuring a 12-year-old passenger in the automobile his car struck after bouncing off the tree. The girl suffered a spinal cord injury that has probably left her without the ability to walk. Dr. Rollins was distraught at this news and unable to work for days, worried that he could have done more for this sad young man and terrified that he might be sued or have an ethics claim brought against him. Ultimately, no lawsuit ensued and no ethics charges were made, and his colleagues and peer consultation group affirmed that he acted appropriately. Still, Dr. Rollins believes it will be a long time before he experiences the same level of satisfaction from this practice that he experienced before Jonathan's suicide and the injury to the innocent child in the car accident.

Ms. Donnell, a licensed clinical counselor in a community mental health center, recently worked with a client diagnosed with a paranoid delusional disorder. Treatment had been effective, and the client was stable and making progress in managing his life more effectively. One aspect of this client's delusion is the belief that his 26-year-old stepson is trying to kill him, a belief completely unsupported by any evidence. In this client's last appointment, he was unusually agitated because he had lost his wallet and because his ex-wife was refusing to loan him money. The man voiced explicit threats to harm his stepson before the young man succeeded in killing him. After completing a thorough risk assessment and consulting with senior colleagues, Ms. Donnell determined that this was a high-risk situation in which the duty to the third party was triggered. After evaluating her options under the state statute, Ms. Donnell set the wheels into motion for an involuntary hospitalization of this client. After a 72-hour hospitalization, the man was released for outpatient treatment and was advised to see Ms. Donnell again. She noted that this client appeared on her appointment schedule for the next day and she was very stressed about seeing him again.

Dr. Marisol, a licensed psychologist, works in a community mental health agency providing therapy to individuals with severe and persistent mental disorders. She also maintains a small private practice during evening hours and weekends. During her 15 years of agency work, Dr. Marisol has dealt many times with clients who have made multiple suicide attempts and has had two patients who actually died by suicide. She has also had clients yell at her and threaten to kill her. Although she always took these threats of suicide and violence seriously and dealt with them in a most professional manner, the threats rarely had a profound or lasting emotional effect on her. However, this all changed after one of her private practice clients threatened to kill her after a particularly difficult couple's therapy session. During this session, the husband became increasingly hostile and unable to control his temper, no matter what intervention Dr. Marisol tried. After threatening her, he stormed out of the session, and neither client has returned for the past 3 months. Since that time, Dr. Marisol has been receiving threatening phone calls at home and at work and has seen the client who threatened her following her on several occasions as she left her office. Dr. Marisol now finds herself being much more guarded with all of her clients and has become increasingly hesitant to confront or challenge them. She has started to have strong feelings of being burdened by her clients, and she no longer looks forward to going to work.[1]

Determining when the duty to protect may be triggered, deciding on the most responsible and legally sound procedure for implementing the duty if it is triggered, and living with the possibility that the client's violence may be turned against the therapist are all inherently stressful situations that require the full intellectual and emotional engagement of the professional. This chapter offers guidance for self-care to clinicians who are facing clients who threaten violence. We begin the chapter by presenting the data on the frequency with which mental health professionals (MHPs) encounter clients who threaten self-harm, harm to others, or harm to their therapists. Next, we discuss the potential emotional and personal sequelae for psychologists working with dangerous clients. Finally, we present strategies therapists can use to protect themselves legally, physically, and emotionally from the challenges and dangers of working with violent or suicidal clients. These strategies assist therapists with laying the groundwork for the prevention of distress, burnout, fatigue, and exhaustion in the face of potential duty-to-protect situations.

INCIDENCE OF PSYCHOTHERAPISTS' ENCOUNTERS WITH VIOLENT OR SUICIDAL CLIENTS

The unfortunate reality is that during the course of their career, it is quite likely that therapists will be confronted with clients who will die by suicide or clients who threaten to or actually harm their clinician. In a national survey of psychologists, Pope and Tabachnick (1993) found that 97.2% of respondents had on at least one occasion experienced serious concern that a client might attempt suicide and 28.8% reported having had a client who actually died by suicide. Chemtob, Hamada, Bauer, Torigoe, and Kinney (1988) reported that 22% of psychologists had a client who died by suicide. Among professional counselors, 23% reported having experienced a client who killed her- or himself, with nearly a quarter of the care providers being students at the time (McAdams & Foster, 2000). Surveys of social workers found similar rates, with Sanders, Jacobson, and Ting (2005) reporting that

---

[1]These cases include no client identifying information and no specific case information.

28.2% of surveyed social workers had at least one of their clients die by suicide, and Jacobson, Ting, Sanders, and Harrington (2004) reporting a rate of 33%. Given that it is a virtual certainty that at least one client in every therapist's caseload will threaten suicide and that there is nearly a 33% chance of a client actually dying by suicide, psychotherapists must prepare for such an eventuality in a number of ways, including legal, physical, and emotional self-protection.

In a recent study of psychologists in clinical practice, Pabian and Welfel (2007) reported that the mean number of clients who had threatened violence against a third party was 3.2 in the past 2 years, with 10.1% of the sample reporting more than 10 clients who represented a serious risk of violence to others in that time period. Psychotherapists are also at grave risk of being the target of threats of psychological or physical harm as well as of actually being assaulted by their clients. Pope and Tabachnick (1993) found that 82.8% of surveyed psychologists reported that on at least one occasion they feared a physical attack by a client; as many as 18.9% reported an actual attack. In a survey of MHPs in Georgia, Arthur, Brende, and Quiroz (2003) reported that 29% had feared for their lives because of threats or perceived threats from clients, and 61% had been actual victims of psychologically or physically violent acts by a client.

Stalking is another source of concern for MHPs. In various studies, 6% to 12% of clinicians indicated that they had been stalked by a current or former client (Galeazzi, Elkins, & Curci, 2005; Gentile, Asamen, Harmell, & Weathers, 2002; Romans, Hays, & White, 1996). In inpatient settings, the risk is even higher. Sandberg, McNiel, and Binder (2002) surveyed clinical staff at an inpatient psychiatric hospital and found that 53% had been stalked, threatened, or harassed by clients at some point during their career. Although setting, clientele, or activities appear to influence the likelihood of a therapist being victimized by a client (e.g., Corder & Whiteside, 1996), as Arthur et al. (2003) stated, "No group of mental health professionals has been immune from violence" (p. 23). Thus, all therapists must be prepared for the inevitability that at some point in their career, they will experience some degree of physical or emotional threat from their clients.

CONSEQUENCES FOR THE PSYCHOTHERAPIST WHEN DEALING WITH VIOLENT OR SUICIDAL CLIENTS

Being a therapist comes with a multitude of challenges that can make successful clinical practice difficult and the provider prone to burnout or impairment. Indeed, when psychologists begin practice, "they enter an arena that is at once highly exciting, stimulating, and rewarding, but also intense, strenuous, and emotionally draining. Physical and emotional burn-out are real dangers" (Walker & Matthews, 1997, p. 11). Indeed, in a survey of psychologists, Rupert and Morgan (2005) found that 44.1% of respondents fell into the high-burnout range on emotional exhaustion, often considered a precursor of full-blown burnout syndrome.

Therapists who are frequently exposed to clients who threaten self-harm or harm to others (especially to the clinician) and other verbally or physically abusive behaviors may be at particular risk of professional impairment, personal feelings of failure, and less-than-optimal physical and mental health (Bayne, 1997). Rupert and Morgan (2005) reported that two indexes of professional burnout, namely, level of emotional exhaustion and depersonalization of clients, were positively correlated with negative client behaviors. Gentile et al. (2002) found that all psychologists who said they had been stalked by a client experienced strong emotional reactions, with 71% reporting being anxious; 71%, angry; and 41%, frightened. Moreover, nearly 75% of stalked psychologists indicated that they experienced a physical response as well, with sleep disturbances the most commonly reported symptom.

Burnout often has an insidious onset in that the symptoms involved develop so gradually that they may escape the attention of the person experiencing them. Clues about potential burnout include feeling "less" (Jevne & Williams, 1998): less enthusiastic, less idealistic, less valued, less able, less connected, less involved, less energetic, and less creative. Professionals who are burning out begin to feel a sense of disillusionment, detachment (evidenced as loneliness, isolation, or withdrawal), dread, depression, worry, despair, and hopelessness and begin to complain of a variety of physical symptoms, such as poor or decreased sleep, lowered immunity, increased aches and pains, digestive problems, or sexual dysfunction (Jevne & Williams, 1998). Early warning signs about possible impairment secondary to burnout include changes in thoughts and emotions (e.g., difficulty concentrating, boredom, loneliness), changes in physical well-being (e.g., tics, tight throat, aches), and changes in behavior (e.g., irritability, accidents, eating too much or too little; Bayne, 1997). If these symptoms are ignored, they may quickly translate into distress and impairment, leading to problems with work and life in general.

If clinicians do encounter symptoms of burnout, impairment, or distress, they must take action to help themselves. It is beyond the scope of this chapter to address burnout or impairment intervention. At a minimum, overcoming burnout requires the clinician to go through the distinct stages of grieving the loss of a dream and experiencing the anger, depression, and despair that may be involved. Although the recovery process is not an easy one, coping with burnout will eventually lead to a point of hope and rebuilding that ushers in renewed enthusiasm for the same career or becomes the foundation of a new life challenge (Jevne & Williams, 1998). To help psychologists prevent burnout, in the following section we discuss how to prepare for dealing with difficult and dangerous clients to inoculate against physical, emotional, and legal harm.

PSYCHOTHERAPISTS' SELF-CARE STRATEGIES WHEN WORKING WITH VIOLENT AND SUICIDAL CLIENTS

The most basic level of self-care is self-protection from clients' threats of harm to the clinician; indeed, the right for such self-protection is guaranteed in the American Psychological Association's (APA's; 2002) "Ethical Principles of Psychologists and Code of Conduct." Specifically, APA's Ethics Code clarifies that "psychologists may terminate therapy when threatened or otherwise endangered by the client/patient or another person with whom the client/patient has a relationship" (Standard 10.10[b]), holding therapists harmless for premature termination of services when their physical welfare is threatened. Statutes in many jurisdictions (e.g., the involuntary treatment process) and case law in some jurisdictions (e.g., *Ensworth v. Mullvain*, 1990) also support the legal right of the psychologist to end care to a threatening client and take other steps to protect his- or herself.

Beyond their very basic right to ensure their physical safety, clinicians also need to attend to specific forms of self-care that will keep them healthy during and after a client crisis. First, therapists ought to be ready to deal with threats in terms of professional self-care that serves to protect their integrity as practicing clinicians. Second, therapists should be ready to deal with personal self-care issues that become particularly salient when a client presents challenges that involve potential harm to the clinician. Professional self-care deals with issues of limiting risk of harm to the therapist, legal liability, ethical responsibilities, and use of training, supervision, and consultation. Personal self-care focuses on keeping therapists healthy in mind, body, and spirit.

Self-care can in many ways be viewed as a mandate for practicing clinicians. For example, APA's (2002) Ethics Code specifies that "psychologists refrain from initiating an activity when they know or should know that there is a substantial likelihood that their personal problems will prevent them from performing their work-related activities in a competent manner" and that "when psychologists become aware of personal problems that may interfere with their performing work-related duties adequately, they take appropriate measures, such as obtaining professional consultation or assistance, and determine whether they should limit, suspend, or terminate their work-related duties" (APA, 2002, Standards 2.06[a] and 2.06[b]). APA's Ethics Code most directly addresses the requirement for professional self-care but clearly implies the need for personal self-care in the context of prevention of impairment.

Professional Self-Care to Deal With Threats of Harm

Professional self-care has many elements, all of which require conscious and concerted effort on the part of the therapist. These strategies have been discussed in detail elsewhere for generic situations (e.g., Brems, 2000, 2001); however, they deserve to be explored in the context of threat of harm by clients, especially as directed toward the therapist. We present four categories of self-care: (a) self-protection, including responding to immediate threats, taking any necessary steps to ensure physical safety in the future, good record keeping, and referral, if appropriate; (b) consultation and supervision, both for ongoing support but also for dealing with specific situations in which the therapist is threatened; (c) networking, as an avenue to enhance the therapist's skill and knowledge; and (d) continuing education, as a means to further the therapist's knowledge. Professional self-care strategies do not focus nearly as much on the emotional impact that will be felt by the therapist in situations in which he or she is threatened by a client; such emotional support and recovery is the focus of personal self-care strategies.

Self-Protection

Self-protection in the context of client threats has, at minimum, the following elements: prevention through addressing immediate threats, careful screening, and referral; safety through configuring the physical space of the therapy setting; and record keeping (see also Berg, Bell, & Tupin, 2000). In addressing immediate threats of violence from a client, it is obvious that the most important initial step therapists must make is to take action to ensure their own safety. Depending on the circumstances, immediacy, and severity of the threat, initial actions might necessitate using clinical skills to deescalate the situation, leaving the physical presence of the client, or seeking help from a colleague or neighbor. Once the immediate threat has been addressed, the next steps may include contacting the police, seeking a restraining order, terminating therapy with the client, and implementing other strategies to keep safe.

Equally as important as therapists' self-protection is clients' welfare. Steps must be taken to ensure that clients' therapy needs are met, to the degree possible. If this involves a continuation of the therapy with this client, future sessions should be conducted under more controlled and monitored circumstances and with an explicit understanding and oral or written contract with the client regarding future threats of violence (see also Brems, 2000, for details about behavior contracts). Such continued work needs to take place in a physical setting (described further later in this section) that can provide a greater margin of safety for both psychologist and client, such as may be provided by a room with one-way windows, video equipment for immediate surveillance, and similar safety features. However, circumstances frequently do not permit the therapist to continue seeing the client, and the therapist should carefully consider whether a continuation of such care is warranted. A consultation with a trusted and experienced colleague about the wisdom of continuation is prudent when continuation is an option under consideration because many who advise about risk management discourage such action (Barnett, MacGlashan, & Clarke, 2003). In some situations, a referral to a more experienced or neutral professional may be possible, but the duty to a client ends when that client threatens violence. In essence, by that conduct the client is terminating care (Barnett et al., 2003). When a referral is possible, a release of information should be obtained so the referral agent may be informed of the circumstances of the termination of therapy. Thus, the new therapist will be in a better position to decide whether to take on the client and, if he or she does, will be better prepared to deal with the client's potential for violence. If no referral is advisable, the professional's responsibility to the client may be ended in most jurisdictions by pursuing involuntary hospitalization.

Although prediction of violence combines both art and science, psychologists may take steps to minimize the likelihood of being in a situation in which a client threatens them. Perhaps most important and simple, clinicians can prevent some of the heartache brought on by dangerous or suicidal clients by selecting clients carefully, commensurate with the clinician's physical environment and clinical experience. Although screening or selecting clients may not always be an option, it may be particularly important for private practitioners. Therapists who work in private practice have to give careful consideration to the type of clientele they choose. If they are in a single-office setting, they cannot guarantee their own safety, nor the safety of their clients, if they accept clients indiscriminately. It could almost be considered negligent for such practitioners not to have basic screening rules to attempt to minimize the risk that could come from dangerous clients in a practice setting that allows for no quick and easy support or assistance by others. Given that the best predictor of future behavior is past behavior, crucial in the screening process is gathering information about clients' history of violence and interactions with the legal system. Screening for such history can be incorporated into one's regular intake protocol or can be accomplished through standardized screening tools such as the Historical Clinical Risk–20 (Webster, Douglas, Eaves, & Hart, 1997) or the Hare Psychopathy Checklist—Revised (Hare, 2002). On the basis of this screening, therapists can determine whether the client is suitable for their caseload or needs to be referred to a setting in which the possibility of violence can be better contained.

Even with the most careful screening, therapists may inadvertently include in their caseload clients who will threaten to harm them. Moreover, therapists may work in settings, such as community agencies, where they are assigned clients by intake staff or receptionists and have no choice but to see them. Regardless of the circumstances, given that it is impossible to predict with certainty which clients may become violent, it is important for therapists to configure their therapy setting to maximize their own safety (Berg et al., 2000; Brems, 2000). Ideally, all therapy rooms should have at least two means of egress, and therapists should always have ready access to one of the exits. The therapy setting should not include any easily accessible objects that could easily be turned into weapons (e.g., heavy paperweights, scissors, envelope openers) and should not be isolated from other therapists, staff members, or neighbors. Although it is critical that therapy rooms be sound-proofed so that sessions cannot be overheard, they should not be so quiet that calls for help would go unheard. Therapists who regularly see potentially dangerous clients should take even more precautions, including seeing the clients in a room that can be easily monitored through video or a one-way mirror, that has a window on the door, and that has a crisis button available to obtain immediate help.

The final form of self-protection, namely, record keeping, is not related to physical self-protection but to professional self-protection. Although not foolproof by any means, thorough and accurate record keeping goes a long way to keep therapists safe from legal repercussions related to dangerous situations and helps ensure that review of a case can be conducted if necessary (Mitchell, 2001). Although malpractice suits are rarer than most clinicians fear (Remley & Herlihy, 2005), they do occur, and when they do, a carefully kept record is crucial to showing that the therapist was not negligent in the management of a case. Indeed, any therapist, regardless of how competent, successful, and skilled, may lose a client through suicide. What will distinguish one therapist from another who was clearly negligent, careless, and indifferent to her or his client's suicidal state is the presence of a well-documented, thorough client record (Fremouw, Perczel, & Ellis, 1990, p. 10).

By documenting in a clinical record all dangerous situations experienced with clients, therapists must think through the actions taken and the actions planned. Through this simple act of preparing paperwork, the therapist refocuses on the case and provides a means of review. Preparation of paperwork may lead the care provider to recognize and rectify an oversight or may lead to the awareness that all actions were complete, thorough, and supportive of the client.

Consultation and Supervision

Maintaining competence is a crucial aspect of ethical practice, and one of the best ways to achieve this is through ongoing supervision by a senior colleague with expertise in treating potentially violent or suicidal clients (Falender & Shafranske, 2004). A second valuable resource is a peer consultation network or one-on-one consultation with a highly competent colleague (Falender & Shafranske, 2004; Gottlieb, 2006). Typically, supervision involves formal oversight in which the supervisor has some authority and responsibility to the client being served; therefore, supervisory arrangements require client knowledge and consent for the supervisor to have access to private client information and records (Bernard & Goodyear, 2004). Supervisors are also typically paid. Consultation varies in level of formality and fee arrangement, but typically consultants do not have oversight responsibilities and do not need access to client records or identifying information. They offer the perspective of a well-qualified peer about the course of care and the avenues for enhancing it (Falender & Shafranske, 2004). Having work reviewed by another competent care provider, whether in a supervisory or a consultative arrangement, helps identify issues missed or overlooked and can be useful in identifying subtle warning signs in clients. Therapists may be unaware of danger signals from both new and long-term clients. A supervisor or consultant who enters the picture with fresh eyes and ears may pick up on signals the therapist may have overlooked. It has been argued that nothing affords clients better clinical services than their providers regularly seeking supervision or consultation (Brems, 2000, 2001). Similarly, it can be argued that peer guidance is one of the best avenues to help keep a therapist safe from potentially dangerous clients. That is, by obtaining regular and ongoing supervision or consultation, therapists create a feedback loop that results in better quality service and enhanced self-development, both personally and professionally (Campbell, 2006). One-on-one support may be more detailed and successful in identifying trouble spots in therapy; however, small group support, in which a dyad or triad meets with a senior professional, has its place as well. It is efficient and can be helpful in building professional networks. Therapists with high-risk clientele may need more individual supervision or consultation, whereas therapists with lower risk clientele and who screen clients carefully may benefit most from small group consultation. For the latter, because they are much less at risk, group interaction may be preferable because it may allow those therapists to confront dangerous clients indirectly by listening to other providers talking about their own difficult clients. Should they then encounter a dangerous individual in their own practice, they may be more prepared than they would have been otherwise.

For clinicians with low-risk clientele, group consultation can add a component of collegiality and joint learning that can be stimulating and exciting. Hiring a leader for a consultation group reduces expense and can yield excellent results in terms of exposure to new material. Consultation (individual or group), however, may not suffice for psychologists who regularly see difficult and challenging clients or who already experience distress or impairment. For these individuals, supervision may well represent the safest route to self-protection. Legal consultation with an attorney experienced in mental health law is another valuable option, and such consultation may be available through the clinician's state or provincial psychological association or malpractice insurance provider (see Gottlieb, 2006, for an excellent discussion of the role of peer consultation for ethics issues).

One of the most crucial times to obtain supervision or consultation is after encountering a crisis situation with a client. Timely discussion of the situation can help the therapist talk through the actions that were taken to ensure that the right choices were made, help diffuse personal emotions and self-doubts, and provide alternatives if the situation is still acute. Debriefings are most helpful if they occur very soon after the actual threatening event. It may be tempting for clinicians to call a personal friend or family member to debrief a dangerous situation, but it is most helpful to call another MHP. The friend or family member will, of course, be able to support the clinician emotionally, but cannot validate that correct action was taken. A supportive colleague can serve both functions and be a monitor to ensure that the clinician did not overlook a crucial detail that has yet to be attended to.

It is imperative to reiterate that when engaging in supervision or consultation, therapists must respect and maintain clients' confidentiality. As a general rule, without specific written permission from the client, this involves not disclosing identifying information about the client and conveying only the information needed to meet the purpose of consultation (APA, 2002, Standard 4.05). However, it is equally imperative to note that an exception to maintaining clients' confidentiality arises when it is deemed necessary to disclose information to protect the client, psychologist, or others from harm if permitted by law.

Networking

Making time for "stimulating and enjoyable encounters with . . . colleagues" is considered essential to maintaining well-being (Alexander, 1997, p. 25), and one easy way to do this is through active networking. Networking requires psychologists to take responsibility for reaching out to others who share similar practice characteristics to build a more or less formal support group. There are infinite ways of creating supports; each therapist needs to decide what is best and most desirable. Some networks may be based in social activities; others may be founded on professional issues. Some therapists may choose to develop a network of colleagues that revolves around going to dinner once a month; others may choose to join a professional association. Becoming a member of a professional association is an excellent way of introducing oneself into a professional network that is guaranteed to address the issue of challenging or dangerous clients.

Continuing Education

No matter where a therapist chooses to work and no matter how a practice setting is set up, knowing how to deal with clients who are dangerous to self or others is the best protective device. One way of gaining this knowledge is by reading books such as this one; another ongoing means is continuing education (CE). Generally speaking, one of the best ways to maintain skills at the highest and most professional level is by seeking out opportunities for CE. This is particularly important with regard to skills needed to deal with clients who may harm themselves or others. CE activities are particularly helpful in the context of preventing impairment or dangerous situations arising from threats by clients in that the careful and targeted selection of relevant CE events helps clinicians stay in touch with the most up-to-date strategies for dealing with such crises. Psychologists, especially those working with high-risk clientele, are well served by seeking out CE events centered on suicide prevention (e.g., gatekeeper training or training using motivational interviewing for working with suicidal ideation), violence prevention (including workshops and seminars on verbal and physical self-defense), and even stalking or harassment. Ethics workshops, mandated for maintaining licensure for MHPs in many U.S. states and Canadian provinces, are also excellent opportunities to learn more about dealing effectively with suicidal and violent clients, as these individuals generally warrant careful ethical attention.

Participating in workshops and other training options is not the only way psychologists can keep abreast of new developments in dealing with potentially dangerous clients. Staying current with the peer-reviewed literature by reading journals and books and participating in online training can be equally helpful (although these means do not provide the social supports and networking opportunities inherent in in-person CE events). Some of the most relevant publications that often cover issues of threats of harm by clients include but may not be limited to *Professional Psychology: Research and Practice; Clinical Psychology Review; Psychotherapy: Theory, Research, Practice, Training; American Journal of Psychotherapy; Journal of Counseling & Development*, and *Clinical Social Work Journal*. More and more online services are available that allow professionals to turn article and book reading into home-study courses for CE credits (e.g., http://www.apa.org/ce/ and http://www.psychceu.com).

Personal Self-Care to Deal With Threats of Harm

Encountering violent or suicidal clients is perhaps one of the most powerful stressors clinicians will ever face. As discussed previously, the emotional aftermath of such a client encounter can be significant, regardless of whether the situation was resolved positively or negatively. What Voltaire wrote centuries ago still rings true today: "I was never ruined but twice, once when I lost a lawsuit and once when I won one." The emotional fallout can be so intense as to lead to practitioner burnout or impairment if not attended to carefully and quickly. The healthy practitioner takes time for self-care and attends carefully to personal emotional and physical needs. The range of personal self-care skills is large and varied, and each therapist needs to develop a set of self-care skills that fits with his or her personal lifestyle and practice demands. Following is a quick overview of personal self-care skills (based on Brems, 2000, 2001) that are useful in the aftermath of dealing with a dangerous client and that are powerful preventive agents that need to be in place at all times to be most effective in inoculating psychologists against burnout and impairment.

Self-Exploration and Awareness

The personal self-care strategies most relevant in the context of preventing burnout and impairment because of difficult or dangerous clients are related to self-exploration and self-awareness. Maintaining self-esteem, self-efficacy, and a basic sense of personal competence is critical during periods of challenge (Wheeler, 1997). One way to achieve emotional stability is through the development of self-awareness. The more self-aware, congruent, and centered psychologists are, the less likely they are to judge their clients and the more likely they are to be empathically accepting of and positive about them (Johns, 1996). Self-awareness leads to better professionalism and helps therapists "flourish as human beings" (Johns, 1996, p. 61), making them more capable of dealing with difficulties and challenges.

Burnout is most easily prevented when the therapist is committed to remaining self-aware and capable of recognizing early symptoms of stress or impairment. Strategies that may be tried include personal psychotherapy, meditation, journaling, and dream work. Some of these self-exploration strategies (e.g., meditation) are most beneficial if used on an ongoing basis; other strategies (e.g., journaling, psychotherapy) may be amenable to use in response to a specific situation. Regardless of which strategy is used and how often it is used, the primary point of these strategies is that therapists need to remain acutely aware of personal reactions to their clients and work and need to make an effort to maintain a routine of self-exploration. Good additional resources in this category of self-care are Kabat-Zinn (1994), Kornfield (1993, 1994), and Pennebaker (2004).

Relaxation and Centeredness

A great way to fortify oneself against stress is an ongoing routine of self-care related to relaxation and centeredness. Many versatile and easy-to-use strategies exist that can help clinicians maintain calm during difficult situations, and they work best if they have become second nature. For example, breathing exercises can be incorporated easily and frequently into a busy practitioner's day (Farhi, 1996). Guided imagery tapes or routines take a bit more effort and time but can be extremely helpful during stressful times in a clinician's life (e.g., http://www.academyforguidedimagery.com, http://www.breathing.com, http://www.mindfulnesstapes.com). Mindfulness is perhaps the most easily applied and most useful of the centering strategies (Hanh, 1975; Rinpoche, 1995; Rosenberg, 1999). Mindfulness is the practice of stillness, centeredness, and full awareness in the present moment. It involves conscious living and alert presence of mind; it helps bring awareness into focus and directs attention to present actions and thoughts (Das, 1999). Progressive muscle relaxation is a strategy that can be used on an ongoing basis or to help cope with a situational stressor. Of course, no one strategy will fit each therapist; thus, a variety of strategies should be tried to identify one that will work.

Healthful Personal Habits

No discussion of personal self-care is complete without some attention to personal health habits such as nutrition, exercise, and rest. Although these strategies may not appear to be very relevant in the context of dangerous or threatening clients, they deserve mention, if only because they provide a solid foundation on which all other self-care strategies rest. Diet and nutrition are an essential part of a person's functioning and well-being. Food choices affect physical, mental, and emotional health, a connection many people do not seem to make (e.g., Null, 2000; Somer, 1999; Werbach, 1999). Individuals who are interested in shifting to more natural ways of eating can find good advice in many resources, including Crayhon (1994), Hyman (2006), and Robbins (2001).

Just as diet is related to a person's emotional well-being, so too is regular exercise. Physical activity has four elements: stamina (or aerobic capacity and endurance); strength (or muscular power); suppleness (or flexibility); and sensitivity (or balance, rhythm, and timing). A good physical fitness program incorporates all four aspects to some degree. Getting plenty of sleep is a most important self-care habit and one that needs extra attention during times of stress or overwork when rest is often a low priority. The number of hours of sleep required varies from about 7 to 9 hours per night, but everyone is best served by exploring their own personal needs for sleep. The development of routines best follows the dictates of the body rather than some external criterion of what "should" or "should not" be done.

CONCLUSION

Most therapists are at risk from a client at some point in their careers, and most experience situations in which clients threaten third parties or themselves with harm. Complicating the picture even further is the real risk of ethical or legal consequences for professional misjudgment about whether the duty to protect has been triggered and how to carry it out competently. In essence, the professional has the triple burden of taking all reasonable professional actions to protect the client from harm, protect third parties from harm, and in the process keep him- or herself physically safe and mentally focused. It is crucial to acknowledge these realities, to take the necessary steps to prevent crises, and to be prepared in case they do occur. Accomplishing this degree of preparation, both personally and professionally, requires planfulness on the psychologist's part. Such preparation can range from screening clients, structuring the therapy setting, and identifying resources to assist with and prevent these situations to more personal protections such as being centered and calm when a crisis arises. Therapists need to be equipped with self-care strategies to deal with any emotional, physical, and legal sequelae of working with clients who threaten them, other people, or themselves. It is far better to be prepared for situations in which clients make violent threats and never have this happen than to face such situations unprepared if they do arise.

REFERENCES

Alexander, M. B. (1997). Caught in the maze, aghast with this phase. In J. A. Kottler (Ed.), *Finding your way as a counselor* (pp. 25–28). Alexandria, VA: American Counseling Association.

American Psychological Association. (2002). Ethical principles of psychologists and code of conduct. *American Psychologist, 57,* 1060–1073.

Arthur, G. L., Brende, J. O., & Quiroz, S. E. (2003). Violence: Incidence and frequency of physical and psychological assaults affecting mental health providers in Georgia. *Journal of General Psychology, 130,* 22–45.

Barnett, J. E., MacGlashan, S. G., & Clarke, A. J. (2003). Risk management and ethical issues regarding termination and abandonment. In L. VandeCreek & T. Jackson (Eds.), *Innovations in clinical practice: A source book* (Vol. 18, pp. 231–245). Sarasota, FL: Professional Resource Exchange.

Bayne, R. (1997). Survival. In I. Horton & V. Varma (Eds.), *The needs of counsellors and psychotherapists: Emotional, social, physical, professional* (pp. 183–198). London: Sage.

Berg, A. Z., Bell, C. C., & Tupin, J. (2000). Clinician safety: Assessing and managing the violent patient. *New Directions for Mental Health Services, 86,* 9–29.

Bernard, J. M., & Goodyear, R. K. (2004). *Fundamentals of clinical supervision* (3rd ed.). New York: Pearson.

Brems, C. (2000). *Dealing with challenges in psychotherapy and counseling.* Pacific Grove, CA: Brooks/Cole.

Brems, C. (2001). *Basic skills in psychotherapy and counseling.* Pacific Grove, CA: Brooks/Cole.

Campbell, J. (2006). *Essentials of clinical supervision.* Hoboken, NJ: Wiley.

Chemtob, C. M., Hamada, R. S., Bauer, G., Torigoe, R. Y., & Kinney, B. (1988). Patient suicide: Frequency and impact on psychologists. *Professional Psychology: Research and Practice, 19,* 416–420.

Corder, B. F., & Whiteside, R. (1996). A survey of psychologists' safety issues and concerns. *American Journal of Forensic Psychology, 14,* 65–72.

Crayhon, R. (1994). *Nutrition made simple: A comprehensive guide to the latest findings in optimal nutrition.* New York: M. Evans.

Das, L. S. (1999). *Awakening to the sacred: Creating a spiritual life from scratch.* New York: Broadway Books.

Ensworth v. Mullvain, 224 Cal.App.3d 1105, Cal. Rptr. 447 (1990).

Falender, C. A., & Shafranske, E. P. (2004). *Clinical supervision: A competency-based approach*. Washington, DC: American Psychological Association.

Farhi, D. (1996). *The breathing book: Good health and vitality through essential breath work*. New York: Owl Books.

Fremouw, W. J., Perczel, M., & Ellis, T. E. (1990). *Suicide risk: Assessment and response guidelines*. Boston: Allyn & Bacon.

Galeazzi, G. M., Elkins, K., & Curci, P. (2005). Emergency psychiatry: The stalking of mental health professionals by patients. *Psychiatric Services, 56,* 137–138.

Gentile, S. R., Asamen, J. K., Harmell, P. H., & Weathers, R. (2002). The stalking of psychologists by their clients. *Professional Psychology: Research and Practice, 33,* 490–494.

Gottlieb, M. C. (2006). A template for peer ethics consultation. *Ethics & Behavior, 16,* 151–162.

Hanh, T. N. (1975). *The miracle of mindfulness*. Boston: Beacon Press.

Hare, R.D. (2002). *Hare Psychopathy Checklist—Revised*. Toronto, Canada: Multi-Health Systems.

Hyman, M. (2006). *Ultra-metabolism: The simple plan for automatic weight loss*. New York: Scribner.

Jacobson, J. M., Ting, L., Sanders, S., & Harrington, D. (2004). Prevalence of and reactions to fatal and nonfatal suicidal behavior: A national study of mental health social workers. *Omega: Journal of Death and Dying, 49,* 237–248.

Jevne, R. F., & Williams, D. R. (1998). *When dreams don't work: Professional caregivers and burnout*. Amityville, NY: Baywood.

Johns, H. (1996). *Personal development in counsellor training*. London: Cassell.

Kabat-Zinn, J. (1994). *Wherever you go, there you are*. New York: Hyperion.

Kornfield, J. (1993). *A path with heart*. New York: Bantam.

Kornfield, J. (1994). *Buddha's little instruction book*. New York: Bantam.

McAdams, C. R., III, & Foster, V. A. (2000). Client suicide: Its frequency and impact on counselors. *Journal of Mental Health Counseling, 22,* 107–121.

Mitchell, R. (2001). *Documentation in counseling records* (2nd ed.). Alexandria, VA: American Counseling Association.

Null, G. (2000). *The food–mood–body connection: Nutrition-based and environmental approaches to mental health*. New York: Seven Stories.

Pabian, Y. L., & Welfel, E. R. (2007, August). *Psychologists' knowledge and application of state laws in Tarasoff-type situations*. Paper presented at the 115th Annual Convention of the American Psychological Association, San Francisco.

Pennebaker, J. W. (2004). *Writing to heal*. Oakland, CA: New Harbinger.

Pope, K. S., & Tabachnick, B. G. (1993). Therapist's anger, hate, fear and sexual feelings: National survey of therapist responses, client characteristics, critical events, formal complaints, and training. *Professional Psychology: Research and Practice, 24,* 142–152.

Remley, T. P., & Herlihy, B. (2005). *Ethical, legal, and professional issues in counseling.* Upper Saddle River, NJ: Pearson.

Rinpoche, A. T. (1995). *Taming the tiger.* Rochester, VT: Inner Traditions.

Robbins, J. (2001). *The food revolution: How your diet can help save your life and our world.* San Francisco: Conari.

Romans, J. S. C., Hays, J. R., & White, T. K. (1996). Stalking and related behaviors experienced by counseling center staff members from current or former clients. *Professional Psychology: Research and Practice, 27,* 595–599.

Rosenberg, L. (1999). *Breath by breath: The liberating practice of insight meditation.* Boston: Shambhala.

Rupert, P. A., & Morgan, D. J. (2005). Work setting and burnout among professional psychologists. *Professional Psychology: Research and Practice, 36,* 544–550.

Sandberg, D. A., McNiel, D. E., & Binder, R. L. (2002). Stalking, threatening, and harassing behavior by psychiatric patients toward clinicians. *Journal of the American Academy of Psychiatry and the Law, 30,* 221–229.

Sanders, S., Jacobson, J. M., & Ting, L. (2005). Reactions of mental health social workers following a client suicide completion: A qualitative investigation. *Omega: Journal of Death and Dying, 51,* 197–218.

Somer, E. (1999). *Food and mood: The complete guide to eating well and feeling your best* (2nd ed.). New York: Holt.

Walker, C. E., & Matthews, J. R. (1997). Introduction: First steps in professional psychology. In J. R. Matthews & C. E. Walker (Eds.), *Basic skills and professional issues in clinician psychology* (pp. 1–12). Boston: Allyn & Bacon.

Webster, C. D., Douglas, K. S., Eaves, D., & Hart, S. D. (1997). *HCR-20: Assessing risk for violence.* Lutz, FL: Psychological Assessment Resources.

Werbach, M. R. (1999). *Nutritional influences on mental illness: A sourcebook of clinical research* (2nd ed.). Tarzana, CA: Third Line Press.

Wheeler, S. (1997). Achieving and maintaining competence. In I. Horton & V. Varma (Eds.), *The needs of counsellors and psychotherapists: Emotional, social, physical, professional* (pp. 120–134). London: Sage.

15

EMERGING ISSUES IN THE DUTY TO PROTECT

ELIZABETH REYNOLDS WELFEL

As scientific knowledge and technological applications of treatment expand, so too do the possible applications of the duty to protect. The first emerging area is the application of the duty when a client discloses threats of harm to self or others via e-mail or another electronic medium. The next is the increasing visibility of suicidal intent coupled with intent to harm others, and the last (and the most distant on the horizon) is the dilemma of mental health professionals when clients refuse to disclose to family members their risk of life-threatening illness because of a genetic anomaly. This chapter introduces the discussion of each issue with a case situation that illustrates the dilemma and continues with an explication of the ethical and legal responsibilities embedded in each situation.

SCENARIO 1: ELECTRONIC COMMUNICATIONS OF HARM TO SELF OR OTHERS

Bernard, a Utah psychologist and Army veteran with expertise in post-traumatic stress, offers e-therapy (i.e., via e-mail exchanges and weekly online chat groups) to clients with loved ones serving in combat zones. Late one night, an online client sends him an e-mail in which she discloses imminent suicidal intent. Two weeks earlier, the client had learned that her husband suffered serious head trauma and the loss of both legs in a roadside bomb attack near Baghdad. When she visited her husband the previous day for the first time at his Virginia hospital, she learned the full scope of his neurological damage. At midnight that night, she wrote to Bernard, "My husband is nearly brain dead and will never function normally or even recognize me. I have lost all purpose to my life and the pain of watching him live in a condition that he would hate is too much for me to bear. So I have decided to end my life and wish I could end my husband's as well, but he is watched too closely for that to happen. At dawn tomorrow I will be driving to my husband's hospital room to say goodbye to him, and then take an overdose of sleeping pills while watching the sunrise at a nearby park. Thank you for your support during these difficult times." By the time Bernard checks his e-mail the next morning, it is already 10:00 a.m. Eastern time. Bernard immediately contacts law enforcement in the location where she has driven, but by the time they arrive the woman is already dead.[1]

Although this particular scenario is fictional, the possibility that clients would use e-mail to disclose dangerousness to self or others is quite real. Research has suggested that people reveal personal information more quickly and easily in electronic communications than in face-to-face interactions (Joinson, 2001) and that norms for self-disclosure get established quickly in online media (Dietz-Uhler, Bishop-Clark, & Howard, 2005). Suler (2004) referred to this as a *disinhibition effect* of online communication. Thus, the situation that Bernard faces—a client who chooses to communicate intent to self harm via e-mail—is likely to occur, if it has not already happened. (One report of a suicide of a member of an online mental health support group has already appeared in the literature; Hsiung, 2007). Indeed, because e-mail has become such a ubiquitous part of most people's lives, even clients receiving traditional psychotherapy may elect to send the therapist an e-mail about intent to die by suicide instead of calling or making an appointment. Currently, nearly 1 billion people across the planet have Internet access, and 147 million Americans use the Internet regularly (Pew Internet & American Life Project, 2007). The figure is even higher for young adults—87% of those between the ages of 18 and 29 use the Internet (Pew Internet & American Life Project, 2007). Estimates of the number of e-mails sent each day across the globe range as high as 183 billion (Brownlow, 2007). The mean number of daily e-mail communications between mental health professionals and clients is not known, but several hundred Web sites offer online counseling and therapy (Ainsworth, 2002; Heinlen, Welfel, Richmond, & O'Donnell, 2003; Heinlen, Welfel, Richmond, & Rak, 2003), and according

---

[1]Scenarios 1 and 5 are fictional.

to the estimate of one author, at least 5,000 e-mails are exchanged each day between mental health providers and consumers (Freeny, 2001).

Other data suggest that a number of psychologists engage in between-session e-mail communications with traditional clients even if they do not offer e-therapy services (Drude, 2005; Salib & Murphy, 2003; Welfel & Bunce, 2003). In a national survey of randomly selected practicing psychologists, Welfel and Bunce (2003) found that nearly half of their sample (46%) reported at least one e-mail from a client in the past 3 years, with the content of these e-mails equally divided between logistic and therapeutic matters. In parallel findings, Salib and Murphy (2003) reported that 42% of their sample of members of American Psychological Association (APA) Division 42 (Psychologists in Independent Practice) received or transmitted e-mails to clients. Projections also suggest that online communications between mental health professionals and consumers are likely to increase (Koocher, 2007; Norcross, Hedges, & Prochaska, 2002; Wolf, 2003). This trend is not limited to psychotherapists and their clients: Driven by consumer demand, increasing numbers of physicians have e-mail contact with patients. In fact, the desire for this mode of communication is so strong among many medical patients that 90% of them would view e-mail contact with a current physician as a benefit, and 56% of patients would consider changing physicians if the new physician accepted e-mail communications (Recupero, 2005). The American Medical Association (2004) has issued guidelines to assist physicians in responding ethically to these patient requests.

In light of the increasingly prominent role that technology plays in the delivery of services, the question arises about Bernard's ethical and legal responsibilities to protect online clients and third parties from harm either when a client is available to the therapist only through electronic communication or when a client receiving traditional services elects to communicate dangerous intent via e-mail. The professional codes of ethics do not distinguish between electronic and face-to-face communications in regard to the duty to protect, with all of the codes allowing for a breach of confidentiality to prevent harm to clients from any modality. With the exception of APA Standard 4.02(c) that requires psychologists to inform clients about the limits of privacy and confidentiality in electronic media (APA, 2002), only the American Counseling Association's (ACA's; 2005) *Code of Ethics* enumerates unique ethical duties for counselors offering online services. Specifically, it instructs counselors about requirements for competent informed consent for online services, including telling online clients about time zone differences (Section A.12.g.2.), emergency procedures if the counselor is not immediately available (Section A.12.g.9.), and potential compromises to confidentiality and access particular to computer-based communications (Sections A.12.g.1–5.). This code also mandates that counselors determine that clients who are interested in online services are capable of using them appropriately and that these services are likely to meet their needs (A.12.b.). It goes on to state that if clients are deemed inappropriate for online care, counselors should consider delivering services face to face (A.12.c.), although referral to another professional is likely to be the only feasible way to comply with this latter standard if the client lives in a different locale.

APA's Ethics Committee issued a statement on telephone and electronic communication in 1997, which clarified that such interactions are not inherently unethical, that ethical issues arising from such communications will be evaluated on a case-by-case basis, and that

> psychologists considering such services must review the characteristics of the services, the service delivery method, and the provisions for confidentiality. Psychologists must then consider the relevant ethical standards and other requirements, such as licensure board rules. (para. 3)

The statement also referred psychologists to the many sections of the then-current Ethics Code (APA, 2002) that may have relevance and notes that the committee will continue to study this issue.

Consequently, the answer to the question of whether Bernard acted ethically rests largely on three factors: the comprehensiveness of the client's informed consent for e-therapy, the adequacy of Bernard's initial and ongoing assessment of the client as an appropriate candidate for e-therapy (especially once Bernard learned of the seriousness of the injuries to his client's husband), and the quality of the therapeutic service provided.

Appropriate informed consent in this circumstance is defined in the following way by the APA (2002) Ethics Code in Standard 10.01 Informed Consent to Therapy:

> (a) When obtaining informed consent to therapy as required in Standard 3.10, Informed Consent, psychologists inform clients/patients as early as is feasible in the therapeutic relationship about the nature and anticipated course of therapy, fees, involvement of third parties, and limits of confidentiality and provide sufficient opportunity for the client/patient to ask questions and receive answers.
>
> (b) When obtaining informed consent for treatment for which generally recognized techniques and procedures have not been established, psychologists inform their clients/patients of the developing nature of the treatment, the potential risks involved, alternative treatments that may be available, and the voluntary nature of their participation. (p. 1072)

In addition to the lack of evidence as to their effectiveness as a mode of therapeutic intervention, computer-based communications contain some unique risks, including the possibility of technology failure, compromises in the security of online communications, difficulties in confirming the identity of the sender and the honesty of information provided, and misunderstanding of text messages, all of which may prevent a professional from accurately identifying a threat of harm (Mallen, Vogel, & Rochlen, 2005).

Bernard's client ought to have received fully informed consent about these risks and her alternatives to online care. Although as a psychologist, Bernard was not governed by the provisions of the ACA (2005) *Code of Ethics* (unless he was also an ACA member), he would have been wise to also inform the client about the implications of the time zone differences between them and the procedures the client should use in an emergency. He should also have been explicit about how and when online clients ought to contact him about destructive impulses and what other resources they should turn to if he is unavailable. Many online sites include language that warns people not to use the services if they are feeling self-destructive or dangerous to someone else. The sites usually advise people with such impulses to immediately call 911 or go to a hospital emergency room. The inclusion of such language represents a minimum level of compliance with a professional's ethical responsibility to online clients, but additional steps to protect individuals whom the clinician recognizes to be at risk for harm are clearly warranted.

Judging the adequacy of Bernard's assessment and treatment is more complicated. Because the standard of care for online services is not well established, research on outcomes of this form of e-therapy is limited. No well-accepted model for conducting this service has been developed, although Maheu (2003) has presented one model that shows promise. As a result, in the absence of a clear theoretical and scientific basis for this mode of care, it is difficult to determine whether Bernard's assessment and ongoing care itself were competent. E-therapy should be considered an emerging area or experimental form of service; thus, Standard 2.01(e) of the APA Ethics Code applies:

> Boundaries of Competence 2.01
>
> (e) In those emerging areas in which generally recognized standards for preparatory training do not yet exist, psychologists nevertheless take reasonable steps to ensure the competence of their work and to protect clients/patients, students, supervisees, research participants, organizational clients, and others from harm. (APA, 2002, p. 1064)

Consequently, the determination of the adequacy of Bernard's care depends on the degree to which he took reasonable steps to ensure competence in an experimental mode of service and to protect clients from harm. One issue that emerges from this standard is whether Bernard ought to have been offering online services to individuals in distant locales at risk for losing loved ones in battle in the first place. The ethics of online therapy is a vigorously debated issue in the profession, with the strongest cautions about its value centering on situations in which clients may be experiencing significant psychological distress, recurrent psychopathology, or suicidal or homicidal intent (Alleman, 2003; Barak, 1999; Ragusea & VandeCreek, 2003). If Bernard had identified or should have identified any of these problems before his client's final e-mail, then he ought to have referred her to more traditional service, on the basis of the APA Ethics Code and on the ethical principle of nonmaleficence. Second, the purpose and scope of the service should have been clearly defined, including its experimental nature and its distinction from traditional counseling and psychotherapy. Finally, given the predictability of extreme distress when loved ones receive news of such a devastating combat injury, Bernard ought to have intervened to anticipate that distress. At a minimum, he should have considered intensifying services. If Bernard had taken all these actions, the likelihood that he acted unethically or incompetently when that late night e-mail arrived would have been diminished significantly.

Many jurisdictions have no statutes or case law that directly address e-therapy or the responsibilities of professionals who offer such services (Terry, 2002). The few states that regulate e-therapy tend to address eligibility to offer services to residents in their states (Recupero & Rainey, 2005). California, for example, specifies that professionals who offer online services to that state's residents must hold California licenses (California Board of Psychology, 2004). Many other states are considering legislation, and the issue of regulation is far from settled. Thus, clinicians should take a cautious stance when offering electronic communication options to clients. In other words, clinicians would be wise to assess the risk of ethical violations and liability issues and define the level of risk that is acceptable at a very low level. Clinicians should also keep apprised of the guidelines and recommendations of other professional bodies and organizations. For example, the Ohio Psychological Association has developed recommendations for responsible online interactions for its members (Drude, 2005). The California Board of Psychology has posted a notice to consumers to assist them in making decisions about online services (http://www.psychboard.ca.gov/consumers/telepsych.shtml) that professionals may also wish to consult. The International Society for Mental Health Online (http://www.ismho.org) exists for the purpose of providing professional support and guidance to professionals with online contact with clients.

SCENARIOS 2, 3, AND 4: HOMICIDE COUPLED WITH SUICIDE

On May 27, 2006, Dr. Edward Van Dyk threw his two children off a Miami hotel balcony and then jumped himself. His wife heard her children's screams from an adjacent room and saw her husband jumping when she rushed to help her children. The couple had been having marital problems, and Dr. Van Dyk's father reported that he had seemed depressed and rather paranoid lately. He had called to ask his father for help in keeping the boys safe just days before. His father was unsure of the reasons for his son's distress or actions (Anasagasti, 2006).

On April 16, 2007, college student Seung-Hui Cho killed 32 other students and faculty and wounded 25 others at Virginia Tech before turning the gun on himself. Cho had a history of depression and elective mutism and had written several papers with disturbing violent content, but he left no suicide note and made no explicit threats to kill others before the shooting began. He had been referred for court-ordered outpatient treatment but had not appeared (Hauser & O'Connor, 2007).

On the evening of January 30, 2006, at a large postal processing facility in Goleta, California, Jennifer San Marco, a former postal employee, killed six current postal employees before killing herself with a handgun. Police later also identified a seventh victim. According to media reports, the Postal Service had forced San Marco to retire in 2003 because of her worsening mental problems. Her choice of victims may also have been racially motivated; San Marco had a previous history of racial prejudice and tried to obtain a business license for a newspaper called *Racist Times* (Molloy, 2006).

In training, professional practice, and the literature, suicide and homicide are typically discussed as independent events. Recommendations for risk assessment and intervention also diverge significantly (Hillbrand, 2001). In reality, as these scenarios so tragically illustrate, the two risks sometimes coincide, and some people who kill themselves take the lives of others immediately before their suicide. The following paragraphs describe the limitations of viewing homicide and suicide as distinct events and the types of situations that may trigger a professional to need to conduct risk assessments for both types of danger. These comments are aimed at helping professionals understand triggers for violence to others when that violent intent is embedded in a plan for concurrent suicide.

The risk of a homicide–suicide is greater in distressed families but has occurred at an increasing rate in employment and educational settings; hence the development of the slang term *going postal*. In the United States, an estimated 1,000 to 1,500 homicides–suicides occur each year, representing approximately 5% of the homicides that take place (Cohen, 2003), a figure consistent with available data from other countries (Coid, 1983; Marzuk, Tardiff, & Hirsch, 1992). Most perpetrators are male, and most victims are female relatives or consorts. The majority of cases involve a single perpetrator and victim; before the Virginia Tech tragedy the prior record number of deaths was 20 victims (Cohen, 2003). Older people experience the highest risk of homicide–suicide, and within this population, 80% to 90% of homicide–suicides involve spousal deaths perpetrated by a male partner (Malphurs, Eisdorfer, & Cohen, 2001). The ratio of completed homicide–suicides to incomplete or thwarted attempts is 5:1, according to data from Florida (Cohen, Llorrente, & Eisdorfer, 1998), a striking contrast to data that show that suicide attempts outnumber suicide deaths by a ratio of at least 8:1 (National Institute of Mental Health, 2003), highlighting the need for clinicians to conduct careful assessment of co-occurring aggression.

Marzuk et al. (1992) identified several subtypes of homicide–suicide. *Filicide–suicide* involves the killing of a child before suicide, as exemplified in the Van Dyk scenario above. *Familicide–suicide* is the type most commonly reported in the media, in which a person kills several relatives before the suicide. In this type and in the next type, *spousal homicide–suicide*, the perpetrator is likely to be an older man who is depressed, paranoid, and abusing substances (Malphurs et al., 2001; Marzuk et al., 1992). Spousal killings can occur either because of jealousy or because of declining health; the latter is the most common provocation in older men who are caregivers for their spouses (Malphurs et al., 2001). The fourth type is the *extrafamilial homicide–suicide*, in which the perpetrator kills others and self in response to a perceived injustice, as the San Marco and Virginia Tech cases illustrate. Hillbrand (2001) noted that extrafamilial events provoke the most media attention in spite of their infrequent occurrence, and he attributed this attention to the high level of fear these events elicit from the general public. A final entry in Marzuk et al.'s (1992) typology is commonly referred to as *suicide by cop*, in which an individual uses lethal force against a police officer with the express purpose of being shot by the police. Law enforcement data indicate an increase in the frequency of justifiable police shootings when the victim appears to have a suicidal motive (Parent, 1998). Sadly, a perusal of any major newspaper shows that another type that must be added to the list is the politically motivated homicide–suicide, commonly known as a suicide bombing, an all-too-familiar occurrence across the globe.

Nonlethal aggression also accompanies suicidal intent more often than is generally acknowledged (Hillbrand, 2001). Hillbrand (2001) made an important point regarding co-occurring aggression toward others and self. He proposed that homicide–suicide be considered the end of a continuum of actions that couple harm to self and harm to others and that professionals ought to be aware of the real potential for actions on that continuum that are less extreme, such as the coupling of self-mutilation and serious injury to others.

The clinical indicators for homicide–suicide resemble the indicators for suicide more than the indicators for homicide. Depression, especially psychotic depression; prior suicide attempts; paranoia; and substance abuse are common predictors (Marzuk et al., 1992; Milroy, 1993), but a lengthy history of impulsivity and violence are not (Hillbrand, 2001). Both the homicide and suicide are planned, sometimes far in advance of the event, and typically despair and hopelessness are present (Cohen, 2003; Malphurs et al., 2001; Marzuk et al., 1992). According to Dietz (1986) and Hillbrand (2001), individuals who commit homicide–suicide seldom give threats or warnings of their intended actions, but older men who plan to kill their wives before their own suicide may be an exception (Malphurs et al., 2001). If a client discloses some information related to the plan, it is more likely to be the intention to die by suicide. Thus, Hillbrand (2001) especially recommended exploring the possibility of danger to others when clients reveal suicidal intent, although he also urged the exploration of suicidal intent when a threat to others is disclosed.

In his review of the evidence, Hillbrand (2001) reported that biological, developmental, and social factors may influence the likelihood of a homicide–suicide. Specifically, he cited the evidence of a connection between serotonin levels and aggression and a history of comorbid depression and disruptive behavior in childhood and adolescence coupled with current severe levels of impulsive behavior as important risk factors. Rogers (2000) also noted some factors that may function to decrease risk, including intelligence, spiritual beliefs, reasons for living, positive social orientation, a resilient temperament, and healthy beliefs about achievement.

Consequently, this literature encourages mental health professionals to take a comprehensive view of danger to self and danger to others and to avoid dichotomizing these risks. Because the presence of depression is the single strongest predictor of both suicide and homicide–suicide, clinicians should assess danger to others along with suicidal intent whenever significant levels of depression are present. In fact, depression frequently occurs among individuals who are violent even in the absence of an intent to couple the violence with suicide (Hillbrand, Foster, & Hirt, 1988), although most recommended treatments for aggression fail to routinely include assessment for depression. Older men who believe they can no longer care for their wives, depressed and somewhat paranoid individuals who feel aggrieved by an event at work or school, and parents who feel rage at spouses coupled with depression and paranoia over the safety of their children should be monitored with special care. In short, although this phenomenon is relatively infrequent and the body of research on influencing factors is less developed than the research on suicidal intent or danger to others, the devastating impact of homicide–suicide on its victims, loved ones of the victims, and on society demands that clinicians discard the simplistic categorization of homicide and suicide as separate events. The evidence that perpetrators do not act impulsively and have considered this plan for some time before the act provides a small window of opportunity for the astute professional to act to reduce the risk of this violent outcome. Although there is no separate legal duty to protect from homicide–suicide, the responsibility of the professional is to be familiar with the risks for this possibility and to be thorough in assessing whether violence to self and others is possible with a given client.

SCENARIO 5: GENETIC RISKS TO FAMILY MEMBERS

Juanita, a 41-year-old client who sought psychotherapy for depressive symptoms after her divorce, has just learned that she has the same genetic mutation that caused her mother and two aunts to experience aggressive breast cancers that caused their deaths. This news has exacerbated her depressive symptoms and provoked great anxiety about her own health and the risks that her three teenage daughters face. Juanita wishes she had never learned of the genetic mutation and is determined not to inform her daughters of their risk, saying that this news will ruin their young lives. She holds this view in spite of knowing that evidence shows that careful medical monitoring and a healthy lifestyle can reduce the likelihood that they will succumb to the cancer if they get it. Juanita does not change her mind even after several more therapy sessions discussing the issue and the implications of keeping such a secret from her daughters. Because she is the only surviving relative from her family, it is unlikely that her daughters will learn of this genetic vulnerability unless Juanita is also diagnosed with this cancer or the physician, genetic counselor, or psychologist decides to breach confidentiality.

Since the development of a map of the human genome in 2000, scientists have made significant strides in identifying genetic markers that place individuals at high risk of developing serious and life-threatening illnesses. In some cases, the presence of the genetic marker indicates the inevitable development of the disease or disorder, as is the case with Huntington's disease, in which the presence of the single gene on chromosome 4 determines the illness (Falk, Dugan, & O'Riordan, 2003), but in most cases the genetic marker or anomaly represents a substantially increased risk for the disease rather than its inevitability. When people are diagnosed with illnesses predictable from one of these known genes, they usually want to share this information with relatives and offspring so that their loved ones can get tested to evaluate their vulnerability or otherwise take preventive action to reduce their risk. Sometimes people decline genetic testing, particularly when nothing can be done to prevent the onset of the disease. For example, many people with family members who have been struck with Huntington's decline testing because they prefer not to know when they are helpless to change the outcome (Harper, Lim, & Craufurd, 2000).

The situation becomes more complicated for physicians and genetic counselors when patients with one of these disorders refuse to tell relatives at risk about their vulnerability, as is the circumstance in the case of Juanita. Dugan et al. (2003) reported that 46% of the genetic counselors they surveyed had at least one experience of a relative refusing to notify another at-risk relative. Aside from an unremitting, untreatable terminal course, factors that influenced these patients' decisions included estranged family relationships, fears of discrimination in employment or insurance eligibility, and worries about the impact on family dynamics. Australian researchers (Clarke et al., 2005) reported that nondisclosure to relatives happened very infrequently in their small sample (<1%) and that worries about the distress such information would provoke was a more salient factor in the nondisclosure than was family estrangement. In these situations, the confidential nature of the physician–patient relationship (or genetics counselor–client relationship) comes into conflict with the desire to protect the welfare of the patient's relatives. This dilemma is particularly intense when the relatives have no other way of learning of their risk for the development of the disease, as is the case with Juanita's daughters.

Because the burden here falls on physicians and genetic counselors, how is this relevant to psychotherapists? It is quite conceivable that patients facing a genetic disease will bring their worries about disclosing to family members to psychotherapists, who will then be placed in the position of having information about serious, often life-threatening health risks to identifiable third parties. Is there any ethical justification for the psychotherapist to break confidentiality? What is the obligation of the therapist if family members make contact or if they ask to join a client in a family session? Is any duty to protect ever likely to develop in this situation? (Obviously, no such legal duty currently exists in any jurisdiction in North America.)

The health care profession is divided on the question of which ethical obligation takes priority when medical practitioners possess knowledge of a genetic risk to relatives. In a 1998 policy statement on the matter, the American Society of Human Genetics urged physicians to respect confidentiality as much as possible but allowed them to contact relatives at risk of a serious disease under some circumstances. These extenuating circumstances included a level of harm that is serious and foreseeable, a persistent patient refusal to disclose even when early notification and treatment would be likely to reduce the risk of morbidity or mortality for that person, and the presence of a level of harm from nondisclosure that outweighs the harm from disclosure. The American Society of Clinical Oncology (2003) took a more conservative position in its policy statement, advocating that medical professionals encourage patients to disclose the genetic risks of cancer to relatives without endorsing the breach of confidentiality without patient consent. The American Society of Clinical Oncology views a discussion with patients about the importance of open communication with family members as the appropriate way to carry out the responsibility to patients and to the third parties at risk.

On the basis of this policy, Juanita's physician would not be mandated to speak with Juanita's daughters at any point, although he or she would be required to have a frank discussion with Juanita about the importance of such a disclosure at the point of diagnosis and probably at later points during her care when it is possible that her view has moderated. The American Medical Association Council on Ethical & Judicial Affairs (2003) advises physicians to raise the issue in pretesting counseling and to notify patients that they will be expected to inform relatives of the information gained from the testing. This approach allows the professional to get a sense of the patient's willingness to disclose before any findings and provides for a more autonomous decision by the patient about the implications of the testing on the family as a whole.

In three well-known legal cases, the courts have weighed in on this issue with slightly differing results. Two of these cases preceded the publication of the human genome map, but data about hereditary risks from the diseases of these patients were well documented in the literature. In the Florida case, *Pate v. Threlkel* (1995), the question was whether the physician had a duty to inform his patient who experienced medullary thyroid carcinoma that her children were at risk for the disease and should be tested. The physician did not discuss this issue with the patient. Pate's daughter later developed the disease and brought a malpractice suit against her mother's physician. Pate's daughter alleged that had her mother been advised of the risk to her children, she would have had the testing and the daughter might have been able to take preventative steps to reduce her own risk. The Florida Supreme Court focused on two issues: the duty of the physician to disclose the genetic risk at all and the broader question of whether the duty would be discharged by a discussion with the patient or whether a duty was owed to anyone other than the patient (Petrila, 2001). The Florida court ruled that the physician had both a duty to warn the patient about the risk to her children along with a duty to the children, but stopped short of requiring the physician to break confidentiality to tell the children. It argued that the physician could discharge the duty to the offspring through his discussions with the patient.

In the second case, *Safer v. Estate of Pack* (1996), brought by the child of a person who died from metastatic colorectal carcinoma, the New Jersey Supreme Court also ruled that a duty to the children existed, but that court declined to specify how the physician should have carried it out. The ruling stated that a physician should take "reasonable steps" to ensure that the necessary information reached those who needed it.

The Minnesota Supreme Court heard the third case, *Molloy v. Meier*, in 2004. In this case, the plaintiff was suing pediatricians for failure to properly test one of her children for genetic abnormalities after a previous child had been born with these abnormalities. The mother had asked for this testing not only for her child's sake but for her own to decide whether to have additional children. The Minnesota court held that the physicians owed a duty to both the mother and the fetus and that their failure to test for the Fragile X syndrome represented a failure to warn the mother of reasonably foreseeable risks.

In short, all three cases point to some degree of duty to family members beyond the individual patient, although the manner of carrying out the duty to protect or warn has not yet been specified in case law or in statute even for medical personnel.

The physician who discloses information about genetic risks may also refer a patient to a psychotherapist for care related to both the stress of the diagnosis and the role of family dynamics in the patient's decision making about disclosure to family. The likelihood of such a referral will increase as scientists discover more genetic risk information that medical professionals are discussing with patients. Other people facing genetic testing or responding to the diagnosis of an illness with a clear genetic origin will find their way into a therapist's office on their own. Thus, the question arises regarding the duty of the psychotherapist to maintain confidentiality when a client refuses to discuss the genetic risks with family members.

The codes of ethics of the professional associations generally allow for disclosure of confidential information to prevent serious and foreseeable harm when demanded or permitted by law even when the client fails to agree with the disclosure (ACA, 2005, Section B.2.a.; APA, 2002, Standard 4.05; National Association of Social Workers, 1999, Section 1.07[c]). To reiterate, currently no specific statutory obligation exists in any state related to a duty for psychotherapists to disclose genetic information to relatives at risk. Such an obligation is unlikely to develop because psychotherapists rarely have access to medical records or test results that would confirm a diagnosis. The primary duty clearly falls to the medical professionals with access to such records, but the moral and ethical dilemma for the psychotherapist is not entirely erased by the fact that there is no imminent danger and no legally imposed duty to protect. Just as therapists worry over their responsibilities when a client may be a threat to another, so, too, are they likely to worry about their moral obligations to relatives when clients like Juanita tell them of significant future medical risks to family members, risks that the client intends to keep secret.

Patenaude (2005) and Kaut (2006) have written excellent guides to clinical practice in this area, and I refer readers to their work for an in-depth analysis of the clinical and ethical issues of psychotherapy with clients at genetic risk for various conditions such as cancer. Patenaude advised that psychotherapists recognize several important considerations when working with people with genetic risks for cancer. First, as already mentioned, she reminded clinicians that substantial variability exists in the interest of people at risk in obtaining that information (e.g., some individuals would be very displeased). Thus, in the sessions with Juanita, the therapist would be wise to explore what, if anything, the client knows about the children's possible perspective on this issue. Second, in reality, individual susceptibility is not well understood for many diseases, so the presence of a genetic marker in one family member does not necessarily translate into any guarantee of a particular life course in another. Environment, lifestyle, and other factors are likely to influence the level of risk. The early enthusiasm of a direct link between a genetic marker and the emergence of a particular disease has waned, and a more complex understanding of etiology has replaced that notion. Consequently, for some diseases, particularly some cancers, and of course for mental illness, genetic factors may play only a limited role in influencing the onset of disease for any given person. Thus, medical professionals and psychotherapists alike need to be cautious when they consider a breach of confidentiality when the actual role of genetics in the emergence of the disease is not fully understood. In other words, the danger to the family member should be clear and foreseeable. The therapist would be well advised to explore this issue with Juanita.

Third, the history of the family's interactions and communication patterns needs to be understood. Frequently, the refusal to disclose appears to be motivated by a protective impulse and a fear of causing distress in the family members, as is the case for Juanita. At other times, people decline to inform relatives because of a long-term estrangement that would make communication difficult even under the best of circumstances. They may be fearful for their own welfare if they are the bearers of such bad news, or their efforts may be fruitless, with the relative in such denial that the disclosure feels like wasted effort for the client. In fact, it is the complexity of family dynamics that makes a referral for psychotherapy and close working relationships between medical and psychological professionals so helpful.

Psychotherapists may offer clients alternatives for disclosure that are reasonably comfortable and safe and may help them use this difficult development as a way to broach long-standing family miscommunications or estrangements. Psychotherapists can use the power of the therapeutic alliance to assist clients in finding ways to provide genetic information to relatives who may benefit from it. That may mean working with them to develop strategies for discussing the topic themselves with family, or it may involve the physician and/or the psychotherapist in a group explanation of the genetic findings. Throughout this process, professionals need to respect the autonomy of the client as much as they attend to the welfare of the unsuspecting family members. Consultation with knowledgeable colleagues is essential for the psychotherapist who is working with a client with this issue. Mental health professionals also need to establish alliances with genetics counselors and physicians so that these professionals are prepared to be proactive regarding the psychological and familial impact of genetic testing. In many situations, referral to psychological services before the testing would be useful so that the potential impact of test results can be explored before the patient receives them (Kaut, 2006). Psychotherapists can also assist medical professionals in understanding the role of social and cultural issues in the patient's response to and motivation for genetic testing (Kaut, 2006).

In the future, if the link between genetic markers and the development of mental illness becomes clearer, psychotherapists who diagnose clients with disorders such as schizophrenia or bipolar disorder may have to confront the issue of the duty to protect relatives at demonstrable genetic risk more directly (Finn & Smoller, 2006). Understanding of the role of genes in mental illness is changing rapidly, and for this reason clinicians need to keep abreast of new evidence of genetic risk and of its implications for the duty to protect. At a minimum, psychotherapists ought to be knowledgeable enough to anticipate client questions about the genetic risk of family members for mental illness and to address them accurately and have referral sources available for those who seek more detailed genetic information. They also should be knowledgeable enough to explain to clients the limits of current knowledge in this area and the role of environmental and lifestyle factors in the mental status of their loved relatives.

In short, the development of a specific legal duty to protect third parties—that is, a duty to disclose genetic information to family members at risk—is not on the horizon for psychotherapists, but the moral and ethical quandary future psychotherapists may face when dealing with clients who are unwilling to disclose critical genetic information to family members is quite real. The current ACA *Code of Ethics* (ACA, 2005, Standard B.2.a.) allows for the possible breach of confidentiality to protect people from serious and foreseeable harm and thereby appears to open the door for such a disclosure. The code clearly does not mandate release of such information, but it does not prohibit it either because one can argue that vulnerability to a serious genetic disease is harm, especially if medical intervention can reduce or eliminate the negative effects of that genetic vulnerability. The current wording in APA's (2002) Ethics Code is more ambiguous because disclosure without client consent is allowed only where mandated or permitted by law. The National Association of Social Workers' (1999) *Code of Ethics* would allow such disclosure only if the danger was serious, foreseeable, and *imminent*, a standard not likely to apply to information about a genetic risk of disease.

CONCLUSION

In each situation discussed in this chapter, the message to practicing psychotherapists is to stay attuned to research in the field. Our responsibilities to clients and others at risk of harm are not static—they change as advances in psychological and medical knowledge become available and as legal and ethical standards develop. Consequently, the professional most likely to be successful at protecting clients and others from harm is the one who works to keep up to date with these changes and who consults with other well-informed professionals about complex ethical and legal issues.

REFERENCES

Ainsworth, M. (2002). *Information for journalists: Interview with Martha Ainsworth*. Retrieved July 19, 2006, from http://www.metanoia.org/imhs/interview.htm#numbers

Alleman, J. R. (2003). Online counseling: The Internet and mental health treatment. *Psychotherapy: Theory, Research, Practice, Training, 39*, 199–209.

American Counseling Association. (2005). *ACA code of ethics*. Retrieved July 27, 2006, from http://www.counseling.org/Resources/CodeOfEthics/TP/Home/CT2.aspx

American Medical Association. (2004). *Guidelines for physician–patient electronic communication*. Retrieved July 31, 2006, from www.ama-assn.org/ama/pub/category/2386.html

American Medical Association Council on Ethical & Judicial Affairs. (2003). *E-2.131: Disclosure of familial risk in genetic testing*. Retrieved October 15, 2006, from http://www.ama-assn.org/apps/pf_new/pf_online?f_n=browse&doc=policyfiles/HnE/E-2.131.HTM

American Psychological Association. (2002). Ethical principles of psychologists and code of conduct. *American Psychologist, 57*, 1060–1073. Retrieved July 27, 2006, from http://www.apa.org/ethics/code2002.html

American Psychological Association Ethics Committee. (1997). *APA statement on services by telephone, teleconferencing and Internet*. Retrieved January 4, 2008, from http://www.apa.org/ethics/stmnt01.html

American Society of Clinical Oncology, Working Group on Genetic Testing for Cancer Susceptibility. (2003). American Society of Clinical Oncology policy statement update: Genetic testing for cancer susceptibility. *Journal of Clinical Oncology, 21*, 1–10.

American Society of Human Genetics. (1998). ASHG statement on professional disclosure of familial genetic information. *American Journal of Human Genetics, 62*, 474–483.

Anasagasti, S. (2006, May 28). Tourist throws 2 sons off balcony, jumps. *Miami Herald*, p. 1A. Retrieved July 28, 2006, from http://www.miami.com/mld/miamiherald/14686235.htm

Barak, A. (1999). Psychological applications on the Internet. *Journal of Preventive Psychology, 8*, 231–245.

Brownlow, M. (2007). *Email and webmail statistics* (Email Marketing Reports). Retrieved January 3, 2008, from http://www.email-marketing-reports.com/metrics/email-statistics.htm

California Board of Psychology. (2004). *Notice to California consumers regarding the practice of psychology on the Internet*. Retrieved August 4, 2008, from http://www.psychboard.ca.gov/consumers/telepsych.shtml

Clarke, A., Richards, M., Kerzin-Storrar, L., Halliday, J., Young, M. A., Simpson, S. A., et al. (2005). Genetic professionals' reports of nondisclosure of genetic risk information within families. *European Journal of Human Genetics, 13*, 556–562.

Cohen, D. (2003). *Depression and violent deaths in older Americans: An emergent public mental health challenge*. Retrieved July 21, 2006, from http://www.apa.org/ppo/cohentest.pdf

Cohen, D., Llorente, M., & Eisdorfer, C. (1998). Homicide–suicide in older persons. *American Journal of Psychiatry, 155*, 390–396.

Coid, J. (1983). The epidemiology of abnormal homicide and murder followed by suicide. *Psychological Medicine, 11*, 855–860.

Dietz, P. E. (1986). Mass, serial, and sensational homicides. *Bulletin of the New York Academy of Medicine, 62*, 477–491.

Dietz-Uhler, B., Bishop-Clark, C., & Howard, E. (2005). Formation of and adherence to a self-disclosure norm in an online chat. *CyberPsychology & Behavior, 8*, 114–120.

Drude, K. (2005, June). Technology use by Ohio psychologists. *Ohio Psychologist*, pp. 16–18, 20.

Dugan, R. B., Wiesner, G. L., Juengst, E. T., O'Riordan, M., Matthews, A. L., & Robin, N. II. (2003). Duty to warn at-risk relatives for genetic disease: Genetic counselors' clinical experience. *American Journal of Medical Genetics, 119*, 27–34.

Falk, J. M., Dugan, B., & O'Riordan, M. (2003). Medical geneticists' duty to warn at risk relatives for genetic disease. *American Journal of Medical Genetics, 120*, 374–380.

Finn, C. T., & Smoller, J. W. (2006). Genetic counseling in psychiatry. *Harvard Review of Psychiatry, 14*, 109–121.

Freeny, M. (2001). Better than being there. *Psychotherapy Networker, 25*, 31–39, 70.

Harper, P. S., Lim, C., & Craufurd, D. (2000). Ten years of presymptomatic testing of Huntington's disease prediction consortium. *Journal of Medical Genetics, 37*, 567–571.

Hauser, C., & O'Connor, A. (2007, April 17). Virginia Tech shooting leaves 33 dead. *New York Times*. Retrieved January 4, 2008, from http://www.nytimes.com/2007/04/16/us/16cnd-shooting.html?_r=1&oref=slogin

Heinlen, K. T., Welfel, E. R., Richmond, E. N., & O'Donnell, M. S. (2003). The nature, scope, and ethics of psychologists' e-therapy Web sites: What consumers find when surfing the Web. *Psychotherapy: Theory, Research, Practice, Training, 40*, 112–124.

Heinlen, K. T., Welfel, E. R., Richmond, E. N., & Rak, C. F. (2003). The scope of WebCounseling: A survey of services and compliance with NBCC standards for the ethical practice of WebCounseling. *Journal of Counseling & Development, 81*, 61–69.

Hillbrand, M. (2001). Homicide–suicide and other forms of co-occurring aggression against self and against others. *Professional Psychology: Research and Practice, 32*, 626–635.

Hillbrand, M., Foster, H. F., & Hirt, M. (1988). Variables associated with violence in a forensic population. *Journal of Interpersonal Violence, 3*, 371–380.

Hsiung, R. C. (2007). A suicide in an online mental health support group reactions of the group members, administrative responses, and recommendations. *CyberPsychology & Behavior, 10*, 495–500.

Joinson, A. N. (2001). Self-disclosure in computer-mediated communication: The role of self-awareness and visual anonymity. *European Journal of Social Psychology, 31*, 177–192.

Kaut, K. P. (2006). Counseling psychology in the era of genetic testing: Considerations for practice, research, and training. *Counseling Psychologist, 34*, 461–488.

Koocher, G. P. (2007). Twenty-first century ethical challenges for psychology. *American Psychologist, 62,* 375–384.

Maheu, M. (2003). The online clinical practice management model. *Psychotherapy: Theory, Research, Practice, Training, 40,* 20–32.

Mallen, M. J., Vogel, D. L., & Rochlen, A. B. (2005). The practical aspects of online counseling: Ethics, training, technology, and competency. *Counseling Psychologist, 33,* 776–818.

Malphurs, J. E., Eisdorfer, C., & Cohen, D. (2001). Antecedents of homicide–suicide and suicide in older married men. *American Journal of Geriatric Psychiatry, 9,* 49–57.

Marzuk, P. M., Tardiff, K., & Hirsch, C. S. (1992, June 17). The epidemiology of homicide–suicide. *JAMA, 267,* 3179–3183.

Milroy, C. M. (1993). Homicide followed by suicide (dyadic death) in Yorkshire and Humberside. *Medical Science and Law, 33,* 167–171.

Molloy v. Meier, 679 N.W.2d 711, 718 (Minn. 2004).

Molloy, T. (2006, February 2). Death toll at 8 in ex-postal worker's rampage. *Boston Globe.* Retrieved July 28, 2006, from http://www.boston.com/news/nation/articles/2006/02/02/death_toll_at_8_in_ex_postal_workers_rampage/

National Association of Social Workers. (1999). *NASW code of ethics.* Washington, DC: Author. Retrieved July 27, 2006, from http://www.socialworkers.org/pubs/code/code.asp

National Institute of Mental Health. (2003). *In harm's way: Suicide in America.* Retrieved October 2, 2006, from http://www.nimh.nih.gov/publicat/harmsway.cfm

Norcross, J. C., Hedges, M., & Prochaska, J. O. (2002). The face of 2010: The Delphi poll on the future of psychotherapy. *Professional Psychology: Research and Practice, 33,* 316–322.

Parent, R. B. (1998). Suicide by cop: Victim precipitated homicide. *Police Chief, 65,* 111–114.

Pate v. Threlkel, 661 S.2d 278 (Florida 1995).

Patenaude, A. F. (2005). *Genetic testing for cancer: Psychosocial approaches for helping patients and families.* Washington, DC: American Psychological Association.

Petrila, J. (2001). Genetic risk: The new frontier for duty to warn. *Behavioral Sciences & the Law, 19,* 405–421.

Pew Internet & American Life Project. (2007). *Demographics of Internet users.* Retrieved January 3, 2008, from http://www.pewinternet.org/trends/User_Demo_6.15.07.htm

Ragusea, A. S., & VandeCreek, L. (2003). Suggestions for the ethical practice of online psychotherapy. *Psychotherapy: Theory, Research, Practice, Training, 40,* 94–102.

Recupero, P. R. (2005). Email and the psychiatrist–patient relationship. *Journal of the American Academy of Psychiatry and Law, 33,* 465–475.

Recupero, P. R., & Rainey, S. (2005). Forensic aspects of e-therapy. *Journal of Psychiatric Practice, 11,* 405–410.

Rogers, R. (2000). The uncritical acceptance of risk assessment in forensic practice. *Law and Human Behavior, 24,* 595–605.

Safer v. Estate of Pack, 677A. 2nd 1188 (NJ Sup. Ct. App. Div. 1996).

Salib, J. C., & Murphy, M. J. (2003). Factors associated with technology adoption in private practice. *Independent Practitioner, 23,* 72–76.

Suler, J. (2004). The online disinhibition effect. *CyberPsychology & Behavior, 7,* 321–326.

Terry, N. P. (2002). The legal implications of e-therapy. In R. C. Hsiung (Ed.), *E therapy: Case studies, guiding principles, and the clinical potential of the internet* (pp. 166–193). New York: W.W. Norton.

Welfel, E. R., & Bunce, R. (2003, August). *How psychotherapists use electronic communication with current clients.* Paper presented at the 111th Annual Convention of the American Psychological Association, Toronto, Canada.

Wolf, A. W. (2003). Introduction to the special issue. *Psychotherapy: Theory, Research, Practice, Training, 40,* 3–9.

16

PRACTICE AND POLICY RESPONSES TO THE DUTY TO PROTECT

JAMES L. WERTH JR., ELIZABETH REYNOLDS WELFEL,
G. ANDREW H. BENJAMIN, AND BRUCE D. SALES

The duty to protect as it is currently understood began as the result of a state Supreme Court decision that focused on a relatively narrow set of circumstances (*Tarasoff v. Regents of the University of California*, 1976). Although some states and provinces do not mandate this duty, *Tarasoff*'s initial holding (i.e., that psychotherapists have a duty to exercise reasonable care to protect identifiable individuals whom their clients plan to harm, when they know or should know that the client is potentially dangerous) has expanded significantly over the years in other states and provinces. That expansion includes both the scope of the duty and the jurisdictions in which it is applicable. The previous chapters in this book have highlighted that the duty in regard to clients likely to be dangerous to third parties rarely is defined as a duty to warn. Only six states limit the professional's obligation in this circumstance to issuing warning to victims and/or law enforcement. Most statutes include, at a minimum, the option of hospitalization (see earlier chapters in this book and http://www.apa.org/books/resources/dutytoprotect; username: duty2protect; password: appendix).

Although *duty to protect* is the accurate descriptor, the term *duty to warn* has become the shorthand for references in the literature to the broader obligation to protect clients and the public safety. This probably occurred because there were two *Tarasoff* opinions, with the first speaking of the duty to warn (*Tarasoff v. Regents of the University of California*, 1974). That language is even the key term used in PsycINFO to search the literature on this topic. In addition, in states and provinces that legally include options to hospitalize the client or intensify outpatient treatment, and even in states and provinces in which no statutes or case law on the topic exists (see http://www.apa.org/books/resources/dutytoprotect), many professionals seem to view their obligation as one of warning potential victims. For example, in one recent study (Pabian, Welfel, & Beebe, 2007) nearly 75% of psychologists failed to exhibit an accurate understanding of the duty or lack of duty in state law, a finding consistent with prior research (Givelber, Bowers, & Blitch, 1984; Leedy, 1989; Rosenhan, Teitlebaum, Teitlebaum, & Davidson, 1993).

Focusing on warning rather than on other alternatives fundamentally misrepresents both the legal and the ethical duty of clinicians in most jurisdictions and leaves clinicians vulnerable to overlooking the need to protect potential victims with potentially other, more desirable methods than a warning. In addition, it appears that the duty to protect in California has morphed again, now in the instances in which the clinician has obtained information from a third party about the actual dangerousness of the client (*Ewing v. Goldstein*, 2004). To further compound the therapist's dilemma, when there is a duty, it has broadened in some jurisdictions from situations involving potential homicide to those of potential suicide (*Bellah v. Greenson*, 1978), whereas the zone around possible harm to self or others has increased to encompass situations such as stalking, domestic violence, and nonsuicidal self-harm. Thus, therapists are often confounded by how best to understand and respond to their obligations as jurisdictions have implemented myriad approaches to protect the safety of the public.

The purpose of this chapter is to provide therapists with information and a comprehensive set of guidelines that take into account the realities of the present (and possible future) landscape involving the duty to protect, while offering direction about how mental health professionals, their licensing boards, and their associations can act to better serve clients and the public. To accomplish this goal, we first consider background material to place the discussion that follows in context. We then discuss fundamental practice considerations that are essential to successfully responding to the duty to protect. We conclude the chapter with suggestions for how the profession can change the trend in the expansion of the duty to protect while helping students and clinicians who are currently confused by the exact nature of the current duty in their jurisdiction and across the country.

FOUNDATIONAL ISSUES

We begin by reaffirming that the duty to protect makes sense clinically and as public policy. However, the interpretation of the duty has expanded so broadly and so inconsistently across jurisdictions (see chap. 2 and the online appendix, http://www.apa.org/books/resources/dutytoprotect) that clinicians often find themselves in an untenable position when clients represent a risk to themselves or others. On the one hand, clinicians must maintain the therapeutic alliance to be most effective (Hovath & Bedi, 2002). On the other hand, the vagaries of many clinical contexts may trigger clinician actions that would impair the alliance (Pope, Simpson, & Weiner, 1978). It is not surprising, then, that most clinicians are uncertain or uninformed about the exact definition of their duty.

In the face of such uncertainty about the current status and future direction of the law on this issue, the question of a duty to protect has now moved to the forefront of consideration even among professionals who serve populations not traditionally thought to be at high risk of violence to self or others. In other words, the concern about whether a duty to protect exists now extends in some jurisdictions to those professionals who work primarily with people with HIV disease (see chap. 10, this volume), suicidal individuals (see chap. 11, this volume), or people who stalk (see chap. 7, this volume) or are involved in domestic violence (see chap. 6, this volume). The specter of the duty to protect also looms more broadly for professionals who work with a client who drives a car without awareness of being impaired (see chap. 9, this volume) or sends an e-mail to a therapist that discloses suicidal or homicidal ideation (see chap. 15, this volume). In light of how judicial activism has extended the duty to protect (see chap. 2, this volume) throughout many jurisdictions, it appears to be only a matter of time before other courts further expand the duty to protect.

A good informed consent form and adequate disclosure about the duty to protect before evaluation or treatment begins are the best ways to appropriately and adequately educate clients about what they should know regarding the ending of confidentiality within the therapeutic context. In addition, it appears that such an approach best protects the therapeutic alliance and mental health professionals from disgruntled clients (see chap. 2, this volume). Because the duty to protect is only one of many components of a competent informed consent process (Pomerantz & Handelsman, 2004), disclosure clauses within informed consent forms will become more complicated and extensive.

Providing thorough informed consent regarding these issues at the initiation of service risks the client not reading everything or tuning out during the verbal review, not following through with a session, or not feeling comfortable with saying very much because of uncertainty about what is truly confidential (see chap. 13, this volume). These risks should not be underestimated. For example, Marsh (2003) found that a sample of commuters in a Washington, DC, train station would refuse to disclose to a therapist information that would put them at risk of civil commitment or criminal prosecution. Whether this reluctance would be borne out in client behavior in therapy remains unclear, but this finding is consistent with our own clinical experience and with the reasoning behind the U.S. Supreme Court decision in *Jaffee v. Redmond* (1996; see also Shuman & Foote, 1999). Thus, it is reasonable to hypothesize that the duty to protect has evolved to a level that may be interfering with client willingness to enter into the therapeutic process or disclose potentially dangerous ideation and behavior. Indeed, it appears that the recent mass murders at Virginia Tech by Seung-Hui Cho, who was previously evaluated and treated by the mental health system for his dangerous ideation, highlight the issue (Luo, 2007); Cho never returned for further treatment during the following year (NBC, MSNBC, & News Services, 2007). Either cautionary behavior impairs the clinician's capacity to protect both the welfare of the client and the public.

Fundamental Practice Considerations

To assist therapists in their work and protect them from liability in regard to the duty to protect, this section outlines key practice considerations related to clinical work with clients, some of whom may be dealing with issues that engender the duty to protect. The seven practice considerations are (a) the importance of informed consent; (b) the crucial need for thorough, contemporaneous assessment and documentation; (c) the importance of consultation; (d) the realization that context matters; (e) the understanding that, legally, malpractice has four components; (f) the recognition that good clinical care is the best protection against possible legal action; and (g) a summary of recommended practices.

Informed Consent

As we previously noted, informed consent is a crucial part of the therapeutic process, not only for the client's sake but also in terms of risk management. Informed consent includes both written documentation of informed consent, which is signed and dated by the client, who also receives a copy of the form, and verbal review of its contents (see Pomerantz & Handelsman, 2004, for an additional approach to informed consent). Verbal review is particularly important both because many documents are written at a reading level not attained by many clients (Handelsman, Kemper, Kesson-Craig, McLain, & Johnsrud, 1986; Handelsman & Martin, 1992) and because clients are often absorbed with the issues that brought them to treatment at the initial session and are at risk of giving only cursory attention to such documents at that time. The review also creates an opportunity for the development of a positive, collaborative relationship between the clinician and the client as questions emerge about the details of consent. Interactions around the inquiries provide data about whether a therapeutic alliance can be formed in a meaningful manner.

Informed consent is a process, not an event, and it is not concluded at the initial session with the documentation because the direction of therapy typically changes over time. Examples of consent forms are present in a variety of books, including one developed by the American Psychological Association (APA) Insurance Trust (Harris & Bennett, 2006), and on the Internet. The importance of this process is evident in the APA's (2002) "Ethical Principles of Psychologists and Code of Conduct," in which the documentation of informed consent is mandated in Standard 10.01.

Providing the client with the information necessary to provide informed consent protects the client and the clinician. Informing the client of the limitations and risks (as well as potential benefits) of treatment allows the individual to make decisions about whether to enter into therapy and if so, what to say or not say during therapy. The client will also be less likely to make assumptions about what will happen with the information she or he discloses. The therapist, in turn, has protection if the client claims that she or he did not know that confidentiality could be broken or that hospitalization might be attempted. See Miller and Thelen (1986) and VandeCreek, Miars, and Herzog (1987) for discussions of the misunderstandings clients are likely to have about confidentiality.

Whatever the clinician writes or says related to informed consent needs to be accurate. Misunderstandings about the language in ethics codes and state and provincial laws and regulations do occur, and we know many therapists who accidentally misinform their clients about the duty to protect. For example, no ethics code *requires* that confidentiality be broken if the therapist is concerned that the person may hurt her- or himself or someone else, yet some clinicians believe they must disclose and therefore include such language in their written or verbal informed consent. Similarly, only a handful of state and provincial laws or regulations specifically require hospitalization in such circumstances, and even in those jurisdictions additional requirements must be present before such a course of action should be pursued. In addition, some therapists may decide that their value system or morals would mandate breaking confidentiality if a client appears to be planning to hurt her- or himself or someone else. However, therapists need to take ownership of that perspective and not say that "the ethics code" or "state law" mandates a particular action.

Assessment and Documentation

In duty-to-protect contexts, a structured risk assessment to determine whether a threat of violence is significant enough to warrant intervention must occur. Not only must the risk factors be identified, but interventions must be designed to reduce the effects of possible precipitating factors and increase the power of inhibiting factors (see chap. 2, this volume).

Documentation of informed consent and the assessment process is required. In fact, documentation is in general considered to be one of the cornerstones of good risk management and, one hopes, quality care. Malpractice attorneys have told us that a well-documented record is enough to deter them from bringing a case, and court decisions make it clear that poor documentation is enough to infer liability (Soisson, VandeCreek, & Knapp, 1987). The increasing importance of good documentation is illustrated by the fact that the APA just released new record-keeping guidelines (APA, 2007), and this document is several times longer than the previous version.

Several aspects of an adequate record often go unmentioned. The first of these is that the documentation needs to be timely. Falling into the habit of writing case notes weeks after a session is setting oneself up for problems. Part of the reason for 45- to 50-minute sessions is to allow time to complete documentation before the confounding of memory by passage of time or hearing other stories. Any documentation added to a record after something bad has happened is bound to be viewed very skeptically by a jury, licensing board, or ethics committee.

Similarly, the old adage of "if it isn't written down, it didn't happen" is important to keep in mind because the assumption is that anything important will be in the record. Thus, therapists should not only document what they did and why but also what they decided not to do. For example, if a clinician is concerned that a client may be suicidal but does not break confidentiality or attempt hospitalization, then the record should clearly explain why these interventions were not implemented and why other interventions were selected. If there is nothing in the file indicating that the therapist considered these options, the assumption will be that they did not occur to the professional, and any verbal protestation after the fact that these options were considered but rejected for various reasons will likely be viewed suspiciously.

Consultation

One of the best ways a therapist can demonstrate that she or he acted appropriately is to confer with other professionals contemporaneously when duty-to-protect circumstances arise (see chap. 2, this volume). By reviewing the assessment and the intervention with a colleague, especially someone considered knowledgeable by others in duty-to-protect cases, the clinician demonstrates that she or he has acted prudently on the occasion of a threat of violence. This action can demonstrate that the therapist is practicing at or above the standard of care, which is typically defined as having engaged in a course of action that would be viewed as acceptable by reasonable and prudent practitioners with similar training (Bongar, 2002). Consultation with peers and documentation of this consultation will provide some protection against the allegation that the therapist acted outside of professionally accepted behaviors. In fact, Principle B (Fidelity and Responsibility) of the

APA Ethics Code alludes to the value of consultation in meeting a psychologist's professional responsibilities:

> Psychologists establish relationships of trust with those with whom they work. They are aware of their professional and scientific responsibilities to society and to the specific communities in which they work. Psychologists uphold professional standards of conduct, clarify their professional roles and obligations, accept appropriate responsibility for their behavior, . . . *Psychologists consult with, refer to, or cooperate with other professionals and institutions to the extent needed to serve the best interests of those with whom they work* [italics added]. They are concerned about the ethical compliance of their colleagues' scientific and professional conduct. (APA, 2002, p. 1062)

If a professional consults the literature on the issue, a note of the sources he or she consulted should also be included. If a malpractice claim is possible, consultation with an attorney is essential as well.

If a therapist does consult but then does not follow the direction of the consultant or goes directly against the consultant's recommendations, she or he needs to document the rationale for that decision. Ideally, clinicians should seek out consultation with peers who can review the assessment issues and intervention steps in light of the standard of care and the circumstances of the case. Unless the advice of the consultant was inconsistent with ethical and legal standards for practice, the suggestions of the consultation should be pursued. Further consultation must occur if doubts about the original consultation emerge, and the clinician cannot provide an adequate professional rationale for her or his disagreement. Clinicians therefore are well advised to have a network of consultants who can assist with considering options without necessarily telling the clinician what to do.

Context Matters

One of the axioms in the legal arena is "bad facts make bad law," and this seems to be true in cases or legislation involving the duty to protect. An egregious set of facts based on actions or inactions by therapists leave the expert witnesses for the plaintiff and the judge and jury no other option really than to find that the clinician did something wrong; this may then translate into law that is overbroad. However, it is also true that context matters and that although two cases may look similar, a change in the fact pattern may lead to the outcome being very different in one situation versus another.

For example, consider a set of nearly identical cases in which a therapist's client kills or injures someone else. If clinician A did not consult with a colleague, clinician B did not document what interventions were considered, and clinician C consulted and documented the assessment and interventions that occurred in the case, clinician C will be much less likely to be charged with an ethics complaint or subjected to a malpractice lawsuit. Consider also a set of cases in which two therapists have clients who kill someone, but clinician D's client said he was thinking of harming the victim, whereas clinician E's client denied homicidal thoughts; if clinician E can demonstrate not only that did she not know of the homicidal intent but that she also had no reason to suspect any threat of violence, then even though someone is dead at the hands of her client, she has a better case than clinician D. The facts of the case, of which the clinical record and consultation with others are a big part, will influence whether charges are brought and, if so, whether the case results in an ethics complaint or a malpractice lawsuit.

Legal Definition of Malpractice

Malpractice is a form of negligence. The question then is what needs to be found for the therapist to be considered negligent in the professional care provided. Although this chapter is not the place for a full formal legal education, the concept of the "4 Ds" of malpractice is important here. Specifically, to win a malpractice case against a therapist, the plaintiff must show that the clinician had a duty, this duty was breached, and that this breach directly led to damages. A mnemonic for these elements is "Dereliction of Duty Directly causing Damages"—the 4 Ds (Rachlin, 1984, p. 303).

If a clinician accepts a client and begins a therapeutic relationship, then a *duty* is established. Talking to a person on the phone or receiving an e-mail would typically not be enough, but starting a case file would likely lead to an assumption that the person is a client. As an aside, this duty then continues for the duration of the person's status as a client, so a formal termination is important to show that the duty no longer adheres. The next issue is whether there was a *dereliction* of the duty (i.e., whether the clinician's work fell below the standard of care). This is the reason why consultation is valuable. It helps ensure that the therapist's decisions comported with what other professionals would do in a similar case, minimizes the possibility that the clinician will act unreasonably in light of the circumstances of the case, and establishes that the clinician attempted to competently assess and intervene. Documentation also becomes crucial because an expert witness can testify as to whether what is in the record is consistent with standard of practice, but if the record is incomplete or inadequate, then the expert will have little choice but to say that the chart does not indicate that the standard was met.

The third element is whether this alleged dereliction was the *proximate* cause of the bad outcome. Causation cannot be determined merely by looking at the passage of time; months may have passed between the clinician's last meeting with the client, but liability may still accrue. Thus, the issue is whether intervening factors arose that distance the clinician from the client's decision to act in a violent manner. For example, did the client fail to tell the therapist of her or his intentions to act violently? If yes, then the question becomes whether the clinician should have known the client's intentions in light of the circumstances of the case. In other words, the clinical record must also demonstrate that no other indications arose during sessions about the client's potential to act violently.

The last element to be proved in a negligence claim is whether *damages* occurred. In the case of someone being seriously injured or having died because of the client's intentional actions, this element of a malpractice action is readily found.

Thus, the clinician who had an active client involved in an incident would likely argue that although there was a duty and damages happened, she or he was not derelict in the duty and was not directly responsible for the damages. Given this, the importance of the preceding fundamental practice considerations should be clear. Providing clients with informed consent can minimize the likelihood of a successful charge that the client was betrayed by the therapist, and consultation and documentation can minimize the chances that one will be found derelict and directly responsible.

Good Care Is Good Protection

Finally, the best protection against malpractice liability is to focus first on providing good care and second on reducing risk. Although we emphasize the role of informed consent and documentation and consultation in risk management, it should be clear that another, probably more important role of these components is to assist in the provision of the best care possible to the client and, possibly, those around her or him. Providing competent care and being genuinely committed to the well-being of clients and those around them can mitigate much ill will after a negative outcome because it has been said that suits and ethics charges are influenced by bad feelings more than by bad outcomes (Bongar, 2002). Through the provision of good care to the client and, when possible and relevant, collaborative involvement of interested others (e.g., family, friends), those who would have standing to sue are less likely to have bad feelings toward the therapist and believe that incompetent care was provided.

Summary of Recommended Practices

In light of the above discussion, some practice recommendations stand out. Because these are either self-explanatory or have already been discussed in this section of the chapter, we simply list them without commentary (see chap. 2 for more details).

- Know your association's ethics code, and review it instead of assuming you know what it says.
- Know your state- or provincial-specific case law, statutes, and regulations, and review them instead of assuming you know what they say (see the online appendix, http://www.apa.org/books/resources/dutytoprotect).

- Attend ethics and risk management workshops on a regular basis and engage in self-study of the abundant literature on ethics and legal issues in practice.
- Keep up to date on the literature and statutory changes regarding the duty to protect.
- Provide thorough informed consent to all clients, both in written and verbal form.
- Build and maintain a strong therapeutic relationship with clients.
- Thoroughly and contemporaneously engage in assessment and document your decisions.
- Consult with knowledgeable peers when a threat of violence emerges, and document these consultations.
- Involve others (e.g., family members) in treatment with potentially dangerous clients, when clinically appropriate and agreed to by the client.
- Encourage professional associations and licensing boards to take an active role in informing members about their responsibilities to protect clients and the public as the laws evolve over time.

CHANGING THE TREND

As we noted at the outset, we are concerned about the apparent expansion of the duty to protect to a broader array of situations. Although we certainly believe that therapists have some responsibilities in regard to the duty to protect, we do not think that the duty should ever be allowed to evolve to the point that clinicians are held responsible for any dangerous behavior engaged in by a client. Unintended consequences are likely to arise if the duty to protect becomes too broad. For example, the more clinicians become worried about possible liability or licensure board complaints, the less they will be able to focus on the issues and needs of their clients.

The profession needs to address this challenge in multiple ways. First, we echo the sentiments that DeKraai and Sales (1984) voiced 25 years ago when they recommended that APA become actively involved in policy development regarding issues of confidentiality. APA should articulate a clear recommended policy with rationale for the duty to protect to encourage consistent legislation across jurisdictions. This book provides essential background information to stimulate this policy debate.

Second, state and provincial professional associations and licensing boards must educate their members about the legal duties with clients who are dangerous to self or others. Currently, more than 60% of the licensing boards of North America may not provide guidance to psychologists about the law and ethics regarding a potential duty to protect because of a reluctance to provide a legal opinion (see chap. 2, this volume). Who better to provide such an opinion than the licensing board of the jurisdiction that would prosecute ethical violations? If such an abdication of responsibility exists for defining the standard of care with clarity about this complicated area of ethics and the law, the best interests of clinicians or the public are poorly served. Thus, state and provincial associations and licensing boards should alleviate the worry, confusion, and misunderstanding about the duty to protect by including relevant legal and professional updates on their Web sites (e.g., relevant statutes, case law, professional opinions).

Finally, training programs in professional psychology need to become more involved by developing a comprehensive training module for educating students about the duty to protect. Prior research has shown that psychologists tend to view their ethics education as insufficient in regard to responsibilities with dangerous clients or that they believe they know their duties when they are actually misinformed about them (Pabian et al., 2007). Such a concerted effort by national associations, state and provincial associations, and licensing boards, grounded in accurate and thorough training in graduate school, will help protect the public from foreseeable harm, our clients from taking actions that will devastate their lives, and clinicians from providing incompetent practice.

Of course, training can only be as effective as the knowledge base on which it rests. As a result, additional research into the strategies professionals implement when confronted with clients dangerous to others is critical to effective training. To date, research has suggested that the outcome of professionals' decision making about their legal duty is flawed (e.g., Pabian et al., 2007). However, little is known about the process of decision making professionals use and the factors in the case, their training, or their context that influence their choices of strategies for deciding what triggers the duty and what action is needed to implement that duty. Without that knowledge, training is likely to be inefficient or ineffective. So much is at stake when the question of a potential duty to protect arises that it is imperative for researchers, educators, and practitioners to act responsibly to protect third parties from harm and clients from unwarranted disclosures of confidential information.

REFERENCES

American Psychological Association. (2002). Ethical principles of psychologists and code of conduct. *American Psychologist, 57*, 1060–1073. Retrieved May 14, 2007, from http://www.apa.org/ethics/code.html

American Psychological Association. (2007). *Record keeping guidelines*. Retrieved May 14, 2007, from http://www.apa.org/practice/recordkeeping.html

Bellah v. Greenson, 146 Cal. Rptr. 535, 81 Cal.App.3d 614 (1978).

Bongar, B. (2002). *The suicidal patient: Clinical and legal standards of care* (2nd ed.). Washington, DC: American Psychological Association.

DeKraai, M. B., & Sales, B. D. (1984). Confidential communications of psychotherapists. *Psychotherapy, 21*, 293–318.

Ewing v. Goldstein, 120 Cal. App. 4th 807 (2004).

Givelber, D. J., Bowers, W. J., & Blitch, C. L. (1984). *Tarasoff,* myth and reality: An empirical study of private law in action. *Wisconsin Law Review, 1984,* 443–497.

Handelsman, M. M., Kemper, M. B., Kesson-Craig, P., McLain, J., & Johnsrud, C. (1986). Use, content, and readability of written informed consent forms for treatment. *Professional Psychology: Research and Practice, 17,* 514–518.

Handelsman, M. M., & Martin, W. L., Jr. (1992). The effects of readability on the impact and recall of written consent material. *Professional Psychology: Research and Practice, 23,* 500–503.

Harris, E., & Bennett, B. E. (2006). *Sample psychotherapy patient contract.* Retrieved May 14, 2007, from http://www.apait.org/apait/resources/riskmanagement/inf.aspx

Hovarth, A. O., & Bedi, R. P. (2002). The alliance. In J. C. Norcross (Ed.), *Psychotherapy relationships that work* (pp. 37–69). New York: Oxford University Press.

Jaffee v. Redmond, 518 U.S. 1, 116 S. Ct. 1923 (1996).

Leedy, S. (1989). Psychologists' knowledge and application of Tarasoff in their decision about dangerousness. *Dissertation Abstracts International, 50*(10), 4775B.

Luo, M. (2007, April 19). Mental health and guns: Do background checks do enough? *New York Times.* Retrieved June 13, 2007, from http://www.nytimes.com/2007/04/19/us/19weapons.html?ex=1181880000&en=a2d5f50529c43643&ei=5070

Marsh, J. E. (2003). Empirical support for the United States Supreme Court's protection of the psychotherapist–patient privilege. *Ethics & Behavior, 13,* 385–400.

Miller, D. J., & Thelen, M. H. (1986). Knowledge and beliefs about confidentiality in psychotherapy. *Professional Psychology: Research and Practice, 17,* 15–19.

NBC, MSNBC, & News Services. (2007). *High school classmates say gunman was bullied.* Retrieved June 13, 2007, from http://www.msnbc.msn.com/id/18169776/

Pabian, Y. L, Welfel, E. R., & Beebe, R. (2007, August). *Psychologists' knowledge and application of state laws in* Tarasoff*-type situations.* Paper presented at the 115th Annual Convention of the American Psychological Association, San Francisco.

Pomerantz, A. M., & Handelsman, M. M. (2004). Informed consent revisited: An updated written question format. *Professional Psychology: Research and Practice, 35,* 201–205.

Pope, K. S., Simpson, M. H., & Weiner, N. F. (1978). Malpractice in outpatient psychotherapy. *American Journal of Psychotherapy, 32,* 593–602.

Rachlin, S. (1984). Double jeopardy: Suicide and malpractice. *General Hospital Psychiatry, 6,* 302–307.

Rosenhan, D. L., Teitelbaum, T.W., Teitelbaum, K.W., & Davidson, M. (1993). Warning third parties: The ripple effects of Tarasoff. *Pacific Law Journal, 24,* 1165–1232.

Shuman, D. W., & Foote, W. (1999). *Jaffee v. Redmond's* impact: Life after the Supreme Court's recognition of a psychotherapist–patient privilege. *Professional Psychology: Research and Practice, 30,* 479–487.

Soisson, E. L., VandeCreek, L., & Knapp, S. (1987). Thorough record keeping: A good defense in a litigious era. *Professional Psychology: Research and Practice, 18,* 498–502.

Tarasoff v. Regents of the University of California, 13 Cal.3d 117, 529 P.2d 553 (1974), 131 Cal. Rptr. 14, 551 P.2d 334 (1976).

VandeCreek, L., Miars, R., & Herzog, C. (1987). Client anticipations and preferences for confidentiality of records. *Journal of Counseling Psychology, 34,* 62–67.

AUTHOR INDEX

Numbers in Italics refer to listings in the references.

Bowman, Q., 22, *27*
Breitbart, W., 203, *206*
Brems, C., 217, 218, 220, 222, *225*
Brende, J. O., 214, *225*
Briere, J., 183, *191*
British Psychological Society, 49, 53, *56*
Brock, D., 128, *140*
Brown, G. K., 167, 174, *178*
Brown, M. Z., 184, *191*, *192*
Brownlow, M., 230, *244*
Brurer, N. L., 37, *39*
Bryan, C. J., 172, *178*
Buchanan, A., 64, 65, *75*
Buckner, F., 67, *75*
Bunce, R., 231, *247*
Burke, A., *180*
Burris, S., 142, 143, 153, *159*, 200, *206*
Bush, J., 80, *93*
Byock, I., 37, *39*

Calhoun, F., 111, *125*
California Board of Psychology, 234, *244*
Callaway, D., *125*
Camilleri, J. A., 22, *27*, 84, *92*
Campbell, J., 220, *225*
Campbell, J. C., 84, 85, 86, 89, *92*, *93*
Canadian Psychological Association, 48, *56*
Canchola, J., *180*
Carr, D. B., 133, *139*
Catania, J., *180*
Centers for Disease Control and Prevention, 129, *139*
Chamgless, D. L., 67, *75*
Chater, S., *208*
Chemtob, C. M., 213, *225*
Chenneville, T., 154, *159*
Childress, J., 131, 132, *139*
Chiles, J. A., 167, 174, *178*, *179*
Chinese Psychological Society, 48, 54, *56*
Chochinov, H. M., 199, *206*
Choi, S. Y., 71, *76*
Clarke, A., 238, *244*
Clarke, A. J., 218, *225*
Clarkson, P., 44, *57*
Clay, R., 136, *139*
Coggins, M., 111, 114, 119, 120, 121, *125*
Cohen, D., 235, 236, *244*, *246*
Coid, J., 235, *244*
Coker, A. L., 79, *92*
Comprehensive Alcohol Abuse and Alcoholism Prevention, Treatment and Rehabilitation Act, 130, *139*

Comtois, K. A., 184, *191*, *192*
Conrad, S. K., 183, *192*
Conterio, K., 182, 184, 186, 189, *192*
Cook, R. S., *75*
Coon, H. M., 71, *76*
Cooney, L. M., Jr., *140*
Corder, B. F., 99, *108*, 214, *225*
Cormier, C. A., 84, *93*
Cornelius, J. R., 171, *178*
Cornelius, M. D., *178*
Cornell Research Program on Self-Injurious Behavior, 183, *192*
Corvo, K., 80, 81, 83, *93*
Covell, C., *125*
Craufurd, D., 238, *245*
Crawford, M., 168, *179*
Crayhon, R., 224, *225*
Crook, K. H., 63, *77*
Crow, L., 201, *208*
Cruzan v. Director, Missouri Department of Health, 201, *206*
Curci, P., 214, *226*
Czech-Moravian Psychological Society, 48, *56*

Das, L. S., 223, *225*
Davidson, M., 250, *260*
Davies, J., 83, *92*
Davison, S., 64, *75*
de Becker, & Associates, 84, *92*
deGuzman, Isabel Nino, 54
DeKraai, M. B., 11, *27*, 258, *260*
de Moore, G. M., 171, *178*
Dickey, T. O., 176, *178*
Dietz, P. E., 236, *245*
Dietz-Uhler, B., 230, *245*
Dimidjian, S., 68, *75*
Dobson, K. S., *75*
Dominican Psychological Association, 49, *56*
Douglas, K. S., 218, *227*
Downing, V., *179*
Drapeau, M., 98, *108*
Draper, R. D., 68, *77*
Drozd, J. F., 174, *178*
Drude, K., 231, 234, *245*
Dubinsky, R., 133, *139*
Duchek, J., 133, *139*
Dugan, R. B., 238, *245*
Duncan, B. L., 68, *75*
Durham, M. R., 198, *208*
Dutton, D. G., 80, 81, 83, *93*
Dvoskin, J., 111, *125*

D'Zurilla, T. J., 188, *192*

Eaves, D., 84, 93, 218, *227*
Eckenrode, J., 183, 184, *193*
Edleson, J. L., 88, *92*
Ehler, J. G., *178*
Eisdorfer, C., 235, *244, 246*
Eisen, S., *178*
Elkins, K., 214, *226*
Elliot, P., 80, *92*
Ellis, S. P., *180*
Ellis, T. E., 176, *178*, 219, *226*
Enns, M., *206*
Ensworth v. Mullvain, 216, *226*
Estate of Long, *ex rel* Smith v. Brodlawn Med. Ctr., 16, *27*
Eth, S., 19, *27*
European Federation of Psychology Associations, *56*
Evans, E., 183, *193*
Evans, J., 67, 68, *77*
Ewing v. Goldstein, 5, *7*, 250, *260*

Fabrega, H., Jr., *178*
Falender, C. A., 219, 220, *226*
Falk, J. M., 238, *245*
Farberman, R. K., 38, *39*, 200, *206*
Farhi, D., 223, *226*
Farrenkopf, T., 199, *207*
Favazza, A., 182, 183, 184, 185, 186, 190, *192*
Fein, R., 103, *108*, 111, 112, 114, 115, 116, 118, 121, *125*
Feldman, S. B., 19, *27*
Ferrada-Noli, M., 168, *180*
Finn, C. T., 242, *245*
Firestone, M., 67, *75*
Fisher, R., *39*, 3637
Fitzgerald, A., 88, *92*
Foa, E. B., 190, *192*
Foley, D., 128, *140*
Follette, V. M., 190, *192*
Foster, H. F., 237, *245*
Foster, V. A., 213, *226*
Fouad, N. A., 34, *40*
Fowers, B. J., 70, *75*
Francini, K., *179*
Frank, J. B., 68, *76*
Frank, J. D., 68, *76*
Freeny, M., 231, *245*
Fremouw, W. J., 219, *226*
Friedman, M. J., 190, *192*

Fuchs, B., *180*
Fulero, S. M., 154, *159*
Fuller, K. M., 151, *159*

Galeazzi, G. M., 214, *226*
Galfalvy, H., *180*
Gallop, R. J., *192*
Garb, H. N., 118, *125*
Garlow, S. J., 168, *178*
Garner v. Stone, 67, *76*
Gauthier, J., 42, 55, *56*
Geffner, R. A., 81, *92*
Gelles, M., 115, 120, *125*
Gentile, S. R., 214, 215, *226*
German Psychological Society & Association of German Professional Psychologists, 46, *56*
Gerstein, L. H., 34, *40*
Gibson, C. A., 203, *206*
Gil, E., 183, *191*
Givelber, D. J., 4, *7*, 32, *39*, 250, *260*
Glass, N., 89, *92*
Glass, T. A., *140*
Glosoff, H. L., 11, 20, *27*, 43, *56*
Gold, J., 66, *76*
Goldberg, J., *178*
Goldfried, M. R., 188, *192*
Golding, S., 118, *125*
Goodstein, J. L., 167, *179*
Goodyear, R. K., 219, *225*
Gordon, J. R., 201, 203, *208*
Gothard, S., 101, *108*
Gottleib, M. C., 34, *39*, 219, 220, *226*
Gottman, J. M., 65, *75*
Graham, I. D., *208*
Gratz, K. L., 183, 188, *192*
Green, C. E., 81, *92*
Greenberg, L. S., 68, *76*
Grudzinskas, A. J., 87, *93*
Grunebaum, M. F., *180*
Gunderson, J. G., 188, *192*
Guralnik, J., 128, *140*
Gutheil, T. G., 25, *27*
Gutierrez, P. M., 183, *193*

Haggard-Grann, U., 5, *7*
Halliday, J., *244*
Hamada, R. S., 213, *225*
Hamberger, L. K., 82, 83, 89, *92*
Handelsman, M. M., 20, *27*, 251, 252, *260*
Hanh, T. N., 223, *226*
Harbin, J. J., 41, 43, 45, 47, 55, *57*

Hare, R. D., 218, *226*
Harley, K., 128, *140*
Harmell, P. H., 214, *226*
Harmon, R. B., 101, 104, *108, 109*
Harper, P. S., 238, *245*
Harrington, D., 214, *226*
Harris, E., 253, *260*
Harris, G. T., 22, *27*, 63, *76*, 84, 85, 92, *93*
Hart, S. D., 84, *93*, 104, *108*, 218, *227*
Hastings, J. E., 82, *92*
Hatch Mailette, M., *125*
Hauser, C., 235, *245*
Hawton, K., 183, *193*
Hays, J. R., 214, *227*
Health Insurance Portability and Account-
    ability Act, 170, *178*
Heard, H. L., *192*
Heath, N., 183, *193*
Hedges, M., 231, *246*
Heilbrun, K., 22, *27*
Heimovitz, H., 128, *140*
Heinlein, K. T., 230, *245*
Helenius, H., 184, *193*
Helms, J. E., 70, *76*
Heninger, M., 168, *178*
Henriques, G. R., *178*
Herlihy, B., 11, *27*, 219, *227*
Herlihy, S. B., 11, *27*
Herrell, R., 168, *178*
Herschler, J. A., 98, *108*
Herzog, C., 20, *28*, 253, *261*
Hillbrand, M., 64, *76*, 235, 236, 237, *245*
Hilton, N. Z., 84, 85, *93*
Hirsch, C. S., 235, *246*
Hirt, M., 237, *245*
Hjern, A., 168, *178*
Hofstede, G., 71, *76*
Hollander, E., 181, 184, 185, 186, *193*
Hollander, J. E., *178*
Hollon, S. D., *75*
Holtzworth-Munroe, A., 80, 83, *93*
Hong Kong Psychological Society, 49, *56*
Horvath, A. O., 21, *27*, 68, *76*, 251, *260*
Houghton, A. B., 84, *94*
Howard, E., 230, *245*
Hsiung, R. C., 230, *245*
Huprich, S. K., 151, *159*
Hyman, M., 224, *226*

Iannelli, R. J., 36, *40*, 146, *159*
Ibrahim, F. A., 71, *76*
Ising, M., *180*

Israel, T., 34, *40*
Israel Psychological Association, 46, 50, *56*

Jackson, A. M., 129, *140*
Jacobson, J. M., 213, 214, *226, 227*
Jacobson, N. S., 65, *75*
Jaffe, P., 83, *93*
Jaffee v. Redmond, 30, *39*, 87, *93*, 252, *260*
Jevne, R. F., 215, *226*
Jobes, D. A., 165, 166, 167, 169, 170, 173,
    174, 175, *177, 178, 179, 180*
Johns, H., 223, *226*
Johnson, M. P., 80, 83, *93*
Johnson, R. R., 203, *208*
Johnsrud, C., 252, *260*
Joiner, T. E., 170, 171, 172, 174, *179, 180*
Joinson, A. N., 230, *245*
Juengst, E. T., *245*

Kabat-Zinn, J., 223, *226*
Kagitçbasi, Ç., 71, *76*
Kaljonen, A., 184, *193*
Kallio-Soukainen, K., 184, *193*
Kane, K., 131, *140*
Karmel, M. P., 174, *179*
Kaut, K. P., 241, 242, *245*
Keane, T. M., 190, *192*
Keith-Spiegel, P., 45, *56*
Kelly, B. D., 102, *108*
Kemmelmeier, M., 71, *76*
Kemper, M. B., 252, *260*
Kern, N., *180*
Kerzin-Storrar, L., *244*
Kessler, R. C., 171, *179*
Kesson-Craig, P., 252, *260*
Kettlewell, C., 185, *192*
Khan, N. L., 102, *108*
Kim, U., 71, *76*
King, C. A., 174, *180*
Kinney, B., 213, *225*
Kitchener, K. S., 42, *56*, 142, 143, 151, *159*,
    200, *206*
Kleespies, P. M., 198, 199, 200, *206*
Knapp, S., 128, 131, 132, 138, *140*, 254, *261*
Knish, S., 67, *77*
Kohlenberg, R. J., *75*
Kokaliari, E. D., 183, *192*
Koocher, G. P., 45, *56*, 231, *245*
Koppel, M. S., 37, *39*
Kornfield, J., 223, *226*
Kosinski, A., 203, *206*
Kovacs, M., 167, *179*

SUBJECT INDEX

International Society for Mental Health Online, 234
Internet, therapy via, 229–234
Intervention
    client's theory of change, 68–69
    with client threatening harm to others, case example, 69–70, 72, 73–74
    with client who threatens public officials, 121–123, 124
    with client with communicable disease, case examples of, 145–157
    clinical supervision, 72–73
    court-ordered, 98
    cultural considerations, 70–72
    documentation, 25–26
    harms of inappropriate disclosure, 33, 34
    with impaired vehicle operator, 132
    peer consultation in, 24–25
    with perpetrators of partner violence, 80–81, 86–87, 91
    risk assessment and, 24, 64–65
    risks to therapist, 98–99
    self-injurious behavior, 188–191
    with stalking offender, 101–102, 107
    suicidal patient, 169–176
    terminally ill client's end-of-life decisions, 37–38
    See also Assessment; Effectiveness of psychotherapy; Therapeutic alliance
Intimate partner violence
    among same-sex couples, 80
    assessment instruments, 84–85
    case example, 81–82
    child abuse and, 83, 88–89
    child exposure, 88
    confidentiality issues, 81, 87, 90
    duty-to-protect obligations, 88–90
    gender differences, 80
    identification, 80
    perpetrator entry into treatment, 82
    prevalence, 79, 80
    risk assessment, 82–86
    risk factors, 86
    role of MHPs, 79–80
    safety planning for victim, 83
    spousal homicide–suicide, 236
    standard of care, 87–88
    therapeutic alliance in perpetrator treatment, 91
    therapist qualifications for intervention, 83

treatment challenges, 86–87, 91
treatment effectiveness, 81
treatment for perpetrators of, 80–81
typology, 83
victim safety concerns, 90
victim's perception of risk, 86, 90, 91
Iterative Classification Tree, 22–23

Jaffee v. Redmond, 30–31, 252
Jurisdictional variations, 5–6, 26
Justice
    ethical principle of, 42
    working with client with communicable disease, 151–152

Kingston Screening Instrument for Domestic Violence, 84, 85

Law
    client privacy rights, 30–31
    end-of-life decisions, court cases and legislation, 201–202
    ethical practice obligations and requirements of, 30, 32
    mandatory reporting of HIV status, 36
    partner violence risk assessment, 85
    protection of public officials, 113
    suicidal client, reducing liability in work with, 169–176
    See also Malpractice claims; Mandatory reporting; State law

Malpractice claims
    context considerations, 255–256
    essential elements, 256–257
    importance of documentation, 254
    liability under duty-to-protect statutes, 9–10
    peer consultation in defense against, 72, 254, 255
    prevention, 257
    society's expectations of MHP responsibility, 63
    suicide-related, 169
Mandatory reporting
    exceptions to ethics code requirements, 31–32
    informing client of pending disclosure, 35, 47–53
    informing clients of duty-to-protect obligations, 20
    intimate partner violence, 88–90

therapist fears and, 98–99

therapist self-assessment in work with client with communicable disease, 146–147, 148

Universal Declaration of Ethical Principles for Psychologists, 42–43

Violence Risk Appraisal Guide, 84, 85

Violent behavior or threat of violent behavior

assessment goals, 22

assessment techniques and instruments, 22–24

associated variables, 23

case example of therapy with, 61–62, 66, 67, 69–70, 72, 73–74

challenges for therapists working with, 79

client expressions of, in therapeutic setting, 34

continuing education for therapists working with, 221–222

co-occurring homicide–suicide, 234–237

disclosure decision, therapist's responsibility, 44

documentation of therapy with threatening client, 25–26, 219

goals of risk assessment, 63

likelihood of MHPs encountering client with, 214

MHPs as targets of, 214, 216–222

obstacles to predicting, 64–65

predictability, 63–64

prior threats as predictor of, 102

stalking and, 97

therapeutic alliance and, 21–22

therapist's disclosure decision, 44

therapist self-care strategies in work with, 215–225

See also Homicidal ideation or threats of violence; Intimate partner violence; Public officials, threats against

Warning third parties

alternative to, in duty-to-protect compliance, 4–5

client with communicable disease, 148, 150–154

contact information, 106

decision in stalking cases, 105–106

psychologists' understanding of duty to protect, 250

risk of genetic disease transmission, 237–243

See also Confidentiality; Duty to protect; Failure to protect third parties

ABOUT THE EDITORS

James L. Werth Jr., PhD, is professor of psychology and director of the PsyD program in counseling psychology at Radford University and is a licensed psychologist in Virginia, although the first part of this book was completed while he was an associate professor in the Department of Psychology at The University of Akron. In addition to ethical and legal matters, his primary areas of research and practice are HIV disease and end-of-life issues. He has written, edited, or coedited several books and journal special issues on the latter topics. He served on the American Psychological Association's (APA's) Ad Hoc Committee on Legal Issues and Ad Hoc Committee on End-of-Life Issues and currently serves as the federal advocacy coordinator for the Society of Counseling Psychology (Division 17 of the APA). He received his doctorate in counseling psychology from Auburn University in 1995, his master of legal studies from the University of Nebraska—Lincoln in 1999, and served as APA's HIV Policy Congressional Fellow in the office of Senator Ron Wyden (D–OR) from 1999 to 2000.

Elizabeth Reynolds Welfel, PhD, is codirector of training in counseling psychology and professor at Cleveland State University, where she has been teaching graduate students in counseling and counseling psychology for 20 years. Before her appointment at Cleveland State, she was on the counseling psychology faculty at Boston College. She has authored numerous articles on the ethics of professional practice, and her book *Ethics in Counseling and Psychotherapy: Standards, Research and Emerging Issues* is in its third edition. Her current research projects focus on ethical issues in the use of technology in professional practice and psychologists' understanding of their legal responsibilities with violent clients. Along with Dr. Elliott Ingersoll, she coedited the *Mental Health Desk Reference.* Her third book, *The Counseling Process,* coauthored with Lewis Patterson, is in its sixth edition. Dr. Welfel has conducted numerous continuing education programs on professional ethics across the nation. She received her doctorate in counseling psychology from the University of Minnesota in 1979 and has been a licensed psychologist in Ohio since 1986.

G. Andrew H. Benjamin, JD, PhD, is an affiliate professor of law at the University of Washington and director of the Parenting Evaluation/Training Program (PETP; http://depts.washington.edu/petp). While working with families engaged in high-conflict litigation and lawyers and law students with various mental health and drug abuse problems, he was named "Professional of the Year" by the Washington State Bar Association's Family Law Section. He was elected president of the Washington State Psychological Association, and his colleagues in that association created an award named after him for "outstanding and tireless contributions." Dr. Benjamin was honored by the Puyallup Indian Nation's Health Authority as a "modern day warrior fighting the mental illnesses, drug–alcohol addictions" of the people served by the Nation's program. The American Psychological Association (APA) gave him the Heiser Award in recognition of his record of public service and advocacy. He has published 41 peer-reviewed articles in psychology, law, and psychiatry journals. He also is the author of two other books published by APA: *Law and Mental Health Professionals: Washington* (1995, 1998) and *Family Evaluation in Custody Litigation: Reducing Risks of Ethical Infractions and Malpractice* (2003).